The Long Climb:
From Barber-Surgeons to Doctors of Dental Surgery

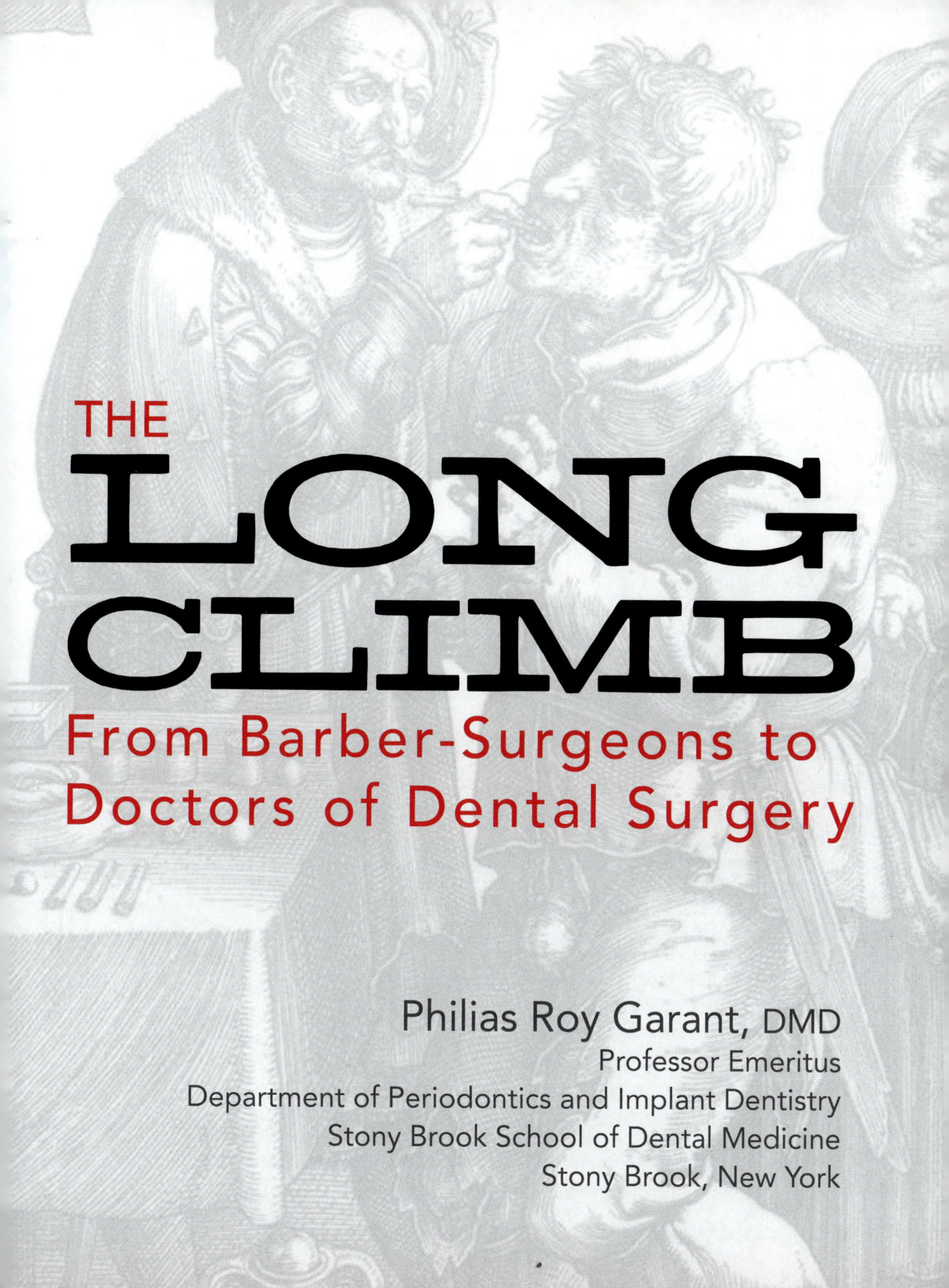

THE LONG CLIMB

From Barber-Surgeons to Doctors of Dental Surgery

Philias Roy Garant, DMD

Professor Emeritus

Department of Periodontics and Implant Dentistry

Stony Brook School of Dental Medicine

Stony Brook, New York

Quintessence Publishing Co, Inc

Chicago, Berlin, Tokyo, London, Paris, Milan, Barcelona, Beijing, Istanbul, Moscow, New Delhi, Prague, São Paulo, Seoul, Singapore, and Warsaw

Dedication

This work is dedicated to my wife, Jeanne, and our six wonderful children.

Library of Congress Cataloging-in-Publication Data

Garant, Philias R., author.
The long climb : from barber-surgeons to doctors of dental surgery / Philias R. Garant.
p. ; cm.
Includes bibliographical references and index.
ISBN 978-0-86715-649-2 (hardcover)
I. Title.
[DNLM: 1. History of Dentistry. WU 11.1]
RD533
617.009--dc23
2013033497

quintessence books

Quintessence Publishing Co Inc
4350 Chandler Drive
Hanover Park, IL 60133
www.quintpub.com

5 4 3 2 1

Editor: Leah Huffman
Design and production: William Jotzat

Printed in the USA

Contents

Preface

As a dental educator and scientist, I found special pleasure in studying the history of medicine and dentistry. From my readings (often at the expense of more pressing issues), I obtained a better sense of how dentistry evolved and how it became separated from medical practice. Throughout this journey, I have been inspired by the courage and determination of dentistry's pioneers. From Pierre Fauchard to G. V. Black, there is much to appreciate. On the other hand, there have been episodes of weakness and dishonesty that tarnished the image of the dentist. From consideration of both the good and the bad, we form a true picture of who we are.

There are excellent general histories of dentistry and several recent books on specific periods in the development of dentistry, so why publish another book of this nature? It was my belief that a new narrative, highlighting some of the personalities and the controversies particularly related to developments in the United States, would be instructional as well as enriching for dentists and dental students who might otherwise find a void in their education when it comes to understanding the history of their profession.

The obscure beginnings of dentistry are uncovered in the work of barber-surgeons and surgeons during the Middle Ages and Renaissance. Italian surgeons are credited with early attempts to restore teeth with gold fillings. Following two centuries of slow progress, the dawn of a new era was marked by the apparent sudden arrival of the surgeon-dentist, epitomized by Pierre Fauchard. The rapid growth of dental practice and dental science in Europe and England during the 18th century provided a foundation for the development of an independent dental profession in the American colonies.

This book relates the events that led to the formation of dental schools and dental societies in the United States with the role that these institutions played in promoting laws to regulate dental practice. The pioneering practitioners who led the professionalization of dental practice and the growth of dental science receive special focus. Controversies such as the use of gold versus amalgam filling materials, operative versus mechanical dentistry, the relationship between medicine and dentistry, and the restriction of practice imposed by patents give the story life. Attention is given to how, in the face of growing commercialism, the new dental profession sought to improve its image by adopting a code of ethics. The riveting and tragic story of the discovery of inhalation anesthesia is presented as a tale of ambition, greed, and deceit.

The beginnings of dental research, mostly in microscopic anatomy and microbiology, gave rise to controversy, rivalry, and a brief adherence to vitalism long after it had been dismissed by mainstream science. Recognition of the need for a standardized dental curriculum and the correction of deficiencies in equipment, standards, and research, mainly in the proprietary schools, engendered the Gies Report, a widespread study of dental education resulting in numerous recommendations for change. Implementation of the Gies Report elevated dentistry to its legitimate position within the modern university, alongside medicine, and within the scientific community at the national level by the formation of the National Institute of Dental Research. We end our peregrination through times past with dentistry's acceptance as a legitimate university discipline.

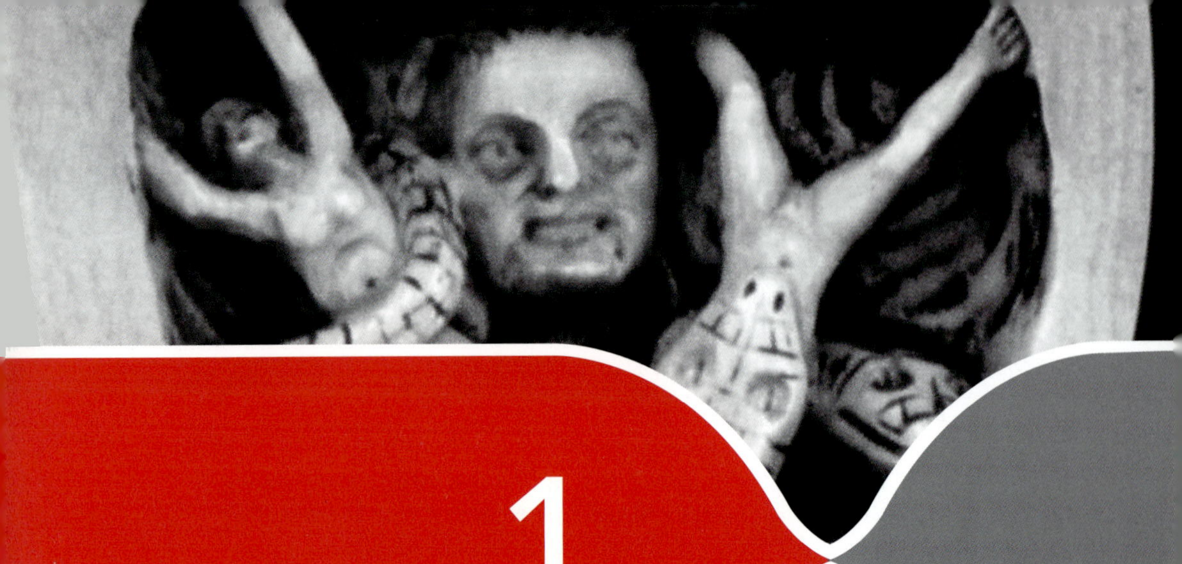

1

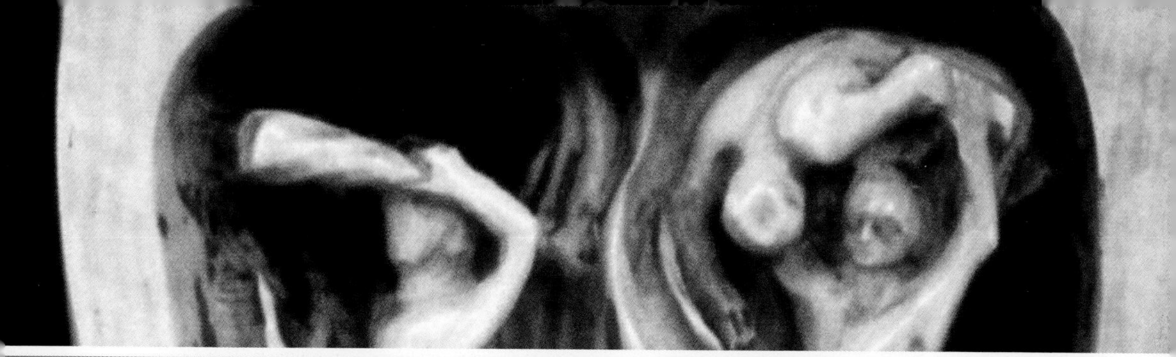

Antiquity to the Early Middle Ages

Dental diseases have been a part of human existence since the days of earliest man. Paleolithic human remains contain evidence of advanced dental attrition and periodontal disease.[1] Ancient Egyptian skulls contain evidence of dental caries and bone destruction from periodontal infection.[1] Toothache is among the common ailments described in the earliest known textbooks of medicine. How did man cope with the excruciating pain of toothache and how did he accommodate to the loss of teeth? How did the practice of dentistry develop and flourish as a separate profession from medicine? To answer these questions and uncover the origins of dentistry, we must examine the records of ancient civilizations.

[1] Dinosaurs and Pleistocene cave bears show evidence of dental caries and periodontal disease.

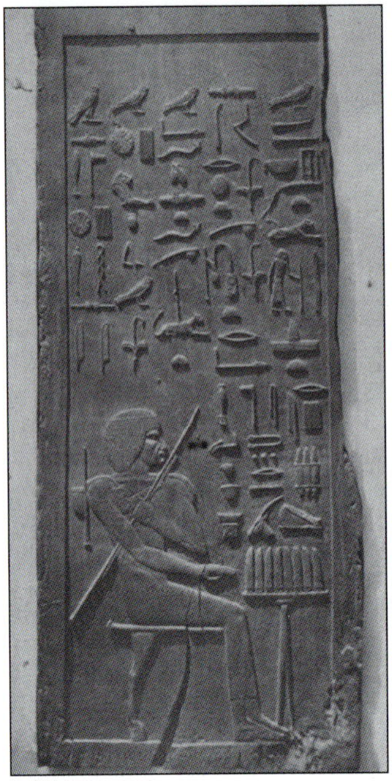

Fig 1-1 Wooden panel recovered from an Egyptian burial chamber depicting Hesyre and identifying him as a physician and a dentist.

Ancient Egypt

The Egyptians created numerous tomb inscriptions and papyri that have allowed us to form a vision of their way of life, including their approach to maintaining health and dealing with disease. The healing arts were closely integrated with their religious beliefs, and practitioners of medicine were members of the priesthood. Tomb inscriptions and early histories have suggested that Egyptian medicine may have been diversified. Herodotus, the Greek historian who traveled through Egypt, described the country as rich with practitioners, some specializing in diseases of the eyes, some for the heart, some for the gut, and some for the teeth.[2] Egyptian tomb inscriptions have revealed that approximately 150 individuals practiced medicine; at least three of them, and perhaps as many as nine, appeared to have treated dental problems.[3,4] The earliest dentist, Hesyre, is depicted on carved wooden panels recovered from excavations at Saqqara near Cairo (Fig 1-1). The panel inscription shows that he held the titles of both physician and dentist.[4]

Egyptian medical practice was dominated by the use of herbal remedies concocted in the form of emetics, diuretics, purgatives, and palliative dressings.[5] The Egyptian pharmacopeia consisted of mineral, plant, and animal products, often in the form of powders or salves. Egyptian surgeons were adept in the use of the knife and cautery for excision or ablation of diseased tissues.

Examinations of the skeletal remains recovered from Egyptian burial sites have shown that 10% of teeth had dental decay, and 20% contained evidence of periodontal disease. Dental calculus (tartar) was present on 50% of all teeth.[6] Radiographs of two royal mummies, Amenhotep III and Ramesses II, revealed extreme tooth abrasion, periodontal disease, and periapical abscesses but no evidence of dental treatment.[4] From thousands of Egyptian mummies that have been examined, there is no evidence that Egyptians performed any dental operations. Although instruments that may have been used in medical practice have been recovered in burial chambers, none appear to have been specifically designed for use in dental procedures.[4]

In his studies of Egyptian skulls, F. F. Leek concluded that excessive attrition of occlusal surfaces was the greatest cause of death of the dental pulp, leading to abscess formation, osteomyelitis, and the spread of infection into the jaws.[1] Erosion of enamel and dentin was caused by the consumption of coarse bread and fibrous vegetables.[7] The masticating (grinding) surfaces of the first molars exhibited the most severe wear, with the crowns often eroded to the gum line.

Tooth erosion and dental abscesses affected all classes, including members of the royalty.[8] Loss of alveolar bone from periodontal disease is a common finding in ancient Egyptian skulls. The cause of the bone loss appears to have been an excessive accumulation of tartar on the roots of the teeth. No toothbrushes or instruments for scraping tartar have ever been found among Egyptian artifacts. Although dental decay was relatively rare in ancient Egypt, it became more prevalent at the time of the construction of the Great Pyramids. Excavation of 500 skeletons of aristocratic families at gravesites of the Giza pyramids revealed that the prevalence of tartar, caries, and dental abscesses were equal to that found among modern Egyptian populations. This decline in dental health may have been the result of changes in the quantity or form of carbohydrate intake. In 1920, paleoanthropologist Sir Armand Ruffer concluded, "Carious human teeth from ancient remains have been discovered in so many places that it is legitimate to doubt whether there was ever an epoch when the human species was not cursed by toothache."[7]

From the archaeologic record, it appears that Egyptians did not practice operative dentistry.[1] No tooth filled with gold or any other metal has ever been found within Egyptian tombs. Evidence suggests that severely infected and loose teeth were not extracted.[8] It would seem that a suffering dental patient had nothing but herbal remedies and magical incantations to afford relief from the pain of toothache and infection.

Among the papyri that have been recovered from Egyptian gravesites, the Ebers Papyrus and the Edwin Smith Papyrus are special sources of medical information. The ability to decipher the hieroglyphic script of the papyri and tomb inscriptions was made possible by the discovery of the Rosetta Stone during Napoleon's ill-fated expedition to Egypt in 1799. The stone fragment found in the village of Rosetta in the Nile Valley was inscribed with a message written in the three writing systems used in Egypt: the hieroglyphic (or picture form), the hieratic (religious form), and the demotic (used in everyday communication). In 1822, Jean-Francois Champollion, a master of Greek and eastern languages, translated the demotic text into French and thereby was able to decipher the hieroglyphic sign text. Some hieroglyphics suggest that there may have been physicians for the teeth, as depicted by the juxtaposed symbols of an eye (for *he who cares for*) and a tusk (for *teeth*). Similarly, the juxtaposition of a bird (signifying *the greatest*), a tusk (*teeth*), and an arrow (a *medical practitioner*) was translated to mean the "greatest of those who deal with teeth" (upper right corner of Fig 1-1). However, not all experts of Egyptian hieroglyphics are in complete agreement on these interpretations.[1]

The Ebers Papyrus, dating from around 1500 BC, is significant because of its description of the heart and its blood supply, evidence of the relatively advanced knowledge of the vascular system as well as the major organs of the human body, believed to have been gained in the practice of embalming and mummification. Dental diseases such as gumboils, pulpitis, and alveolar abscesses are described in the Ebers Papyrus and confirmed by the pathologic findings of the skeletal remains.[9] Recipes for powders and ointments for tooth and mouth ailments are contained among the 700 formulas listed in the Ebers Papyrus.[1]

The Papyrus Anastasi is of interest to dental science in that it contains the idea that toothache was caused by worms that had burrowed into the tooth's interior (Fig 1-2). The earliest version of this myth can be traced to a Mesopotamian clay tablet, dating back to 1800 BC, discovered in the ancient city of Sumer (now Nippur), Iraq.[2] The myth of the tooth worm continued to be popular well into the late Middle Ages and was accompanied by the prescription that toothache could be treated by fumigating the infected tooth with the fumes from burning henbane seeds.

The Edwin Smith Papyrus, an even older text dating back to 2700 BC, contains 48 medical case histories of Egyptian medical practices

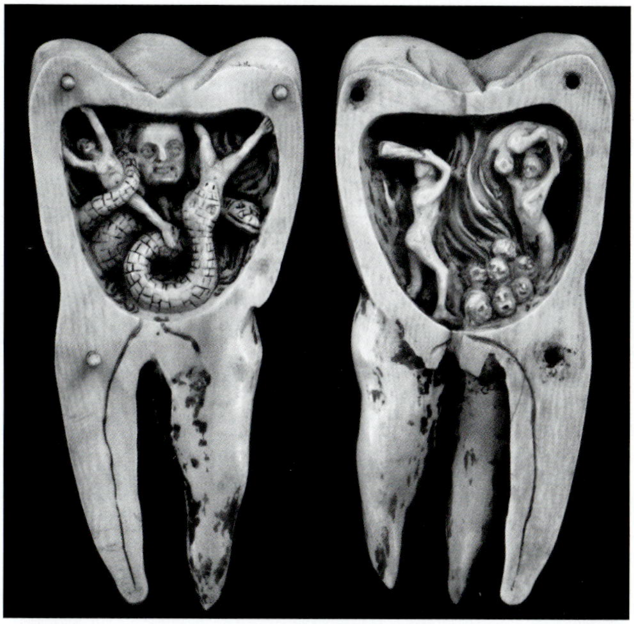

Fig 1-2 Ivory carving depicting worms and demons as the cause of toothache.

for dealing with various injuries, including a description for reducing fractures of the mandible.[2] The level of anatomical and physiologic knowledge contained in the Edwin Smith Papyrus is superior to other known papyri. Its emphasis on surgical technique suggests less reliance on the healing power of magic and religious incantation. However, with the exception of the mandibular fracture description, there are no other references to oral diseases in the Edwin Smith Papyrus.[1]

Based on research and critical examination of the literature, Thomas Nickol concluded that there was no evidence of any prosthetic work being carried out on the dentition or of any surgical treatment of teeth by medical practitioners in ancient Egypt.[10] The only treatment of dental disease and mouth ailments was by herbal preparations applied to the problematic sites by either physicians or, more likely, artisans of a lower, nonpriestly class. According to Guerini, there is no proof that any fillings or artificial teeth were ever found in mummies.[11] In the thousands of Egyptian skulls excavated at burial sites, there are only two examples of attempts to secure loose teeth with gold wire. These were recovered from a burial chamber at Giza in 1914.[2]

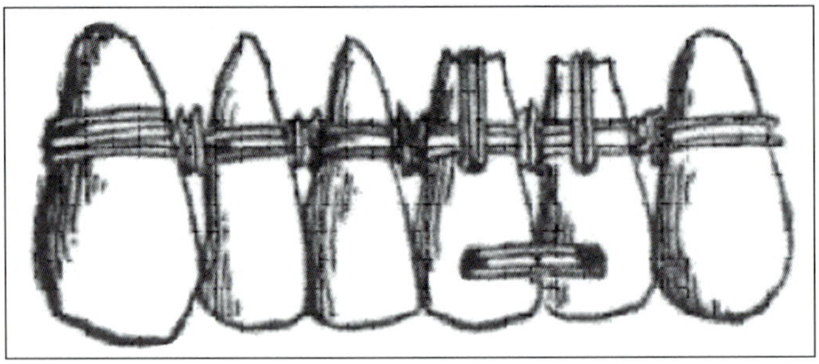

Fig 1-3 Primitive dental prosthesis recovered in the Phoenician city of Sidon.

Guerini wondered why the Egyptians, talented in the craftsmanship of gold and other plastic arts and fond of beautifying the human body, did not undertake dental restorative work.[11] The artisans who fabricated the exquisite burial masks and other ornamental objects recovered from the pyramids had the necessary talent for making dental restorations. Why there is no evidence of such work remains a mystery.

Phoenicia and Mesopotamia

The first evidence of the replacement of missing teeth was discovered in the Phoenician city of Sidon, now part of Lebanon.[12] A dental segment consisting of two canines and four incisors, wired together with gold wire, was recovered from a burial chamber dating back to the 5th or 4th century BC. Two of the incisors had been sectioned to remove the apical end, thereby creating a flat surface for vertical wiring of these teeth to the main horizontal wire network[2,12] (Fig 1-3). These teeth were part of the skeletal remains of a man of high rank judging by his gold ring, linen wrappings, and the marble anthropoid sarcophagus that contained his body (Fig 1-4). Bone resorption of the jaws indicated that the individual suffered from advanced periodontal disease and that he had undoubtedly sought dental treatment for loose teeth. This gold wiring method allowed for replacement of two teeth and stabilization of all six. This artifact is believed to be the first partial denture ever discovered. Despite its primitiveness, it is ingenious in its design of incorporating the two canines for stability and in the method of attaching the two replacement teeth.

A second sarcophagus within the same burial chamber contained the body of a woman believed to be the man's wife (see Fig 1-4). The sarcophagi were of Parian marble and thought to be the workmanship

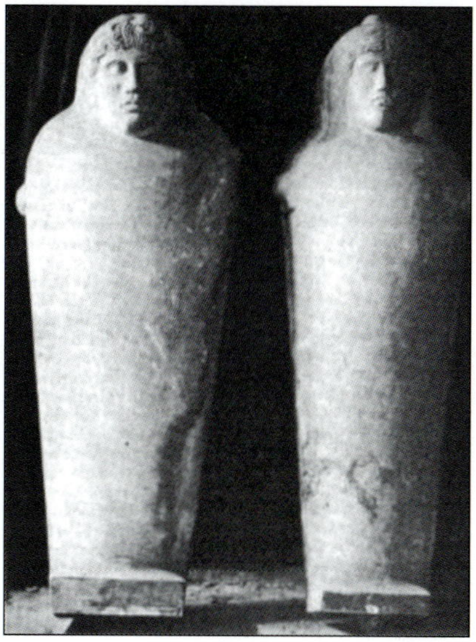

Fig 1-4 Anthropoid sarcophagi from Sidon.

of Greek sculptors. Burial vaults of this type were contracted during life only by the wealthiest citizens of Phoenicia. Sidon was reputed to have numerous skilled metal workers who fabricated a variety of art objects. It would seem that among them were artisans who found the courage to venture into the care of ailing dental patients.

Knowledge of medical and dental diseases and their treatment in ancient Israel are contained in the Bible and the Talmud.[13] Although it is suggested that oral diseases were treated by herbal regimens, as in adjacent cultures, and that gold teeth may have been fabricated, there is no paleoanthropologic evidence for such activity. But judging from the skills in metallurgy of the contemporaneous Phoenicians, one cannot rule out that such dental craftsmanship existed. The single most important medical contribution of the Israelites was the set of laws put forth by Moses for maintaining the public health through improved sanitation.[13]

The records of ancient civilizations of Sumeria, Assyria, and Babylonia, located in the land of the Tigris and Euphrates Rivers (Mesopotamia), provide another source of information on the origins of medical practice.[14] Evidence points again to the priestly class as the guardians of magical and herbal remedies for all types of ailments, including toothache and other diseases of the mouth. Knowledge of their medical culture has been retrieved from clay tablets and votives recovered from archaeologic sites.[13] More than 800 medical tablets (some in fragments) have been partially translated from their cuneiform language. Tablets now preserved in the British Museum describe incantations and herbal remedies for toothache. The overriding belief in Babylonian medicine was that diseases were the result of possession by demons (each disease its own demon).[15] Incantations and magic as means of driving demons out of the body were major elements in the cure of diseases.[14] One tablet, now held in the British Museum, contains the myth of tooth worms as the agent of toothache (see Fig 1-2), along with incantations for their expulsion. The most extensive Babylonian medical text, the *Diagnostic Handbook*, written by the physician Esagil-kin-apli during the reign of the Babylonian King Adad-apla-iddina (1069–1046 BC), contains a list of medical symptoms and empiric observations with logical rules to be used in making a diagnosis and prognosis. A major contribution of this civilization was the civil Code of Hammurabi (King of Babylonia, 3123–2081 BC). Among its laws were rules for the practice of medicine, including the setting of fees and penalties for malpractice, such as loss of a hand for a botched surgery.[14]

Ancient Greece

It was not until the development of the Greek civilization that rational remedies began to replace the reign of superstition in medical and dental practice. Nevertheless, the oldest Greek medicine continued to be based on religious superstition and was administered by priests in health temples or spas (asclepiads). An excellent description of these extensive health temples, and the curious rites that took place within, are described by Richard Caton.[16] Cures were mainly the result of the combined effects of suggestion, empiric remedies, and minor surgeries. Medical knowledge was passed on, generally from father to son, within families over many generations.

Asclepius, a mythologic Greek physician believed to have existed around 1200 BC, became the central figure of a religious cult of medicine practiced by priests at temples[2,14] (Fig 1-5). An Asclepian cure was obtained by overnight rest in a spalike setting where treatments were often made when the patient was in a semihypnotized state. The patient's complaint and the method whereby a cure was made were recorded on clay votive tablets and kept within the temple. At the ruins of the asclepiad of Epidaurus, votive tablets of teeth and jaws were discovered. Evidence that tooth extraction was performed in ancient Greece is also supported by the discovery of a pair of forceps (odontagra) in the ruins of an asclepiad. Aristotle described the use of this instrument for extracting teeth.[11]

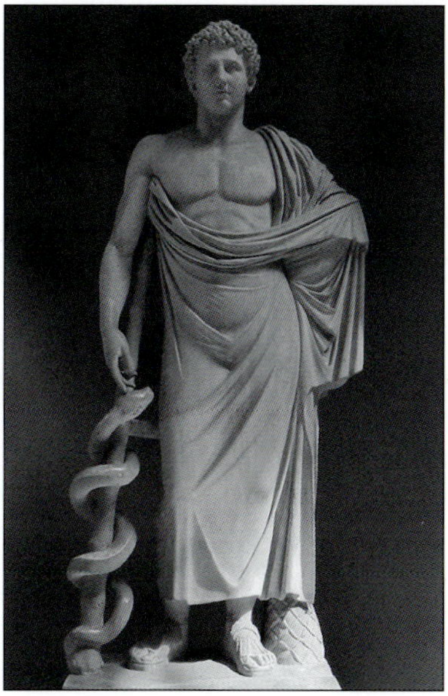

Fig 1-5 Asclepius.

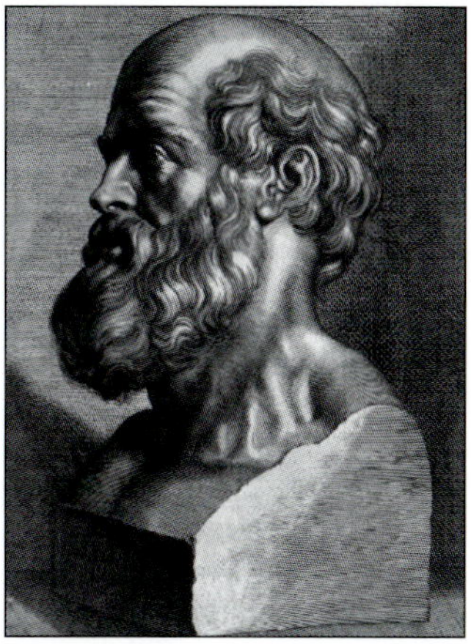

Fig 1-6 Hippocrates.

Greek philosophers developed the theory of the four elements—fire, air, water, and earth—and associated them to the four qualities that formed the earliest idea of a chemical universe (hot with fire, cold with air, moist with water, and dry with earth). The humoral theory of health and disease was developed by Empedocles, the founder of a Greek medical school in Sicily in the 5th century BC. Empedocles believed that health was the result of a balance of the elements and that imbalance led to disease. This theory of the four elements became the standard dogma for nearly 2,000 years.

Hippocrates

Hippocrates, born in 460 BC on the Greek island of Cos, became the leader of the rational school of Greek medicine, a system based on careful observation of the patient and treatment of the observable problems (Fig 1-6). His clinical medicine was based on centuries of accumulated knowledge gained in the temple medicine of Asclepius.[17] But Hippocratic medicine was less reliant on magic or religion and more nature based, advocating herbal and dietary approaches to better health.[18] Hippocrates extended the ideas of Empedocles by postulating the existence of four principal fluids (the cardinal humors: blood, phlegm, black bile, and yellow bile) to correspond with the four chemical elements (hot, cold, moist, and dry). In addition, there were four corresponding temperaments: hematic (excitable), phlegmatic, melancholic, and bilious. For the followers of Hippocrates, health existed when these four humors and elemental conditions were in balance.[5] Disruption of the balance was the cause of disease. His writings (and those of his associates and pupils) became known as the "Corpus Hippocraticus."[18]

Guerini described the many references to dental and oral diseases that are scattered within the Corpus Hippocraticus.[11] For example:

> *In cases of toothache, if the tooth is decayed and loose it must be extracted. If it is neither decayed nor loose, but still painful, it is necessary to desiccate it by cauterizing. Masticatories also do good, as the pain derives from pituita (phlegm) insinuating itself under the roots of the teeth. Teeth are eroded and become decayed partly by pituita, and partly by food, when they are by nature weak and badly fixed in the gums.*

In the seventh book, on Epidemics, a case of scorbutus (scurvy) is described:

> *Large tubercles, of the size of grapes, had formed on the gums close to the teeth, black and livid, but not painful, except when the patient took food. For the mouth, incense powder mixed with some other ingredients proved useful. The internal use of the decoction of lentils also did good to the ulcers of the mouth.*

According to Hippocrates, the extraction of firmly embedded teeth was fraught with danger; therefore, he advocated the extraction of loose teeth only and the use of leaden forceps to minimize fracturing the crown from the roots.[9] Brief discussions of gingival overgrowth, dental abscess, caries, and jaw luxation are found in the Hippocratic writings.[2]

Examination of 1,500 teeth recovered from Greek cemeteries established around 1500 BC revealed similar dental diseases as those found at Egyptian sites, namely extensive dental attrition, periodontal bone loss (28%), and a relatively low level of caries (9%).[19] In the Hippocratic writings, toothache was thought to arise by accumulation of phlegm draining down from above for the maxillary teeth and up from the internal organs for the mandibular teeth. Treatment consisted of bloodletting, purging, and application of various herbal remedies. Teeth were extracted only if these remedies were unsuccessful. It was the practice to extract only loose teeth. Various dressings were applied to teeth and gums to degrade the periodontal tissues and loosen the teeth in advance of the extraction. As a precautionary step, cavities were filled with lint and lead to strengthen the crown before applying the forceps in order to minimize the chance of breaking the crown from the root. This practice persisted into the Middle Ages in Europe.

Hippocrates believed that doctors should possess social responsibility and high ethics.[20] They must avoid unkindness and offer their services free when necessary. Greek practitioners who embraced the Hippocratic method held themselves to a higher social responsibility and pledged to avoid all unkindness and to offer their services free when necessary. The Hippocratic Oath, taken by all who entered the medical profession, may be summarized by the dictum "help the patient and do no harm."[21] The oath directs the physician to respect the patient's personal information and to avoid taking advantage of the patient's dependence and vulnerability. The admonition in the oath that "I shall not use the knife even upon sufferers from stone, but will leave the operation to the technicians" has special meaning for understanding how the manual practices of surgery and dentistry developed in separation from the intellectual exercises of diagnosis, prognosis, and prescription, responsibilities of the physician class. Over the ensuing centuries, this led to the unfortunate separation of surgery and dentistry from medicine, with physicians in a supreme position by virtue of their knowledge of Latin and their university education.

The Etruscans

The Etruscans of northern Italy are considered to have produced the earliest examples of prosthetic dentistry. The Etruscan civilization flourished before the Christian era and the establishment of the Roman Empire. The Etruscans spoke a separate language and practiced advanced decorative arts, largely influenced by their extensive cultural and commercial ties with Greece and Egypt. Prosthetic dental appliances constructed with teeth carved from bone, animal teeth, or with human teeth removed from cadavers and fastened with gold bands have been found in Etruscan and Roman gravesites (Fig 1-7). Twenty Etruscan dental appliances have been documented, but only nine survive. All appear to have been used as decorative bands or to support replacements to one or both maxillary central incisors in women from whom healthy teeth may have been removed deliberately.[11] This evidence seems to confirm that gold dental appliances were worn only by

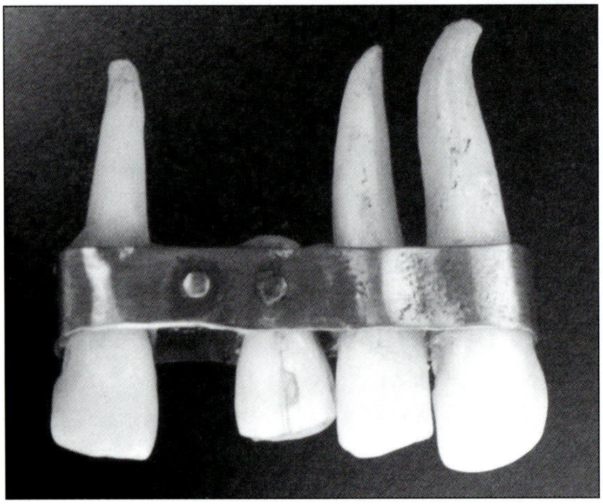

Fig 1-7 Etruscan dental prosthesis.

Etruscan women, suggesting that cosmetic concerns were paramount in their creation.

The Roman Empire

Greek, Egyptian, Phoenician, and Persian civilizations influenced the growth of medical knowledge and technology through the intercourse of commerce in the eastern Mediterranean Sea. The Egyptian city of Alexandria became a center of learning, where a great university and library were developed.[5] Greek medical lore was translated into Arabic and preserved for centuries before translation to Latin in the Early Middle Ages. The Roman civilization, beginning with the foundation of the city of Rome in 753 BC, absorbed a great deal of what was known from the establishment of Greek communities within its territories. The Greek medical system of health spas (temples) spread its influence among the Romans. The humoral theory of diseases fundamental to Greek medicine was accepted in Rome.

Medicine in the Roman Empire became less philosophic and more practical out of the necessity of maintaining large armies and meeting the demands of an increasingly wealthy urban population. Roman armies spread throughout the Empire were accompanied by

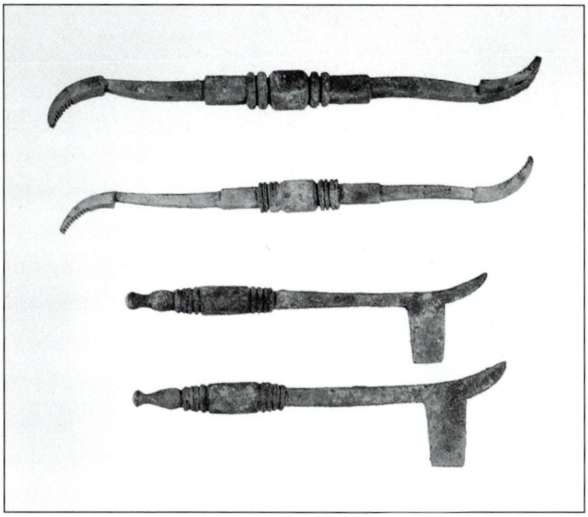

Fig 1-8 Roman surgical instruments. (Courtesy of Historical Collections & Services, Claude Moore Health Sciences Library, University of Virginia.)

surgeons to repair wounded soldiers and physicians who tended to the illnesses common to marching armies and large encampments of men. Although medical remedies were still mostly herbal, there was an increasing place for surgical treatment of wounds. Surgical instruments recovered from Roman graveyards reveal advanced designs and a wide array of implements[22] (Fig 1-8). During the Roman Empire, the profession of medicine became very profitable, and soon it became overstocked. This may have led to a subdivision of medical practice, with specialists becoming common in the latter half of the first century of the Christian era.[23]

Celsus

The two giants of Roman medicine were Celsus (25 BC–50 AD) and Galen (129–200 AD). Celsus, independently wealthy after the death of his father, studied Hippocratic medicine in the Greek islands and later at the medical school of Alexandria.[21] Celsus was a prolific writer, a compiler who assembled most of what was known of Greek medicine into his eight-book *De Re Medicina*. Book 6 dealt with diseases of the eyes, ears, nose, throat, and mouth. Celsus accepted the four classic signs of inflammation as rubor, tumor, calor, and dolor. His *De Re Medicina* served as a basic compendium of medical and dental knowledge into the Middle Ages. He was an empiric in his belief that it was not very important to know what caused a disease but only what cured it or alleviated the suffering. According to Celsus, a man was not qualified for his profession by theory but by practice (experience).

Celsus considered toothache to be numbered among the worst of tortures. He recommended the application of poultices, purgatives, and fumigations for the relief of toothache.[24;2] Periodontal suppuration and carious teeth were best treated by cauterization with a hot iron and/or boiling oil. The later technique was carried out with small pellets of lint attached to a probe or toothpick and dipped in boiling oil before applying to the tooth. Tooth extraction was considered dangerous, to be performed only as a last resort. A finger technique, used after application of loosening agents, was preferred to the use of forceps. Celsus recommended, as others had before him, to pack

---

[2] "IX. In TOOTH-ACHE, which may be justly ranked among the most excruciating affections, wine is most decidedly to be interdicted: even food, at first ought to be denied, and afterwards employed sparingly, choosing such as is tender, that it may not irritate the teeth during mastication; externally the steam of hot water must be applied by means of a sponge, and a cerate prepared with cypress or orris oil, spread on wool, is to be laid over the part, while the head itself ought to be covered. Should the pain become more severe, benefit may accrue from opening the bowels by clyster, laying hot poultices upon the jaw, and retaining in the mouth warm water impregnated with any proper medicines, and repeatedly renewing the liquid. For this purpose cinquefoil root is boiled in diluted wine, and henbane root either in posca or mixed wine, adding to both these liquors a small portion of salt; so also poppy-heads, not too dry, and the root of mandragore. But especial care must be taken lest either of these three be swallowed. A decoction of the bark of the root of the white poplar is also a proper medicine for the same purpose; so also hartshorn shavings in vinegar; and catmint with a fat teda, or with a ripe fig either in mulse or vinegar and honey; after boiling the fig the fluid must be strained; also a probe enveloped in wool is to be immersed in hot oil, and with this the tooth itself is to be fomented. There are certain applications acting upon the tooth itself like a cataplasm: such is the pulp of the rind taken from a sour and dry pomegranate, rubbed up with a like portion of galls and pine-bark, with which minium is mixed; these, after trituration, are beat up with rainwater; or equal portions of panaces, opium, peucedanum and stavesacre without the seeds, are rubbed together; or three parts of galbanum to one of opium. Be the local application to the teeth what it may, one should be equally exact in the use of the cerate for the jaw, covering it, as I said before, with wool. Some also mix together of myrrh, cardamom, of each p. x. I. saffron, pellitory, figs, pepper, of each p. x. IV. mustard p. x. VIII.: having rubbed them together, they smear them on a piece of linen rag, and apply them on the shoulder of that side where the tooth aches; if in the upper jaw on the scapula, if in the lower on the breast. and that alleviates the pain; and after it has produced the proper effect, it is to be immediately removed. Even if the tooth be carious, unless there be urgent occasion, there is no need to be in a burry to extract it; but to each fomentation above mentioned other stronger compositions are to be added, of a nature calculated to allay pain, such as is that of Hera. It contains of opium p. x. I. pepper p. x. II. Sory p. x. x.; these when powdered are formed into a mass with galbanum, and that is applied round the affected tooth."[24]

the cavity of a carious tooth with lead or linen prior to applying the forceps lest the crown fracture away. All bone and root fragments must be removed to minimize any postsurgical infection. Hoffmann-Axthelm considered the exodontia technique of Celsus to be remarkably modern in concept.[2]

Celsus advocated the use of files to smooth jagged edges and to remove tartar from teeth. A mixture containing poppies in the form of a paste was recommended for treating the pain of oral ulcers and toothache.[11] Another remedy for toothache and oral ulcers consisted of application of papyrus paper impregnated with arsenic and other caustic substances to the diseased area. Dental abscesses were to be lanced and drained. Jaw fractures were treated with tooth banding and jaw bandages to immobilize the bony fragments. Paulus Aegineta, a 7th-century Greek physician and author of an encyclopedic survey of Greek and Roman medicine, gave these instructions for tooth extraction:

> *Having scarified around the tooth down to the socket, we must by degree shake the teeth with a tooth-extractor, and draw it out. But, if it is carious, we must first plug up the hole with a small tent, that it may not break when compressed by the instrument. After the extraction we may consume the flesh that is left by sprinkling it with finely levigated salts, and afterwards gargles of wine oroxycrate may be used until the completion of the cure.*[25]

In his many commentaries, Aegineta noted that Celsus disapproved of the extraction of teeth except in cases of extreme necessity. Celsus warned of the danger of fracturing the jawbone during tooth extraction, citing cases that led to death of the patient.[25]

Galen

The most famous of all Greek/Roman physicians and teachers was Galen (Fig 1-9). Born in Pergamum in 129 AD, Galen went on to achieve fame second only to Hippocrates. Like Celsus, he studied Greek medicine at Pergamum, Corinth, and Alexandria. Galen practiced medicine in Rome and for a time with the Roman army under Marcus Aurelius. While at Pergamum, he was surgeon to the gladiators. Galen wrote extensively, leaving a body of medical knowledge that controlled the medical curriculum and practice into the 16th century.[5] In dental medicine, he followed the chief remedies proposed by earlier Greek and Roman physicians. He was the first to recognize that a toothache could be derived from inflammation of the pulp and that dental pain could also arise from an inflammation of the radicu-

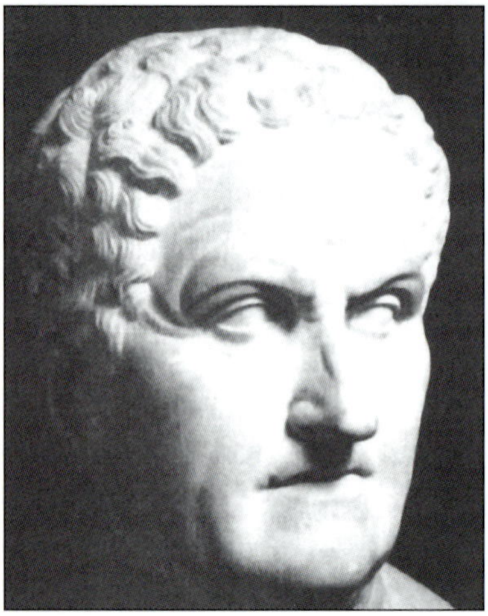

Fig 1-9 Galen.

lar (root) portion of the tooth. Guerini gives us the most complete account of the contributions of Greek and Roman physicians to the treatment of oral and dental diseases. Despite ample references in the medical texts of Greek and Roman physicians to dental and gingival diseases and their surgical and herbal treatment regimens, there is no evidence that any restorative or prosthetic dentistry was actually performed by medical practitioners.[11]

But evidence of a different nature, along with the dental artifacts recovered from Etruscan graves, suggests that there were artisans who carried out dental services for the wealthy classes. Martial, a Roman satirist of the 1st century AD, in writing of daily life makes several references to dental practitioners and false teeth. In speaking of the practitioner Cascellius, Martial writes that he "extracts or repairs an aching tooth." Elsewhere he notes, "and you, Galla, lay aside your teeth at night, just as you do your silken dress" and, to Leila, "You wear bought teeth, and bought hair."[26]

Other influential Romans

Two notable Roman physicians of the first and second Christian centuries were Archigenes and Adromachus. Archigenes's notable achievement was his approach to treating toothache by drilling into the pulp with a trephine to allow the escape of morbid substances and his introduction of medicines. Andromachus, physician to Nero, achieved fame with his concocted mixture called *theriac*. Andromachus claimed that theriac cured all sorts of diseases, including toothache. Its beneficial effect was probably due to its chief component, opium.[11]

Dioscorides, a Roman herbalist of the 1st century, classified hundreds of plants to be used as remedies for most ailments, including toothaches, oral ulcers, and abscesses.[13] His book *De materia medica* was translated into Arabic and later into various European languages. It contained recipes for preparations to be inserted into the cavities of decaying teeth. It also contained formulas for medicines that were reported to loosen teeth and aid in extraction. This book remained in use for about 1,500 years.

Islamic Medicine

The downfall of the Roman Empire was followed by a long decline in the growth of knowledge throughout the Western world. During this period, the Arabian peoples expanded their influence by conquering the Mediterranean and extending their culture into Spain and southern France. In their great cities of Baghdad, Damascus, Seville, Toledo, and Cordova, they established new centers of learning, incorporating the medical knowledge of the Greeks, Romans, and Egyptians through translation into Arabic. Knowledge of Greek and Roman medicine came to the Arabs through Christians who were driven out of the Byzantine Empire. Displaced scholars translated Greek medical manuscripts into Semitic languages and then into Arabic. By adding their own experiences to the Hellenic and Roman corpus of medicine, Arabs developed an Islamic medicine exemplified by its leading practitioners, Rhazes (865–925 AD), Albucasis (936–1013 AD), and Avicenna (980–1037 AD).

Rhazes

Rhazes (Abu Bakr Muhammad ibn Zakariya ar-Razi) was born in northeastern Persia and studied medicine in Baghdad before becoming a court physician and a leading figure in the field of medicine, ranking with Hippocrates and Galen as one of the founders of clinical medicine. The *Al-Mansuri*, one of Rhazes's many writings, consisted of ten parts (books) and is an encyclopedic review of contemporary Islamic medicine, used in teaching until long after the Renaissance. As in all previous compendiums of medical knowledge, attention was given to the care of the teeth and to the treatment of dental and oral diseases much in accord with previous ideas of Galen. For the care of teeth, Rhazes recommended cleansing powders combining abrasive and whitening substances such as the ashes of ocean crabs and mussels.[2] To protect the teeth from caries, he advocated oiling the teeth before going to bed and avoiding sweets. Toothache was treated by filling the cavity with mastic (a resin or gum) and alum (a mineral salt of sulfate of aluminum and potassium).[11] If pain persisted, Rhazes recommended entering the tooth with a drill and applying cauterization with a hot iron or boiling oil.[2] Opium and myrrh were used as topical remedies and in dressings. Extraction, a last resort, was said to be aided by first applying loosening agents such as arsenic paste or the juices of a boiled frog. In general, Arab physicians were cautious about extracting teeth, preferring to firm tissues with astringents, cauterizing and ligating loose teeth to healthier abutment teeth. Diseased gums were treated by scarification and application of leeches. Hoffmann-Axthelm has noted that in 19th-century Baghdad, a metallic substance called *tancar*, similar to that used by tin smiths and plumbers, was used to fill carious teeth.[2]

Albucasis

Albucasis was born in Cordoba, Spain, in 936 AD and is believed to have died after 1009 AD. This university-educated physician wrote an encyclopedic treatise on medicine and surgery called the *Al-Tasrif (The Method)*. It covers the advantages and disadvantages of cautery and the tools for treatment of wounds, venesection (phlebotomy), and cupping, as well as various kinds of needles and threads for stitching wounds, including about 150 depictions and drawings of tools, surgical instruments, droppers, and syringes[11] (Fig 1-10). Albucasis, a foremost oral surgeon, warned of breaking crowns and leaving stumps in the jaw, complications that often occurred when untrained practitioners extracted teeth.[2] For extraction, he advised detaching the gingiva and loosening the tooth before applying the forceps. Like Celsus, he advocated filling the cavity of a carious tooth with linen thread to minimize crushing of the crown. His coverage of dental and oral diseases was rather extensive. He recognized tartar to be the cause of periodontal disease and placed great importance on scaling.[2] He designed numerous types of scalers and other dental instruments.[11] Albucasis advocated ligating loose teeth with silver and gold wires and replacing missing teeth with artificial teeth carved from bone. According to Hoffmann-Axthelm, Albucasis must be considered the most important practitioner of dental medicine up to that time and one that would not be surpassed for several centuries to come.[2]

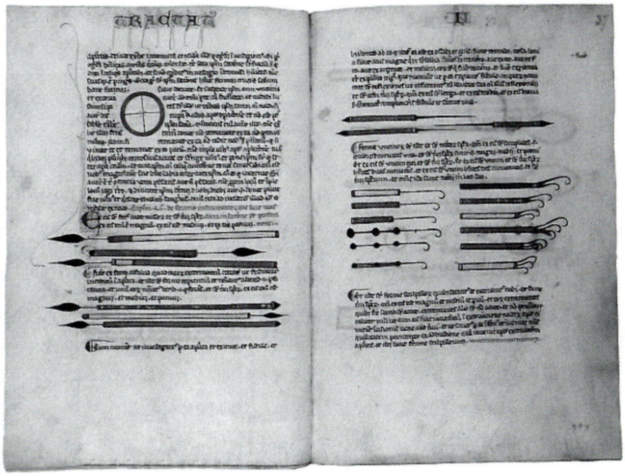

Fig 1-10 Page from Albucasis's *Al-Tasrif* depicting instruments for scraping tartar from teeth.

Avicenna

Avicenna, (Ali al-Husayn ibn-Sina), an Iranian physician, is considered to be the most famous and influential of the philosopher-scientists of Islam. He composed the *Kitab al-shifa'* (*Book of Healing*), a vast philosophic and scientific encyclopedia, and *The Canon of Medicine*, which is among the most famous books in the history of medicine. Avicenna stressed the importance of oral hygiene. He discussed the causes and treatment of toothache and oral ulcerations. According to Avicenna, the proper treatment for relief of throbbing dental pain was to drill the tooth to drain it of its humors and to introduce various palliative medicaments.[11] He recommended the application of arsenic for treatment of toothache, ulcers, and fistulas. A section of *The Canon* dealt with treatment of fractured jaws and the importance of attaining proper occlusion and stabilization with wires and bandages.[2] Herbal remedies, as in former times, remained the most important aspect of treatment of systemic and dental diseases.

Summary

In ancient times, the medical profession considered toothache, gingival disease, and oral ulcerations as ailments to be treated side-by-side with eye, genital, gastrointestinal, heart, and other regional ailments. Indeed, the mouth was connected to the body. From the beginning of written records, it is clear that tooth abrasion, caries, toothache, and dental abscesses formed significant medical needs. Periodontal disease and inflammation of the gums were common problems. Dental calculus (tartar), recognized as a cause of gingival and periodontal inflammation, was removed with special instruments. Treatment was heavily based on local application and or consumption of herbal remedies, sometimes concocted with added "junk" to drive away demons. Textural evidence suggests that dental cavities were "filled" with herbal preparations, often with opium and arsenic as part of the mixture. Cauterization and extractions were performed when herbals remedies proved ineffective. When extraction was necessary, it was advised to loosen the tooth with application of natural medicines before extraction, and it was suggested to leave the actual extraction to one who had experience with the technique. For the rich, loose teeth were splinted to solid ones with gold wires. In a few cases, missing teeth were replaced with teeth carved from bone or with cadaver teeth. But this again was only for the wealthy. In accord with the humoral concept of diseases, bloodletting, cupping, purging, and cauterization were treatments of choice for suppurating infections. Physicians may have prescribed the treatment of oral and dental diseases, but the actual manual service was assigned to a surgeon or subordinate mechanic.

References

1. Leek FF. The practice of dentistry in ancient Egypt. J Egypt Archaeol 1967; 53:51–58.
2. Hoffmann-Axthelm W. History of Dentistry. Chicago: Quintessence, 1981.
3. Ghalioungui P. Did a dental profession exist in Ancient Egypt? Med Hist 1971;15:92–94.
4. Forshaw RJ. The practice of dentistry in ancient Egypt. Br Dent J 2009; 206:481–486.
5. Osler W. The Evolution of Modern Medicine. New Haven: Yale University, 1921.
6. Hillson SW. Diet and dental disease. World Archeol 1979;11:147–162.
7. Ruffer A. Study of abnormalities and pathology of ancient Egyptian teeth. Am J Phys Anthropol 1920;3:335–397.
8. Forshaw RJ. Dental health and disease in ancient Egypt. Br Dent J 2009; 206:421–424.
9. Densham A. A review of the progress of dental science and literature from the earliest ages. Proc R Soc Med 1909;2:71–98.

10. Nickol T. An examination of the dental state of an Egyptian mummy by means of computer tomography: A contribution to "dentistry in ancient Egypt." Bull Hist Dent 1995;43:105–112.
11. Guerini V. A History of Dentistry from the Most Ancient Times Until the End of the Eighteenth Century. Philadelphia: Lea & Febiger, 1909:188–199.
12. Torrey CC. A Phoenician necropolis at Sidon. Ann Am Sch Orient Res Jerusalem 1920;1:1–27.
13. Shklar G, Chernin D. A Sourcebook of Dental Medicine. Waban, MA: Maro, 2002.
14. Libby W. The History of Medicine in Its Salient Features. Boston: Houghton Mifflin, 1922.
15. Jastrow N. The medicine of the Babylonians and Assyrians. Proc R Soc Med 1914;7(Sect Hist Med):109–176.
16. Caton R. Hippocrates and the newly-discovered health temple of Cos. Br Med J 1906;1:571–574.
17. Adams F. The Genuine Works of Hippocrates. New York: William Wood, 1886.
18. Temkin O. Greek medicine as science and craft. Isis 1953;44:213–225.
19. Carr G. Some dental characteristics of the middle Minoans. Man 1960;60:119–122.
20. Grube GMA. Greek medicine and the Greek genius. Phoenix 1954;8:123–135.
21. Garrison FH. An Introduction to the History of Medicine. Philadelphia: W. B. Saunders, 1913.
22. Milne JS. Surgical Instruments in Greek and Roman Times. Oxford: Clarendon, 1907.
23. Barnes H. On Roman medicine and Roman medical inscriptions found in Britain. Proc R Soc Med 1914;7(Sect Hist Med):71–87.
24. Collier GF. A Translation of the Eight Books of Aul. Corn. Celsus on Medicine. London: Simpkin and Marshall, 1831.
25. Adams F. The Seven Books of Paulus Aegineta. London: Sydenham Society, 1846.
26. The Epigrams of Martial. London: Bell & Baldy, 1871.

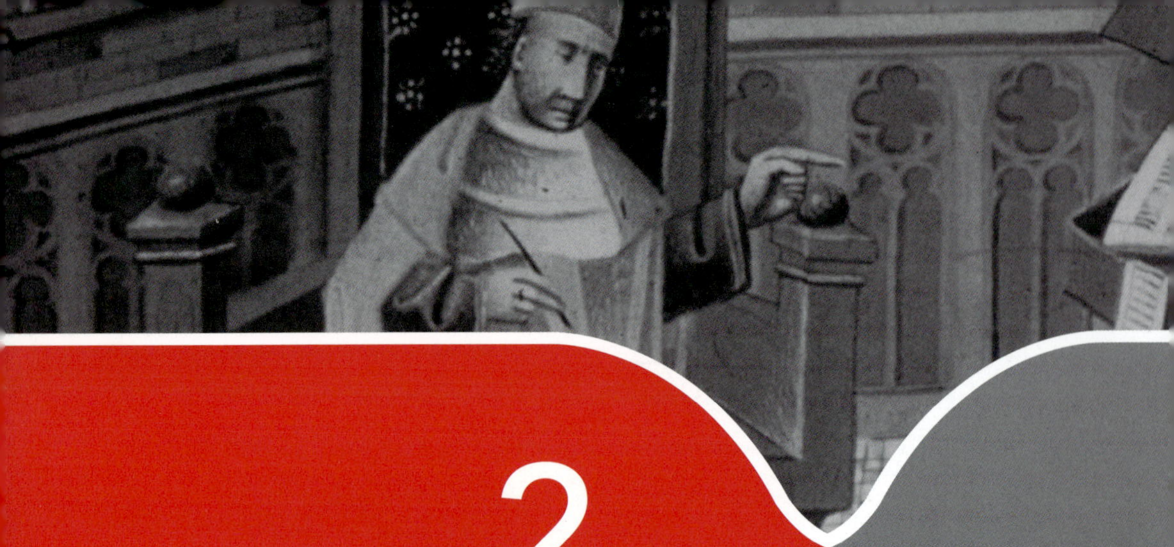

2

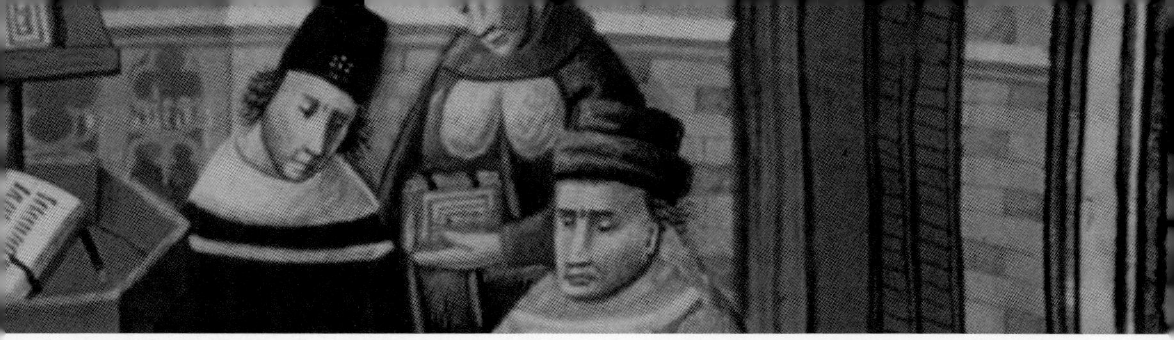

The Middle Ages

The downfall of the Roman Empire in the 5th century AD led to a generalized decline in the stability and organization of society in the Western world. The invasion of barbarians from the northern territories destroyed the established fabric of law imposed by Roman rule, only to be reversed by the subsequent growth of Christian institutions, the rise of kingship and feudalism, and the eventual emergence of commercialism. Centers of learning created by Christian and Islamic scholars in the newly formed kingdoms of Britain, France, Germany, and Spain served to revive social order. The recovery that followed several centuries of relative poverty was halted temporarily by the disruption of commerce in the Mediterranean during the Islamic conquests of the Iberian Peninsula and southern France and by Viking raids in the North. By the 11th and 12th centuries, resurgence in trade of raw materials and manufactured goods was felt in Europe, especially in major cities along the Northern, Atlantic, and Mediterranean coasts and inland along the major rivers.[1] The rise of a rich merchant class was accompanied by increased numbers of affluent clergymen and municipal administrators. By the 13th century, an increasing percentage of the population was employed, organized in guilds, and better educated than before. The rising number of city-dwelling bourgeoisie created a growing, albeit slow, demand for better health care, including treatment of oral and dental diseases.[2,3]

Practice of Medicine

Physicians occupied the top of the health care pyramid in the Middle Ages. They attended university medical schools and upon successful examination earned the right to wear academic robes before entering practice.[4] Having completed the educational program known as the *Articella*, they knew Latin and were steeped in the classical medicine of Galen. In some cities, physicians were required to have passed municipal or university licensing examinations. The few surgeons who held medical degrees were considered to be master-surgeons and to belong to the surgeons of the long robe (a result of their right to wear academic robes). However, most surgeons were uneducated, knew no Latin, acquired their trade by apprenticeship, and were considered to be surgeons of the short robe, or lay surgeons.[5] Barber-surgeons, occupying a still lower place in the hierarchy, were entrusted to carry out minor services such as bloodletting, bandaging, toothdrawing (extraction), and the application of salves. They practiced a manual craft devoid of a theoretic or scientific basis and learned through apprenticeships regulated by the rules of a guild. Both lay surgeons and barber-surgeons, by nature of their manual services and their lack of university education, held a subordinate position to physicians. In their quest for greater social status (ie, equality with university-educated physicians), lay surgeons increasingly delegated manual operations to barber-surgeons.[6]

Medical science was stagnated in the teachings of Galen, still heavily based on herbal remedies, dietary regimes, purging, and bloodletting. The reigning notion that disease was caused by an imbalance in the four elements was made additionally complicated by the belief that sickness was a consequence of individual and collective sin. Good health could only be restored by healing both the soul and the body.[7] The clergy took on this dual challenge, because many physicians and surgeons belonged to monastic orders. In a review of Anglo-Norman practitioners of medicine, E. J. Kealey has reported that around 1160 AD there may have been 90 individuals providing health care in England and Normandy, of which 40% were members of the clergy, and at least 2 appeared to have been engaged in dentistry.[8] In the 6th century, 238 monasteries existed in the Western world. Under the rules established by St Benedict, monks were mandated to provide care to the sick.[7] By the 13th century, nearly 1,000 monasteries had been formed within France.[2] Medical care was based on herbal remedies, magic, prayer, superstition, and astrology. The sick prayed to Christian saints for relief; those suffering from toothache would appeal to St Ursman, because he had suffered from toothache for 9 years, or to St Medardus, who possessed a magnificent set of teeth. If someone had a disease of the tongue, he would pray to St Catherine of Alexandria, famous for her eloquence.[9] On occasion this type of prayer worked, probably because the body was given sufficient time to heal. When the patient was cured, the saint was further glorified for having performed a miracle.

In addition to caring for the sick, monks were employed copying Latin translations of early Arabic and Greek manuscripts. Only university-educated men, chiefly members of the church, were able to benefit from this accumulated knowledge. The practice of medicine and surgery by the clergy was abrogated by the Councils of Reims in 1125 and of Latran in 1139. In 1163, the Council of Tours prohibited monks and priests from conducting any practice that shed blood.[2] These rules drove many clerical surgeons and barber-surgeons to practice outside monastic centers.

A gradual separation of surgery from medicine began when the University of Paris forbade medical graduates from conducting manual operations because it considered them debasing to the status of the physician.[5,10] Medicine had become a text-based discipline taught at universities, while surgery remained a craft of lower social status gained by actual practice. It became increasingly clear to surgeons that they needed a written program of school-based training to achieve equality with medicine. This would begin in the universities of northern Italy during the 12th century.[11] The increasing number and scope of military campaigns in Europe, and the Crusades to the Holy Land, led to an accelerating demand for surgeons. Soon surgeons rose to prominence at court and among generals of the King's armies.

Dentators and apothecaries

As in previous centuries, the practical and speculative aspects of dental and oral diseases were part of the overall body of medical knowledge. Physicians continued to prescribe for oral and dental problems, but they increasingly assigned treatment to technicians of the barber-surgeon class. The use of opium and other herbal remedies continued to be the most commonly applied palliatives. Extractions were considered dangerous and were best left to barber-surgeons with special dental skills (dentators). The Middle Ages brought the first traces of dentists with these *dentators*, a special type of practitioner among the various categories of minor surgeons.[2] The dentator was skilled in tooth extraction (Fig 2-1); the banding of loose teeth together with wire, including replacement of missing teeth with artificial ones carved from bone; excavation of decayed teeth; and the placement

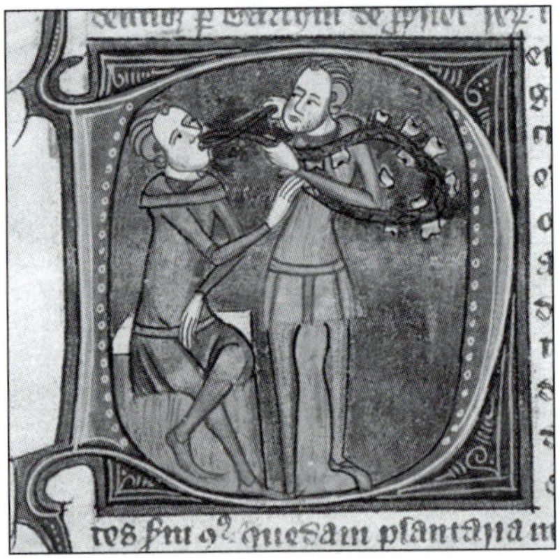

Fig 2-1 Surgeon pulling teeth, from Jacobus's *Omne Bonum* (14th century).

of fillings made of herbal mixtures. Dentators may have been few in number and were of necessity located in major cities where there existed a demand for their services.

Apothecaries, who specialized in concocting the remedies prescribed by physicians, were also prominent members of the health care community. The cultivation of medicinal herbs, mainly by religious orders, was a profitable business ever since the peak of Greek medicine. The Herbarium of Apuleius, dating from 500 AD, is a Latin treatise on medicinal plants that was translated into old English around 1050. Many of the entries are thought to have originated in Dioscorides's *De materia medica*. The following excerpt from an early Anglo-Saxon leechbook, probably belonging to the Glastonbury Abbey, illustrates how toothache was treated:

> *For tooth wark (ache), if a worm eat the tooth, take an old holly leaf and one of the lower umbels of hartwort, and the upward part of sage, boil two doles in water, pour into a bowl and yawn over it, then the worms shall fall into the bowl. If a worm eat the teeth, take holly rind over a year old, and root of carline thistle, boil in so hot water, hold in the mouth as hot as thou hottest may. For tooth worms, take acorn meal and henbane seed and wax, of all equally much, mingle these together, work into a wax candle, and burn it, let it reek into the mouth, put a black cloth under, then will the worms fall on it. For tooth wark, boil in wine or in vinegar the netherward part of ravens foot, sup as thou hottest may.*[12]

Bald's Leechbook contains recipes for preparing remedies for toothache and oral diseases.[13] In the 10th century, Bald's Leechbook recommended that: "For sore and looseness of teeth, take spearwort (*Inula helenium*) [Fig 2-2] give it to eat fasting; it steadieth the teeth"

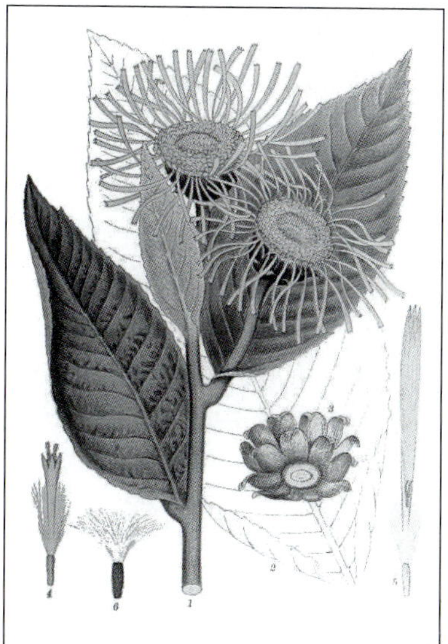

Fig 2-2 *Inula helenium* (spearwort).

and "For toothache, take a root of this wort (plant) which we named rosemary (*Rosmarinus officinalis*) give it to eat, without delay it removes the sore of the teeth; and let him hold the ooze in his mouth; soon it healeth the teeth." Although many of these recipes were ineffective, henbane and nightshade were pain relievers.[14] It has been argued that medieval medical care as described in herbal texts was not only pragmatic but effective. The addition of tables of contents, along with lists of ailments for which the plant may be used as a remedy, gave the user an easy information retrieval system.[15]

Medical curriculum

A significant development in the advance of medicine occurred with the establishment of a medical school in Salerno, Italy, in the 10th century. The seaside town of Salerno was a place frequented by the wealthier class of Romans who came to enjoy its restful setting and thermal spas. Initially, the Schola Medica Salernitana was simply a gathering of successful physicians rather than a formal medical school.[16] Legend is that the school was founded by four men of Arabian, Jewish, Greek, and Roman descent. However, the traditional view that these four cultures were incorporated into the teachings of the school has been viewed with skepticism.[9,16] The teaching at Salerno was based on the works of Hippocrates, Galen, and Dioscorides, much of it translated from Greek and Arabic texts to Latin at the nearby monastery of Monte Casino, founded in 529 AD by St Benedict.[16]

Constantinos Africanos, a Christian native of Carthage skilled in both Arabic and Latin, was encouraged to undertake the work of translation by the Archbishop of Salerno.[17] His first major work was the translation of the *Complete Book of the Medical Art* from the *kitab al-malaki (Royal Book)* of the 10th-century Persian physician Ali ibn al-Abbas, followed by the translation of the *Viaticum* by Ibn al-Gazzar.[18] These 11th-century medical texts became known as the Pantegni or "complete art" and the mainstay of the early medical curriculum. It is of interest that in these books, toothache was treated with arsenic-based fillings to relieve pain and to kill the pulp. Extraction was done only if the above treatment failed.[18]

The philosophy of the school at Salerno was based heavily on dietary rules for good health dictated in the *Regimen Sanitas Salernitanum*, a medical poem dating from the 12th century.[9] Writing the rules of good health in 360 rhyming stanzas made it easier for medical students to memorize long lists of recommendations and admonitions. The *Regimen* contains several references to toothache (and tooth worms) as well as dietary and herbal practices for oral hygiene. Over the ensuing centuries, the *Regimen* was translated into French, Italian, German, and English. The tradition of medical care at Salerno can be traced back to the period of the decline of the Roman Empire, and the influence of Arabian medicine at Salerno has been overemphasized.[19] Salerno maintained its reputation as the center of medical care and teaching during the 11th and 12th centuries. One of its chief contributions was the increased emphasis it gave to *materia medica* (the body of collected knowledge regarding the therapeutic effects of a healing substance) and the introduction of Eastern drugs. For the first time, the use of mercury was advocated in medicinal ointments for treatment of facial eruptions and scabies.[9]

From the 12th to 15th centuries, medicine was based on Greek and Roman texts. A new medical practice based on observation, experimentation, and the publication of case reports was slow to develop. The medical school curriculum of the 10th to 13th centuries continued to be based on the writings of Hippocrates and Galen as translated from the Greek to Arabic in Baghdad around 850 AD by the Christian physician Hunayn ibn Ishag al-Ibadi (known in the West as Joannitius). The Latin compendium, the *Articella*, contained the aphorisms and prognostics of Galen and the manuals on the diagnostic value of urine and the pulse. Typically these books were em-

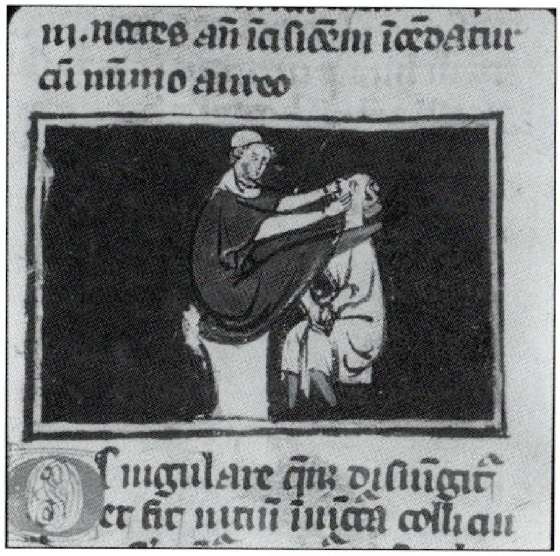

Fig 2-3 Surgeon treating a dislocated jaw, from the *Chirurgiae* of Ruggiero Fugardi (14th century).

bellished with commentary explanations and read to students by the faculty.

The first medieval texts on surgery appeared in Italy around 1180 with the *Chirurgiae Magistri Rogerii (The Surgery of Master Rogerius)* by Ruggiero Fugardi (Fig 2-3), which was later revised by Rolando of Parma.[11] Ruggiero's text was used at the Universities of Bologna and Montpellier, two of the most important early centers of medical education. With the invention of the printing press in 1450, marking the end of the Middle Ages, there was a surge in the production of medical and surgical textbooks, including many in the vernacular languages. The first works exclusively limited to dental and oral diseases made their appearance in the 15th century.

Following the establishment of the medical school at Salerno, new medical schools were established in many of the larger population centers. The schools at Bologna and Padua in Italy and at Montpellier and Paris in France achieved a high reputation, drawing students from all over Europe. The title of Doctor of Medicine was first granted by the college at Asti, in Italy, in 1329.[20] Medical education began at Oxford in the early 13th century, and by the 14th century Merton College was granting the title of Doctor of Medicine.[6]

Physicians, as graduates of medical schools, focused on the more speculative and philosophical natures of the discipline, leaving the

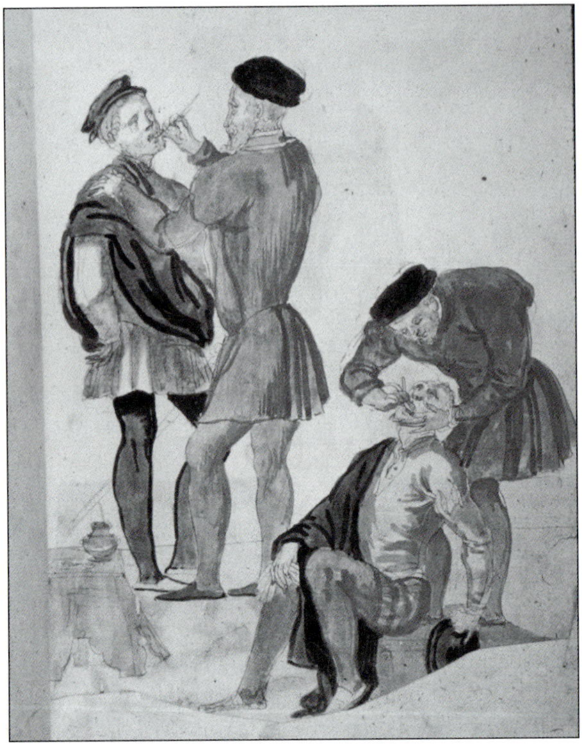

Fig 2-4 Surgeons treating patients, from Albrecht Meher's medical picture book (16th century).

actual application to surgeons (Fig 2-4). Schooled in Latin, they discussed diagnostics, etiologies, and regimens to be used in curing diseases from head to foot, including dental and oral diseases. The rigid adherence to Galen's theories soon led to stagnation in medical thinking, with no real advances made during the long period of the Middle Ages. But in the Renaissance (see chapter 3), university medical schools began a slow movement away from reliance on the traditional Greek-Arab medicine toward more emphasis on investigation and the introduction of chemical remedies.

Illiterate and untrained providers of health care carried out an itinerant trade, moving from town to town. Among these illiterate practitioners, many were charlatans who preyed on the sick, marketing their own concoctions. Henri de Mondeville, writing in the early 14th century, complained of the large number of cheats, forgers, and illiterates who were allowed to practice surgery and of the superstition of the people who were "more disposed to believe those who say they hold their science from God alone, than those who have learned their science from man, by dissection and books."[5]

Practice of dentistry

The little information available concerning the practice of dentistry in the Middle Ages is contained in the surgical writings of Henri de Mondeville and Guy de Chauliac. Both men continued the long tradition of integrating diseases of the teeth and mouth with general medicine and surgery. In discussing dental treatment, they noted that such services were best delegated to assistants or dentators. During the late Middle Ages, the dentator appears to have evolved from among the barber-surgeons or from surgeons of the short robe by acquiring special skills and new techniques. They removed decay and tartar from teeth and filled the cavities with herbal preparations or ground bone. By the early Renaissance period, they employed lead and gold as filling materials. They also practiced stabilization of loose teeth with wire bindings and carved artificial teeth from animal bones.

Although dental surgeries were performed by barber-surgeons or dentators, physicians retained the traditional right to prescribe surgery and/or the application of herbal remedies for oral and dental diseases. Medical and surgical practice continued to depend heavily on herbal concoctions containing opium for internal ailments and for dressing wounds. Practitioners of folk medicine knew that when opium was taken orally, it subdued the senses, making pain disappear. Anesthesia was induced with a concoction of mandrake, henbane, and opium steeped in wine. In the 9th century, the monks of Monte Cassino in Italy described the use of a sponge soaked in the above mixture and allowed to dry until needed. In use, the sponge was moistened and the patient was made to inhale its vapors. Guy de Chauliac described it as the soporific sponge and warned of potential asphyxia and death as complications.

Practice of Surgery

In Italy more so than in France, the practice of surgery remained united to medical practice. The great medieval surgeons—Lanfranc, Guy de Chauliac, and Henri de Mondeville—were trained in Italian medical schools, and their clinical practice combined medical knowledge with surgery.

Lanfranc

Lanfranc of Milan was a pupil of William Salicet (Guglielmo Salicetti), an eminent Italian physician. Lanfranc moved from Milan to Lyons and then to Paris, where he joined a new college of surgery founded in 1279 by Pitard, the surgeon who had accompanied the crusade of St Louis to Palestine. This college was placed under the "protection" of Saints Cosmas and Damianus, two practitioners of medicine who were martyred in the reign of Diocletian (284–305 AD). Graduates of the College of St Come were considered lay surgeons because they knew no Latin and were fully engaged in a manual trade.[5] From the time that Lanfranc lectured at the college, it grew in prominence, attracting students from many parts of France and the continent. At a much later date in the early 18th century, Pierre Fauchard, who became known as the father of dentistry, came to study surgery at the College of St Come.

Henri de Mondeville

Lanfranc's most famous pupil was Henri de Mondeville, First Surgeon to the King of France, Philippe Le Bel. Mondeville taught anatomy and surgery (Fig 2-5) at the medical school in Montpellier from 1304 to 1306 before joining the college of St Come in Paris.[5] Nicaise states that Mondeville taught surgery initially at the medical school of the University of Paris, a practice briefly tolerated until 1350, when the medical faculty established a ban on the practice of surgery by physicians.[21] It was held at that time that the practice of surgery, a manual and bloody exercise, had a demeaning effect on the profession of medicine. The prejudice against surgery dominated French medicine well into the 19th century.

In 1320, Mondeville wrote *The Surgery*, the first compendium on the practice of surgery written in Latin.[21] Among the illustrations in this treatise is a pair of forceps for extracting teeth. Unfortunately, Mondeville died before completing his book. Although his chapters on dental and oral diseases, listed in the table of contents, were never completed, there is much to be learned of his approach to dental disease from his lengthy chapters on incisions, cautery, venesection, and the application of plasters. He recommended cautery of painful teeth and gingiva and venesection on the surface of the lips for gingival abscesses and for stimulating blood flow following tooth extraction. Of a particular note is his bizarre recommendation to perform venesection under the chin for the relief of halitosis.[21]

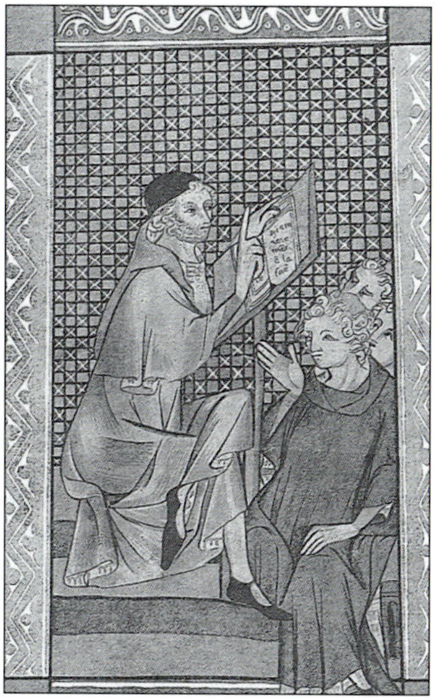

Fig 2-5 Mondeville lecturing to students. (Adapted from Nicaise.[21])

Although much of Mondeville's treatise is of little practical value today, there remains a body of insightful advice on the conduct of surgical and medical practice that rings true today.[21] Mondeville was a firm believer that surgery and medicine were best practiced hand-in-hand and that a good surgeon must possess knowledge of medical science. According to Mondeville, the good qualities of a perfect surgeon are many: He should be audacious, not dispute in the presence of laymen, operate with prudence and knowledge, and not undertake perilous surgeries without anticipating all the potential problems and solutions. The good surgeon must be physically strong and agile. He must give himself totally to his patient. He must comfort his patients with good words and should listen to their just demands only so far as they do not impair the treatment outcome. The surgeon should promise his patients that they will get better while not hiding from them the dangers of their sickness. He should avoid getting involved with hopeless cases. Above all, he must help the poor and not inflate his importance. A surgeon is just to withhold services from those rich men who seek to cheat the doctor, and it is not necessary to treat for charity those who prefer their riches to their health.[21] This remains good advice from a man who practiced his art with apparent dedication and charity.

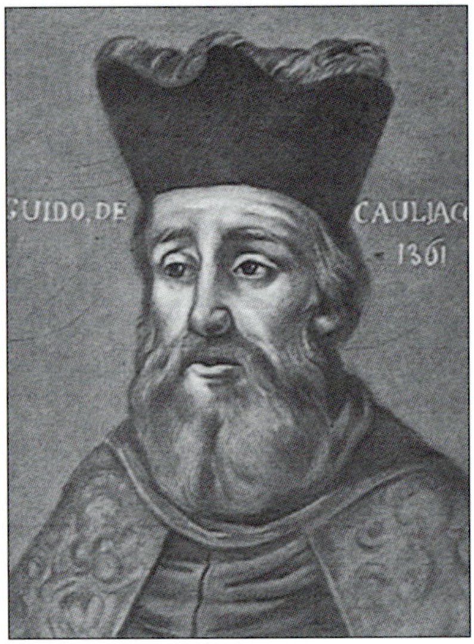

Fig 2-6 Guy de Chauliac.

Guy de Chauliac

Guy de Chauliac (Fig 2-6) was born around 1300 and died in 1368. He studied medicine at the universities of Montpellier, Toulouse, and Bologna. He was held in such high regard that he served as physician to the popes at Avignon. His great book, the *Chirurgia Magna* (Fig 2-7), was written in 1363 but not published until 1478, many years after his death. Its popularity was so great that it was translated into most European languages and underwent 130 editions. It was an encyclopedic work containing an extensive bibliography.[22] As surgeon to the popes, he had access to the vast collection of the Vatican library. Chauliac's theories of disease, *materia medica*, and surgical practice were mainly patterned after Galenic and Arabian medical practice. For example, Densham considers Chauliac's ideas on teeth to be merely a "réchauffé" of Albucasis.[23] While providing a thorough account of Chauliac's treatment of dental problems, Guerini stresses Chauliac's dependence on the prior writings of Galen and the Arabian authors (Ali Abbas, Avicenna, and Rhazes). All of the various dental remedies previously described in the classic literature were repeated by Chauliac. Nevertheless, there is much historical significance regarding the history of dentistry in what Chauliac has to say. According to Guerini, no other book gives a better picture of dental practice in the 14th century.[20]

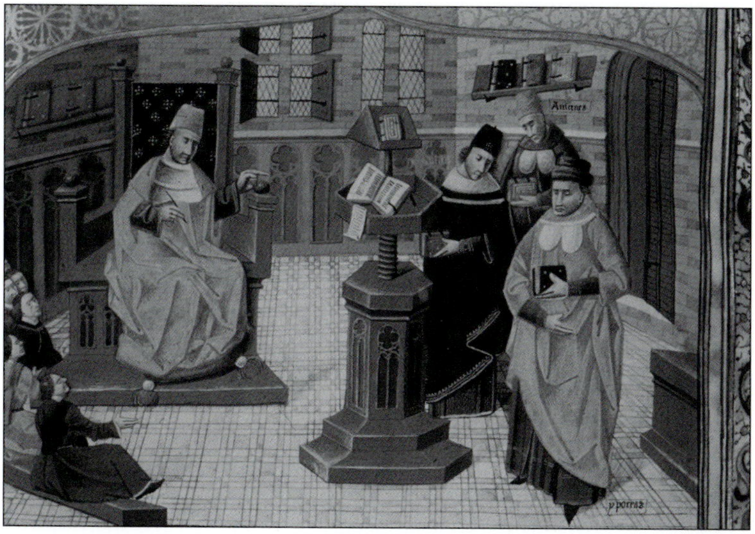

Fig 2-7 Guy de Chauliac seated before a book on a lectern, with Galen, Avicenna, and Hippocrates and their books, from a 15th-century copy of Chauliac's *Chirurgia Magna*.

A key statement in the *Chirurgia Magna* notes that operations on the teeth are performed by barbers or dentators.[2] According to Chauliac, physicians have abandoned dental practice, yet they retain the responsibility to advise and to know the methods to be used to cure dental diseases.[2] The physician, in selecting a dentator, needs to know who among them is experienced and who is equipped with the proper instruments. Also to be noted is the comment that when teeth fall out or are extracted, replacements may be inserted using teeth from another person or with teeth carved from ox bone and secured to the patient's teeth with gold wires, a service again to be delegated to a dentator. It is increasingly clear from the writings of Chauliac that many physicians and surgeons were increasingly recommending that extractions be performed by barber-surgeons and dentators who possessed skills for this type of work.[2] It had become clear that many of the medications prescribed by the ancient Greeks and Arabs for loosening teeth prior to extraction were useless or harmful. Chauliac claims that he had never seen them work. Guerini has suggested that physicians and many surgeons of the long robe may have considered tooth extraction to be a relatively risky procedure with a good chance of hemorrhage and postoperative complications—troubles that they did not want to deal with.[20] Furthermore, Chauliac notes that there were no small number of toothdrawers and barber-surgeons willing to undertake the task. Also to be considered is the reluctance on the part of surgeons and physicians to undertake demeaning tasks that were more appropriately the province of barber-surgeons.[6] Chauliac gave specific rules for treatment of toothache: All mechanical treatments are assigned to barber-surgeons; the role of the physician is to prescribe remedies and courses of action; and barber-surgeons must be equipped with proper instruments and should be supervised by physicians.

Chauliac was clear in his position that surgeons (as well as physicians) must be knowledgeable in dental diseases and their treatment in order to diagnose, delegate, and supervise treatment by a dentator. His book shows what constituted the dentator's instrumentarium and that his scope of practice included making mouthwashes, dentifrices, fumigations, cauterizations, and fillings and scaling tartar. For these services, the dentator needed scrapers, rasps, spatuminae, elevators, scalpels, tooth trephines, files, tenacula, probes, and cannulas (Fig 2-8). Among the procedures described in his *Chirurgia Magna* was the removal of foreign bodies, suturing of separated tissues, control of hemorrhages, treatment of fractures, excision of cancers, cauterizations, bloodletting, cleaning and medicating of dental cavities, ligation of loose teeth, removal of tartar, and extraction of teeth. Repeating much that is contained in Mondeville's treatise, he advocated bloodletting from the veins of the lip close to the teeth in cases of inflamed gingivae and dental abscess.[2] Cauterization applied at the base of the chin or the ear was recommended to ease toothache as well as eye and ear disorders.[2]

Anesthetic inhalations were administered with sponges previously soaked in herbal solutions containing opium, henbane, and mandragora. Extensive use was made of gargles, rinses, medicated fillings, ointments, infusions, dentifrices, and poultices. Among the many ingredients used in treating dental diseases were pumice and bone powders, camphor and opiates for pain, mint, rose oil, camphor, boiled wine and vinegar, and hundreds of other herbal preparations.[20] The treatment of carious or rotten teeth consisted of cleansing the teeth with aqua vitae (eg, brandy) or some other mouthwash and filling the cavities with wax or mastic containing herbal and natural ingredients to relieve the ache and to occlude the cavity. Files were used to gain access to interdental caries and to create interdental spaces that could be more easily cleaned.

There is substantial evidence that dental diseases were considered serious medical matters by professors of medicine/surgery of medieval medical schools and that the methods for dealing with these dis-

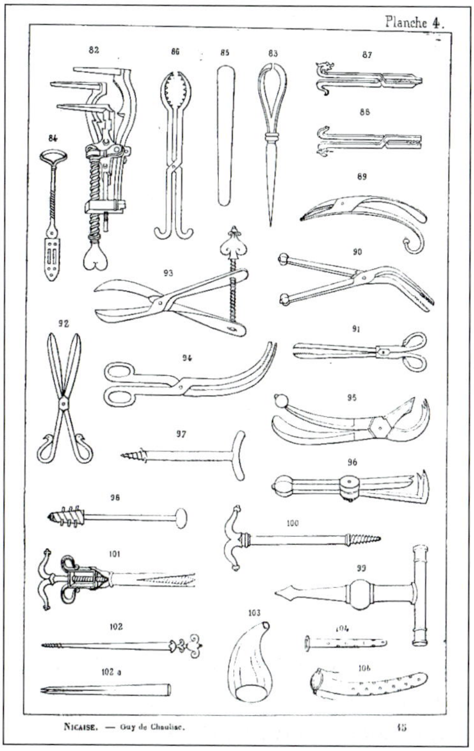

Fig 2-8 Chauliac's surgical instruments. Numbers 95 and 96 are dental forceps. (Adapted from Nicaise.[2])

eases were taught in the curriculum. Guerini cites the work of three 15th-century physicians who commented on dental diseases as part of their writings.[20] The works of Valescon, professor at the University of Montpellier; Pietro of Argelata, professor of surgery at the University of Bologna; and Bartolomeo Montagnana of the University of Padua confirmed the basic methods for dealing with dental diseases as they are outlined in Guy de Chauliac's *Chirurgia Magna*.

Surgeon guilds

Toward the close of the Middle Ages, surgeons formed guilds that were similar to other craft guilds. In Paris, they formed an association with the Church of St Come and later established a college of surgery. In 1311, they held examinations in the presence of the First Surgeon to the King for those seeking licensure. With royal approval, they wore academic robes and assumed the title of surgeons of the long robe. In Paris at that time, surgeons of the long robe were instructed in Latin and studied medicine for 2 years and surgery for an additional 2 years before being received into the guild as Master Surgeons. Barbers who became skilled in minor surgery took on the title of barber-surgeons or surgeons of the short robe.

At about the same time that surgeons and barber-surgeons were organizing in Paris, a guild of Master Surgeons was organized in England in 1368. The Company of Barbers of London was incorporated in 1462. The Royal Commonality of Barber-Surgeons granted by Henry VIII in 1540 united barbers and surgeons and defined their scope of practice. Barbers were forbidden to perform surgery except for extractions, while surgeons were not to shave patrons or operate barbershops. In commemoration of incorporation, the company published the first English translation of a compilation of the works of Galen, the *Questyonary of Cyrurgyens*, in 1542.[24] It was based on an earlier French translation of the same material, containing substantial portions of Chauliac's treatise on surgery in addition to Galen's medical questions.

Summary

The most significant development during the 11th to 14th centuries was the rise of surgery, rivaling and surpassing medicine in successful management of a broad category of illnesses. Along with this process, there arose within the barber-surgeons a group of individuals skilled in dealing with dental and oral diseases, the dentators. The dentator's training was purely practical, by apprenticeship, on-the-job, without schooling or consideration of medical theory. Their rudimentary understanding of and ability to cure dental diseases would develop slowly during the Renaissance period. Because of the tendency to secrecy and the lack of education on the part of practitioners, they left no written record of this advancement. But that it did occur is manifested in the celebrated treatise of Pierre Fauchard, which revealed to the world a new profession.

References

1. Pirenne H. Medieval Cities: Their Origins and the Revival of Trade. Princeton: Princeton University Press, 1952.
2. Nicaise E. La Grande Chirurgie de Guy de Chauliac. Paris: Felix Alcan, 1890.
3. Cantor NF. The Civilization of the Middle Ages. New York: Harper Collins, 1993.
4. Lacroix P. Science and Literature in the Middle Ages and at the Period of the Renaissance. New York: Appleton & Co, 1878.
5. Clarke C. Henri de Mondeville. Yale J Biol Med 1931;3:459–481.
6. Bullough VL. Medical study at mediaeval Oxford. Speculum 1961;36:600–612.
7. Siraisi NG. Medieval and Early Renaissance Medicine. Chicago: University of Chicago, 1990.
8. Kealey EJ. Medieval Medicus: A Social History of Anglo-Norman Medicine. Baltimore: The Johns Hopkins University, 1981.
9. Withington ET. Medical History from the Earliest Times. London: The Scientific, 1864.
10. Allbutt TC. Historical Relations of Medicine and Surgery to the End of the Sixteenth Century. London: The Macmillan, 1905.
11. McVaugh M. Surgical education in the Middle Ages. Acta Hisp Med Sci Hist Illus 2000;20:283–304.
12. Cockayne O. Leechdoms, Wortcunning, and Starcraft of Early England. London: Longman, 1865.
13. Payne JF. English Medicine in the Anglo-Saxon Times. The Fitz-Patrick Lectures for 1903. Oxford: Clarendon, 1904.
14. Anderson T. Dental treatment in Anglo-Saxon England. Br Dent J 2004; 197:273–274.
15. Voigts LE. Anglo-Saxon plant remedies and the Anglo-Saxons. Isis 1979;70: 250–268.
16. Kristeller P. The school of Salerno. Bull Hist Med 1945;17:138–194.
17. Bloch H. Monte Cassino, Byzantium, and the West in the earlier Middle Ages. Dumbarton Oaks Pap 1946;3:163–224.
18. Hoffmann-Axthelm W. History of Dentistry. Chicago: Quintessence, 1981.
19. Daremberg C. L'Ecole de Salerne, et De la Sobriete. Paris: J. B. Bailliere et Fils, 1861.
20. Guerini V. A History of Dentistry from the Most Ancient Times Until the End of the Eighteenth Century. Philadelphia: Lea & Febiger, 1909:188–199.
21. Nicaise E. Chirurgie de Maitre Henri de Montville. Paris: Germer Bailliere, 1893.
22. Bonnichon P. Guy de Chauliac et la "Grande Chirurgie." Quatres siecles de vie universitaire. Memoires de L'Academie Nationale de Chirurgie 2007; 6:39–44.
23. Densham A. A review of the progress of dental science and literature from the earliest ages. Proc Roy Soc Med 1909;2:71–98.
24. Erler MC. The first English printing of Galen: The formation of the Company of Barber-Surgeons. Huntington Libr Q 1985;48:159–171.

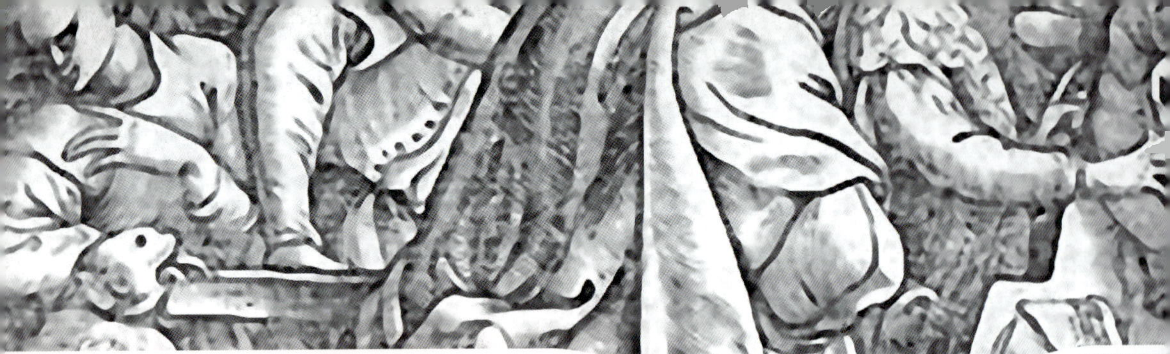

3

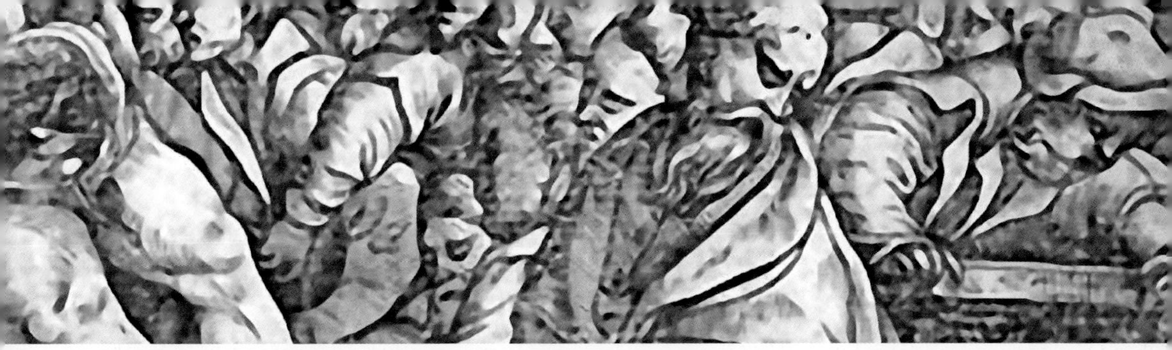

The Renaissance

The Renaissance period started in the 15th century with the invention of the printing press (1450), the fall of Constantinople to the Ottomans (1452), and the discovery of America by Christopher Columbus (1492). It was characterized by a diminishing acceptance of religious and ancient authority, along with a greater reliance on observation and analysis for understanding the world and man's place in it. Latin translations of the natural philosophy and logic of Aristotle had led to a gradual decline in strict adherence to Galen's medicine, bringing with it improvements in medical knowledge and practice.[1] The scientific method was applied to the study of the human body at universities throughout the West. During the Renaissance, medical instruction rose to an important place, equal with religion and law, in the universities of Bologna, Padua, Pisa, Paris, Montpellier, and Basel. With the invention of printing, professors of medicine published compendia describing diseases and their treatment, including diseases of the mouth and teeth. Physicians, surgeons, and scientists, such as Paré, da Vigo, Vesalius, Leeuwenhoek, Paracelsus, and Eustachi, contributed to a growing body of medical and dental knowledge. The art of surgery was perfected through dissection at newly developed medical schools in Italy and France. In spite of improvements in medical science, the actual practice of medicine continued to be based largely on herbal remedies and constrained by superstition and quackery.[2] For the general populace, the everyday care of minor ailments continued to be provided by empirics who had no formal training or regulation by guilds.

It was only through a gradual process, lasting several centuries, that the art and surgical craft of caring for the mouth and teeth were perfected by barber-surgeons, who had become known as *operators for the teeth*, *dentators*, or *surgeon-dentists*. Dental care was no longer confined to the application of herbal remedies and tooth extraction; dental decay was increasingly treated by excavation and/or cauterization and the resulting cavity plugged with lead and/or gold. The growth of commerce and the associated increase in wealth gave rise to a bourgeoisie who expected better medical and dental care. By the end of the 17th century, the practice of dentistry was performed on a full-time basis by a few men in the major cities of Europe. This trend reached maturity in 1728 when Pierre Fauchard outlined the scope of dental practice in his treatise *The Surgeon Dentist; Or, Treatise on the Teeth*.

Significant Medical Texts

Of the many medical books written by the faculty of the new medical schools, Giovanni of Arcoli's commentary on the medicine of Rhazes stands out for the amount of information it contains on the practice of dentistry.[3] Arcoli's book includes brief discussions of dental anatomy and physiology and the treatment of dental diseases. He summarized much of what was then known about oral health into 10 rules for good oral hygiene.[3] To preserve good teeth, he recommended avoiding both the consumption of sweet and sticky foods, acid liquids, and excessively hot or cold foods and the biting of hard objects. Teeth should be cleaned with wooden sticks or a woolen cloth after each meal. Dentifrice should be used before bedtime. Arcoli recognized that toothache could originate either from within the tooth or externally from the gums.[3] As in former times, scarification and cauterization were used for conditions that failed to respond to herbal and mineral-based remedies. Arcoli recommended drilling teeth to gain access to the pulp for application of hot cauterization.[4] In discussing fillings, Arcoli stated that "By means of a drill or file the putrefied or corroded part of the tooth should be completely removed. The cavity should then be filled with gold leaf."[5] However, Guerini points out that gold foil may have been routinely used as a filling material and that the method was not original with Giovanni of Arcoli.[3]

Giovanni da Vigo (1460–1520) (Fig 3-1) was a professor of medicine at Padua and surgeon to Pope Julius II. He published the book

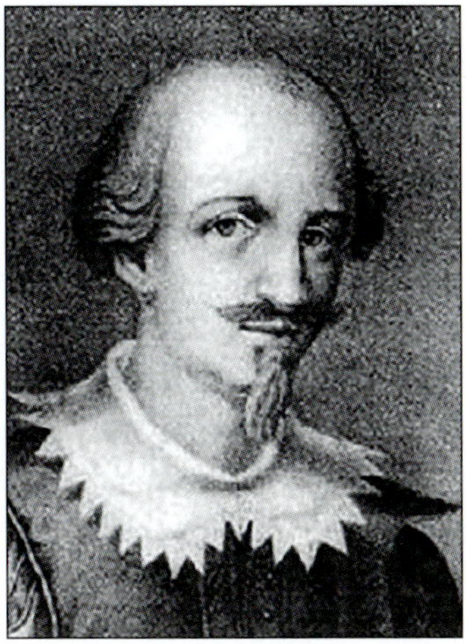

Fig 3-1 Giovanni da Vigo.

Practica copiosa in arte chirurgica, in which he described carious teeth and outlined rules of oral hygiene. He described the removal of tartar, including drilling and scraping to remove dental decay.[3] Dental cavities were filled with gold foil. Many of his methods were derived from previous writers, especially the Arabian physicians. Like Chauliac and Giovanni of Arcoli, da Vigo recommended that when extraction was needed, it was better to seek a barber-surgeon with experience.[3,4] There is no way of knowing whether da Vigo ever practiced dentistry or whether he simply included the care of dental problems in his treatise to be all-inclusive, like other writers before him. From the books of Albucasis, Chauliac, Giovanni D'Arcoli, and Giovanni da Vigo, there is clear evidence that the care of dental and oral diseases was included in the general body of medical knowledge but that the actual manual application of a remedy belonged to the surgeon of the short robe, barber-surgeon, or dentator.

The science of anatomy and the associated practice of surgery made great advances in the universities of northern Italy during the early Renaissance.[6] The practice of dissection took on importance in the curriculum of the medical schools of Bologna, Padua, and other Italian universities. Mondino, of the University of Bologna, wrote the first textbook on dissection in 1316.[7] Mondino's *The Anothomia*, considered by some to be the first modern textbook of anatomy, was criticized for its dependence on Galen's ideas and animal dissection, as opposed to original observations based on human cadavers.[8] Mondino's book underwent 25 editions and served as the most-used work of its kind until the appearance of Vesalius's *De Humani Corporis*

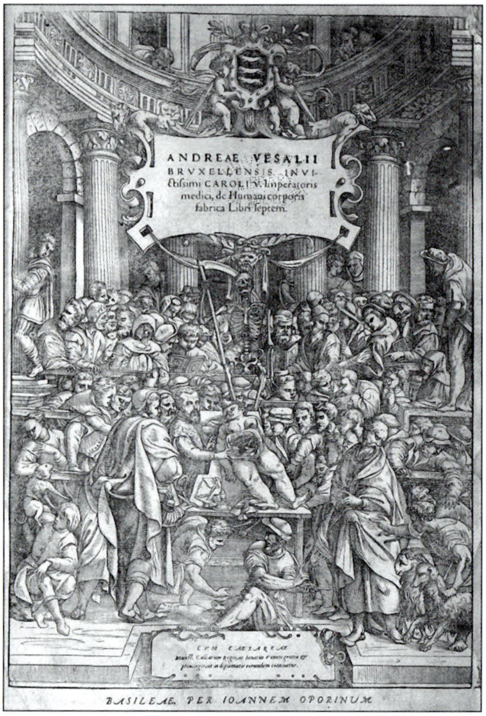

Fig 3-2 Frontispiece of Vesalius's *De Humani Corporis Fabrica.*

Fabrica. Human dissections were performed in anatomical theaters before large audiences, as depicted in the frontispiece to this text (Fig 3-2). These sessions took on a celebratory atmosphere as special social events, often followed with music or a theatrical performance.[2]

A great contribution to the advancement of the study of anatomy was made by Leonardo da Vinci (1452–1519). In over 700 sketches, da Vinci depicted the brain, nerves, blood vessels, lungs, gravid uterus, heart, stomach, bones, and teeth.[4] As an artist, da Vinci trusted his own observations over the traditional anatomy of Galen.[6] But it was not until the great Andreas Vesalius completed his superbly illustrated work *De Humani Corporis Fabrica* that the science of human anatomy achieved perfection.[6] Vesalius's treatise, printed in 1543, was clearly the most influential scientific work in providing impetus for exploring new methods of surgery. It pointed to errors in Galen's anatomy and served to overthrow Galen's authority in medical matters.[9] Vesalius started his studies of anatomy at the University of Louvain, under the tutelage of Jacques Dubois, and completed his work at the University of Padua, where he was a professor of surgery.

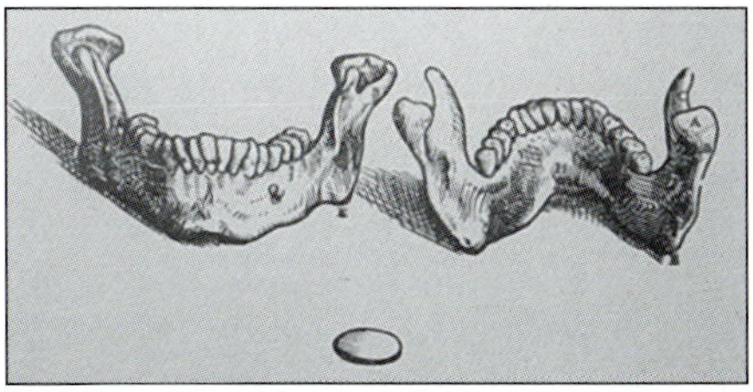

Fig 3-3 Vesalius's sketch of the mandible.

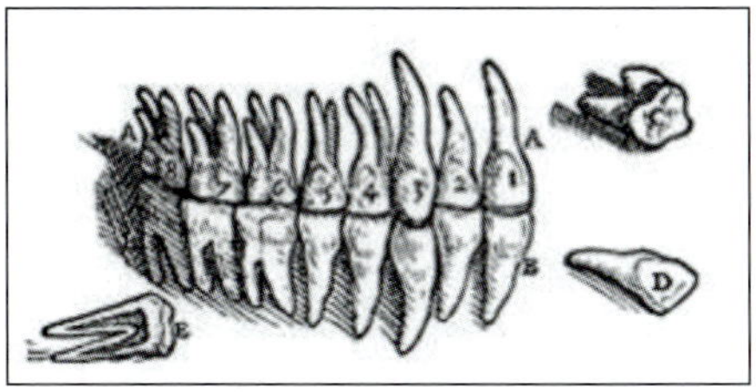

Fig 3-4 Vesalius's sketch of the dentition.

Vesalius described the dental pulp and noted the special character of teeth that made them different from bones.[4] The English translation of Vesalius's *De Humani Corporis Fabrica* has been published by Garrison and Hast of Northwestern University[10] and can be accessed at the following website: http://vesalius.northwestern.edu.

In comparison to his outstanding contribution to the overall anatomy of the human body, Vesalius did not contribute much to the existing knowledge of the structure of teeth beyond describing their number, shape, function, and attachment to the jaws (Figs 3-3 and 3-4):

> *Most often, teeth [dentes permanentes] are thirty-two in number, sixteen in a row on either jaw, arranged like a perfectly aligned row of dancers. Because the first four cut in opposition, they are called incisors, for they are broad and sharp so as to cut away readily by biting, like a knife, food put in their way, and break it up. The Canines Next: a single canine is set on each side, broad at the base next to the gums but sharp at the end, away from the gums, so that if something is not first cut by the incisors because of its hardness, these will break it up. This name is given them because they correspond to the protruding teeth of dogs (in which these teeth are conspicuous). After these, there are five maxillary or molar teeth [dentes premolares et molares] on each side rough, wide, hard, and large, so as to be able to grind to a smoother state things cut by the incisors and broken up by the canines. If they had been made altogether smooth, the molars would not be suitable for, their task, since*

all things are ground better by uneven and diverse surfaces...The teeth not only perform the functions already stated, but they also assist in the modulation of the voice since they are fashioned from a hard and stony substance having small but noteworthy hollows (the tooth marked E) [cavitas pulparis] inside [see Fig 3-4]. These make it possible for teeth to be lighter and more easily to take nourishment. Because of this hollow space, if through an influx of acrid or corrosive humors teeth ever develop cavities which extend to this hollow area, the teeth are very quickly decayed to the bottom of the root...teeth are all fixed in the sockets of the jaws like nails.... These [alveoli dentales] surround and confine each tooth, so precisely holding them in place that thay are not readily moved, not even a little.... Teeth are not fitted to their sockets with the same number of roots: small teeth have a single root [radix dentis], while larger teeth have two and the largest three or four (at the beginning of the chapter we have pictured a typical series of roots). Incisors are attached by single roots. Canines also put forth single roots; which are inserted much more deeply than the incisors' roots and are larger in proportion to the greater strength of the canines. Among the incisors, the two in the middle are attached by more prominent roots than the two lateral incisors next to the canines, no doubt because the middle pair are wider and larger. Molars vary in respect to their roots: those that are affixed to the lower jaw generally have two roots; those in the upper jaw regularly have three. Yet even these sometimes differ, upper molars having four roots apiece; those below are sometimes discovered to be embedded by three roots, especially the two next to the innermost tooth. Quite often you will see the two upper molars [dentes premolares] next to the canine tooth inserted with only two roots and the three remaining [dentes molares] with three each; similarly, the two lower molars [dentes premolares] next the canine have a single root, and the other three [dentes molares] two roots. You will also observe that the innermost [molaris tertius] are attached by smaller roots than those next to them.[10]

Vesalius's successor in the chair of anatomy at Padua, Realdo Columbo, is attributed to have been the first to describe the periodontal membrane and report that when infiltrated by "humoral" fluids, it could become a source of excruciating pain.[4] Columbo's anatomical knowledge was gained mainly from vivisection experiments on dogs, an exercise he is accused of having performed for the amusement of his colleagues.[2] Garrison is critical of Columbo not only for vivisection but also for having plagiarized from Jacques Dubois (Sylvius) in regard to his claim of having discovered the pulmonary circulation.[2]

Gabriel Fallopius (1523–1562) of Modena, Italy, published *Observationes anatomicae* at Venice in 1562. This work is of significance to dental anatomy in so far as it contains accurate descriptions of tooth development. Fallopius was the first to describe the tooth follicle and to dispel the idea proposed by Vesalius that the permanent teeth de-

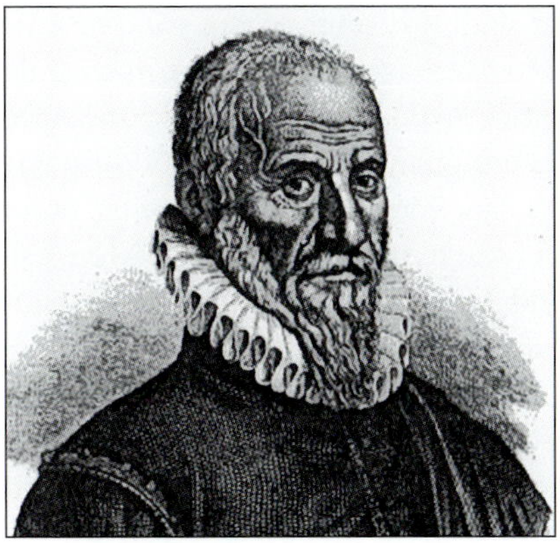

Fig 3-5 Ambroise Paré.

veloped from the roots of the primary teeth.[3] He was also the first to identify a "string" of tissue, later called the *gubernaculums dentis* by subsequent anatomists, which created a path through the alveolar bone through which the permanent tooth erupted into the oral cavity. Fallopius is especially remembered for his discoveries of the chorda tympani, trigeminal, auditory, and glossopharyngeal nerves.[2]

Ambroise Paré

The premier surgeon of the Renaissance was Ambroise Paré of Laval, France (1510–1590) (Fig 3-5). Of all the physicians and surgeons of the Renaissance period, Paré epitomizes the spirit of the age by his courage, skill, and practical application of new methodologies. His books, written in French for the common surgeon and barber-surgeon rather than in Latin for the universities, revealed a life of unusual energy and service.[11]

Paré was apprenticed as a young man to Vialat, a local master barber-surgeon. From 1529 to 1532, he increased his education in surgery at the Hotel Dieu, the only public hospital in all of Paris. As a hospital resident, he attended to patients suffering from every human disease and practiced dissection during postmortem examinations. At the completion of his "internship" at the Hotel Dieu, Paré enlisted as a military surgeon in the army of the Duke of Montejean. His first exposure to combat was at the battle of Pas de Suse in 1537. It was there that Paré made his famous observation that gunshot wounds were best treated with dressings of egg yolk, rose water, and turpentine, as opposed to cauterization with hot irons and boiling oil.[12]

In military service again in 1542 with Monsieur de Rohan's forces at the siege of Perpignan, Paré gained additional fame for developing a technique for locating and removing bullets from gunshot wounds.[12] During the battle of Perpignan, Monsieur De Brissac was shot in the shoulder, and after several surgeons had searched in vain to locate the bullet, Paré instructed De Brissac to assume the same position he had been in at the time when he was shot. By taking into account the line of fire, Paré was able to determine the path of the bullet and thereby locate and successfully remove it. This technique was described in 1545 in his first book, *The Method of Treating Wounds Made by Arquebuses and Other Firearms as Well as Those Made by Arrows, Darts, and Similars with Powder Burns from Canons.*[12]

During military campaigns in Germany, Paré began to stem the bleeding of amputation wounds by using ligatures instead of cautery by hot irons.[11] Paré's success in preserving the King's experienced soldiers by the use of this more compassionate method for treating wounds not only made him beloved by the troops at the frontlines but also won him esteem at the Court of Versailles. Paré's reputation grew while in the service of four Kings of France (Henri II, Francis II, Charles IX, and Henri III), as well as surgeon to the Queen Mother, Catherine de Medici. Possessed of a wealth of experience on human diseases, Paré was often called upon at court for his advice over and above that of the King's physicians, in disregard of official protocol. He had gained so much respect from Catherine de Medici that she insisted he write a treatise on the treatment of the plague, smallpox, and measles.

Paré's inventive mind led him to make significant contributions to nascent prosthetics sciences, such as his design of upper and lower prosthetic limbs that embodied new ideas in basic prosthetic function. He also invented an above-the-knee prosthesis, which served as both a kneeling peg leg and a foot prosthesis. Perhaps his most complex prosthetic device was "Le Petit Lorrain" (Fig 3-6), a prosthetic hand operated by springs and catches that was used in battle by a French army captain.[12]

After several years as a military surgeon, Paré returned to Paris for additional study of anatomy under Jacques Dubois of the Faculty of Medicine. Dubois (also known as Sylvius), a proponent of Galen's anatomy, was later challenged by the fresh discoveries of Vesalius, his former pupil. Paré completed his anatomical studies and passed qualifying examinations by the Faculty of Medicine and was certified as a master barber-surgeon.[12] In Paré's lifetime, medical practice was

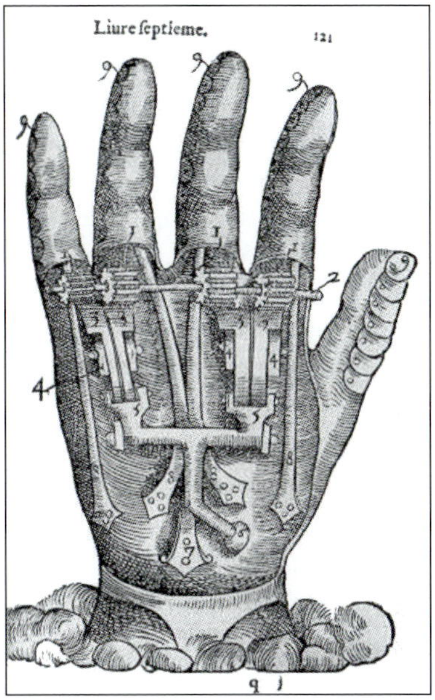

Fig 3-6 Prosthetic hand developed by Paré.

controlled by physicians of the Faculty of Medicine of the University of Paris. By tradition, the practice of the physician was involved solely in the diagnosis of disease, formulation of treatment plans, and the prescription of medications and surgeries, because manual procedures were beneath their status. Surgeons of the long robe, occupying a lesser position in the hierarchy of medical care, were responsible for treating wounds and abscesses with plasters and ointments but opted to leave manual operations to the third level of practitioners (ie, surgeons of the short robe or barber-surgeons).[12] Patients suffering from dental problems sought help from members of the guild of barber-surgeons and dentators or were left to the care of untrained itinerant quacks.

In 1554, Paré became a member of the College of St Come, France's first college devoted to training surgeons. By admission to the faculty, he earned the new title of master surgeon (a surgeon of the long robe rather than a surgeon of the short robe or barber-surgeon).[12] Paré was accused by the Faculty of Medicine of having been fraudulently admitted to the College of Surgery, because he knew very little Latin and was unqualified to sit for entrance examinations. But as a favorite of King Henri II and a famous military surgeon, he was a positive acquisition for St Come and an advantage to them in their long-standing battle for equality with the Faculty of Medicine. In 1564, Paré, as First Surgeon to the King, published his work on surgery, *Ten Books of Surgery: with the Magazine of the Instruments Necessary for It.*

In publishing a collected edition of his writings in 1575, Paré set off a controversy with the Faculty of Medicine. Shortly after his treatise appeared in print, the Faculty of Medicine of the University of Paris demanded a halt to its distribution on the basis that it had not been submitted to them for approval.[13] The Faculty of Medicine complained that Paré was meddling in medicine and that, being ignorant of Latin and Greek, he was unqualified to write on medical topics. His book, written in French, broke the custom to publish in Latin as a way of restricting medical knowledge to graduates of medical schools. It has been suggested that Paré employed an assistant schooled in Latin to embellish his work with references to the older, Latinized medical books, such as those by Galen and Hippocrates.[2] The employment of a Latin scribe to embellish one's writing was a common and acceptable practice in the Middle Ages. The case against Paré was tried in the Parliament of Paris, where the position of the Medical Faculty was upheld. However, it was too late, because Paré's work was already being widely circulated.

Malgaigne stated that Paré's surgical treatise marked an epoch in surgery: "It was the first real surgical treatise which had appeared since that of Gui de Chauliac,—the latter writing at the time when the Arabian influence was predominant, the other at the epoch of the Renaissance."[14] Malgaigne praised Paré's attempt to bring medicine and surgery into closer alliance by stressing the need for medical training for all surgeons. Francis Packard, MD, former dean of the Harvard Medical School, wrote that Ambroise Paré "did for surgery what his great contemporary Vesalius did for anatomy."[12] Guerini, in his *History of Dentistry*, states that Paré treated the subject of dental maladies and their cure very thoroughly, and he attributes this "to his having first been simply a barber (and, therefore, also a toothdrawer) and afterward a surgeon-barber, which placed him in very favorable conditions for acquiring experience in the practice of dentistry."[3]

Dental anatomy and dental diseases were covered in several chapters of Paré's surgical treatise, assembled and reviewed by Fay.[15] Paré described the dental pulp and its nerves and blood supply, stating that dental pain was due to the pulp's rich nerve supply.[15] He described the dental foramen, cautioning surgeons to use extra care not to sever the mental nerve when making incisions in this area. Paré noted that the tooth was anchored to the alveolus by a ligament and that teeth that were accidentally avulsed should be replanted and

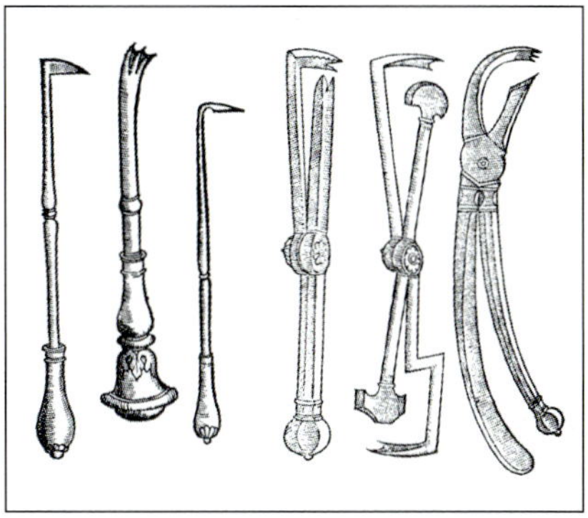

Fig 3-7 Pelicans for drawing teeth *(left)* and elevators and lances for gingival surgery and exodontia *(right)* by Paré.

secured by gold thread to adjacent teeth. Teeth that were loosened as a result of disease or age should be similarly ligated to adjacent teeth and the occlusion adjusted. Guerini states that Paré was the first to describe a case of tooth transplantation.[3]

Paré recommended that gingival overgrowth (epulis) should be removed by cautery or surgical extirpation. He described the treatment of dislocated jaws and the removal of calculus with special instruments. Tooth extraction was seen as a source of complications and to be undertaken only as a last resort. He advised that tooth extraction should be delegated to an older, experienced barber-surgeon or dentator. Fay is surprised that Paré, so experienced in amputations and repairing battlefield wounds, would avoid extractions, preferring to delegate them to experienced barber-surgeons. Paré stressed that one must guard against extracting a sound tooth mistaken for the source of pain. Nor should the surgeon pull a tooth from its alveolus too forcefully or abruptly for fear of rupturing the jaw bone, a complication he had observed numerous times.[15]

Paré gave formulas for making dentifrices, mouthwashes, and whitening agents. Although he gave no evidence that carious teeth should be filled, he did advise the placement of medicaments and opiates into cavities for the relief of toothache.[15] Among the instruments he employed in dental operations were pelicans, elevators, and lances (Fig 3-7). He recommended the use of files to remove dental caries from interproximal areas. He advocated several remedies, including gingival incision, to treat the pain and fever experienced by infants during tooth eruption. There is also much in his writings that shows that he still accepted older erroneous ideas, such as the continued growth of teeth to compensate for tooth erosion, the presence of tooth worms in dental decay, and the application of venesection and cupping to alleviate dental pain.

Paré was the first surgeon to describe the fabrication and use of obturators to replace lost palatal tissue, a complication of tertiary syphilis.[3] Paré's writings clearly state that he treated broken jaws and dislocations of the temporomandibular joint and that he surgically removed tumors, yet it is not known how much operative dentistry he actually performed. Did he delegate most dental procedures to experienced dentators? He most likely performed some dental operations in his early career, but as he progressed from a barber to a barber-surgeon to a surgeon of the long robe, he may have delegated more of that type of work.

Overall, there is little that is new in Paré's recommended treatments for dental and oral diseases. He often refers back to Hippocrates and Celsus for appropriate remedies, such as for mouthwashes, dentifrices, and opiates. Toothache, gingival disease, calculus removal, and oral hygiene are presented as they had been for centuries. In fact, Fay makes the observation that Paré copied sections of Chauliac's treatise on surgery.[15] Yet Ambroise Paré must be included among the leading figures in the development of dentistry by virtue of the fact that he considered the treatment of dental diseases an integral part of the surgeon's overall responsibility. Furthermore, by his appreciation of the importance of medical science in diagnosis and surgical practice, he elevated surgery to the same plane as that of medicine. Garrison concluded that Paré, along with Paracelsus and Vesalius, "shouldered past other men, literally blazed the way, not only for the general advance of medicine, but for keen and liberal thinking in all its branches."[2]

Other Noteworthy Practitioners and Publications

Jacques Guillemeau succeeded Paré at the Hotel Dieu hospital in Paris. In his treatise on surgery, *Oeuvres de Chirurgie* (1598), he described a paste containing resin and powdered coral to be used for filling tooth cavities that had been appropriately cleaned of decay. He claimed to have been the first to make artificial teeth using this coral-based resinous paste.[4] A plate in this book illustrates a variety of forceps for extracting teeth (Fig 3-8). Guillemeau is best known for his *Traite des maladies de l'oeil* (*Treatise of Eye Diseases*, 1584), which is considered to be one of the best Renaissance-era works in ophthalmic medicine.

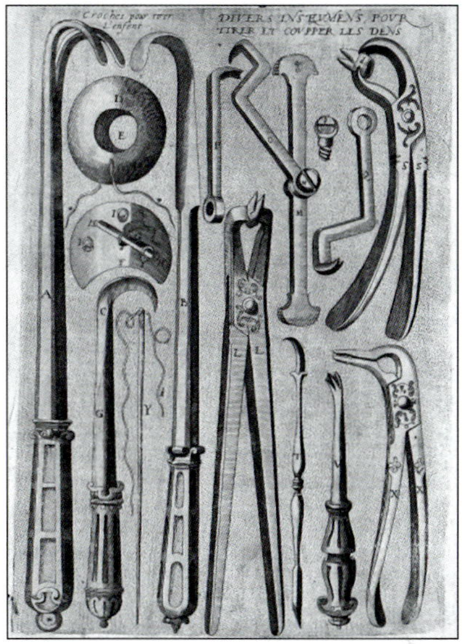

Fig 3-8 Guillemeau's instruments for exodontia from his *Oeuvres de Chirurgie*.

Girolamo Fabrizio d'Acquapendente (1537–1619) wrote his *Opera Chirurgica* in 1570. He was a professor of anatomy and medicine at Padua, Italy. He is remembered for his description of the valves of the veins and for his studies of the embryology of the digestive system. In his *Opera Chirurgica*, he described dental treatments consisting of cavity cleansing, filling with gold leaf, removal of tartar, filing of sharp edges, extractions, and the fabrication of obturators.[3] Of additional interest is the fact that William Harvey, the discoverer of the circulation of the blood, was one of his pupils at Padua.

Bartolomeo Eustachi is considered the first dental anatomist. In 1563, he published *Libellus de dentibus (Pamphlet on the teeth)*, the first book to deal exclusively with the anatomy of teeth. In this pamphlet, he describes the macroscopic anatomy, physiology, and development of the teeth, including the penetration of blood vessels and nerve fibers into the apex of the roots; the number of roots, their variations in length and form, and the presence of the periodontal ligament[3]; and tooth bud development, differentiating the enamel from the dentin. He drew his own anatomical plates (Fig 3-9), which remained unprinted in the Vatican Library until they were discovered in 1714.[2,16]

Johannes Scultetus, a pupil of Fabrizio d'Acquapendente and a graduate of the medical school at Padua, published a book of surgery

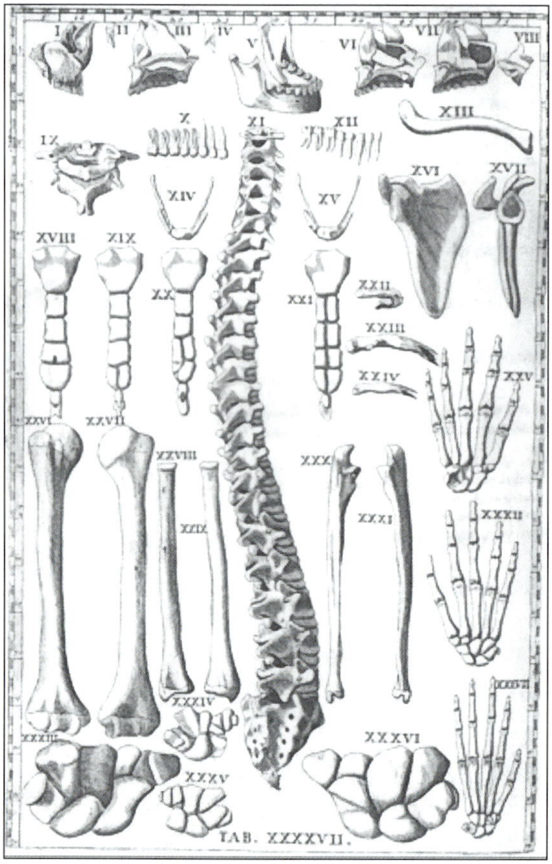

Fig 3-9 Drawing from Eustachi's *Tabulae Anatomica*, depicting the teeth, jaws, and bones of the spinal column and limbs.

especially significant for its large number of illustrations of the surgeon's armamentarium. His book gives the best picture of early 17th-century surgical practice, illustrating such procedures as amputation of the breast, reduction of dislocations, forceps delivery, and neurosurgery, among others.[3] Of particular interest to dentists are Scultetus's descriptions and illustrations of dental surgery, including some of the first illustrations of dental instruments[4] (Fig 3-10). The popularity of the work was such that new editions and translations, many with additional illustrations, kept being published well into the 18th century. He was critical of the average barber-surgeon's treatment of wounds, which often led to infection and gangrene.[17] Scultetus's publication was responsible for an improved standard of education for the nonacademic barber-surgeons, who treated the majority of the population.

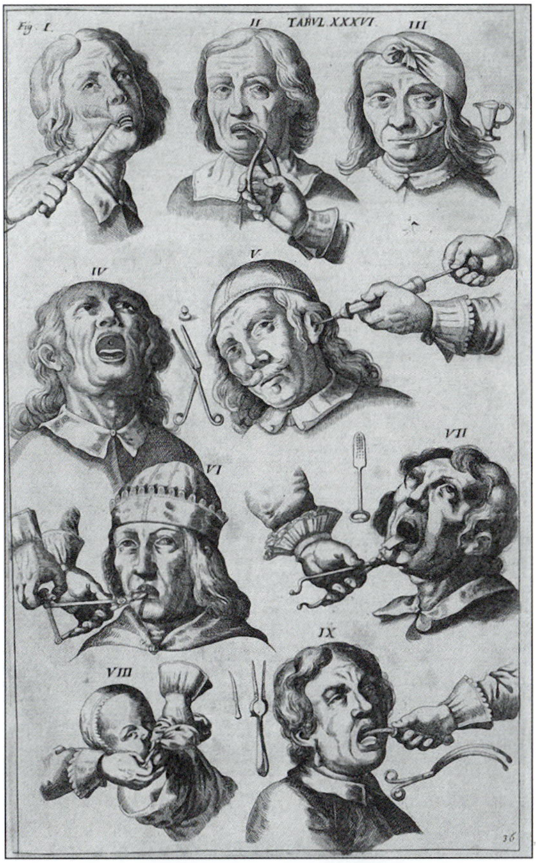

Fig 3-10 Johannes Scultetus's drawings of stomatologic operations (I–IV, VI, VII, IX): cauterization of a tooth (I), tooth extraction (II), feeding via a funnel (III), placement of an obturator (IV), opening of the jaws (VI), use of a speculum for examining the throat (VII), and removal of a foreign object from the throat (IX). (Adapted from Guerini.[3])

Peter Lowe, a member of the Royal College of Physicians and Surgeons of Glasgow, wrote the first book on general surgery in the English language, *A Discourse on the Whole Art of Chirurgerie*, in 1597. Lowe had studied in Paris and knew the work of Paré. Although teeth are mentioned only a few times in his book, Lowe rejected the idea that tooth decay was caused by worms and accused barber-surgeons of extracting too many teeth that could be saved by appropriate treatment.[3] Lowe practiced cauterization of painful teeth and described the use of artificial teeth carved from bone and fastened with gold wires.[18] The instruments used in dental surgery—scalpels, files, forceps, and pelicans—are illustrated in his book.

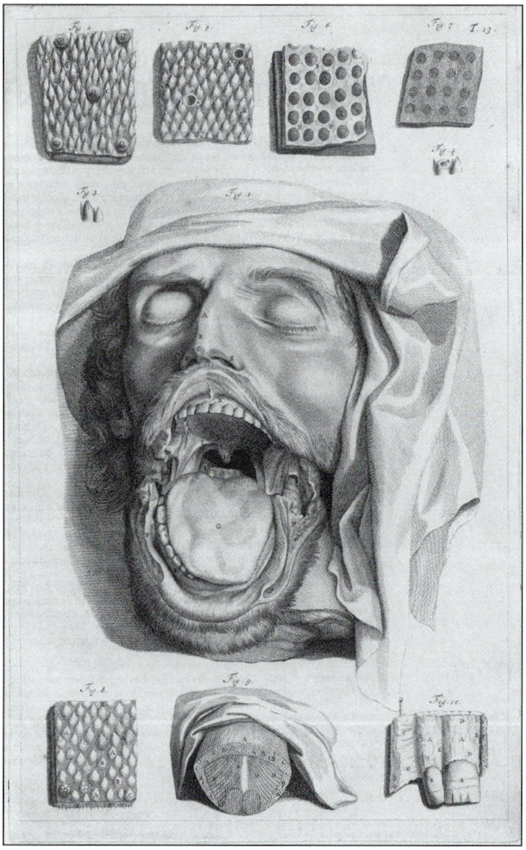

Fig 3-11 Bidloo's depiction of the surface anatomy of the tongue.

Govard Bidloo, a Dutch contemporary of Leeuwenhoek, was born in Amsterdam in 1649. He was a professor of anatomy at The Hague from 1688 to 1694. Bidloo served as a physician to William III of England. His great work is the *Anatomia Corporis Humani* of 1685. This atlas was illustrated with 105 copper-engraved plates showing the human figure both in living attitudes and as dissected cadavers. In one illustration, the surface of the tongue is shown to comprise an infinity of "little tongues." The various papillae of the tongue are illustrated as many oval, pointed, and bicipital bodies (Fig 3-11).

Fabricius Hildanus (William Fabry) (1560–1634) was a German surgeon who, like Paré, had risen from the ranks of the barber-surgeons. In his *Observationum et curationums chirurgicarum centuriae sex*, or *Six Hundred Case Reports*, there are many case reports pertaining to oral surgery. He described the relationship between infected teeth and trigeminal neuralgia. He advised that dental fistulas could be traced to infected roots and teeth and were readily cured by extraction of the offending tooth.[3] As a general surgeon, Hildanus is renowned for his contributions to amputation technique and lithotomy and for improving the training of surgeons. He stressed the need for a thorough knowledge of anatomy, decrying the frivolousness of young surgeons: "While the young surgeons should apply themselves to the study of anatomy, they make music, read the owl-glass, drink, fornicate, enjoy themselves or adorn their rooms and waste their time."[19]

Lazare Riviere (1589–1645), a professor at Montpelier, wrote the *Opera Medica Universal*, in which he devoted considerable attention to stomatologic problems. He considered the cure for toothache from a medical viewpoint, recommending bloodletting, cupping, blistering, and cauterization.[3] Riviere advised filling cavities with mixtures containing opium and camphor. Rubbing the teeth with tobacco ash was prescribed for whitening teeth. In 1640, he introduced oil of cloves for sedative treatment of dental pulp (eugenol, a widely used dental anodyne, is made from essence of cloves).

Dental books

Books exclusively devoted to dental practice were first published in the 16th and 17th centuries, providing clear evidence that the specialization and separation of dentistry from the general practice of medicine and surgery had begun to take place at this time. A comprehensive study of the early dental literature was performed by Bernard Weinberger.[20] The *Artzney Buchlein*, published in Leipzig in 1530, is a 44-page work summarizing dental diseases and their remedies, based entirely on the old practices of Galen, Avicenna, and da Vigo. Other dental books written in German were by W. H. Ryff (1548) and J. Digitus (1586).[20] Francisco Martinez, a Spanish physician, wrote a treatise devoted to dentistry in 1557 in which he advised that extractions and scalings should be left to barbers.[21] Urbain Hemard, a physician of Lyon, France, published the first dental book in French, *Recherche de la vraye anathomie des dents*, in 1582. Hemard also shared the view that tooth extractions were dangerous and should be left to those with experience.[22] The first dental book in English, *The Operator for the Teeth*, written by Charles Allen, an English barber-surgeon, was published in London in 1685.[20] Allen repeated the old methods of removal of decay and the filling of teeth without providing any details as to procedure.[4] One redeeming aspect of Allen's treatise was his condemnation of the practice of tooth transplantation on humanitarian grounds.

Summary

Guerini noted that the number of publications of importance to the science and practice of dentistry jumped from 20 in the 16th century to 100 in the 17th century.[3] However, not all of these contained advances in theory or clinical applications; many continued to recommend old and useless remedies. Superstitions, such as the worm theory of tooth decay, continued to be repeated. Most books were written by physicians and surgeons who had little direct hands-on experience. The barber-surgeons or dentators who did the dental work were unschooled, and thus it was left to physicians and physician-surgeons to write the books.

References

1. Siraisi NG. Medieval and Early Renaissance Medicine. Chicago: University of Chicago, 1990.
2. Garrison FH. An Introduction to the History of Medicine. Philadelphia: W. B. Saunders, 1913.
3. Guerini V. A History of Dentistry from the Most Ancient Times until the End of the Eighteenth Century. Philadelphia: Lea & Febiger, 1909:188–199.
4. Hoffmann-Axthelm W. History of Dentistry. Chicago: Quintessence, 1981.
5. Walsh JJ. Old-Time Makers of Medicine. New York: Fordham University, 1911.
6. Libby W. The History of Medicine; In its Salient Features. New York: Houghton Mifflin, 1922.
7. Walsh JJ. The Popes and Science. New York: Fordham University, 1908.
8. Infusino MH, Win D, O'Neill YV. Mondino's book and the human body. Vesalius 1995;1:71–76.
9. Ball JM. Andreas Vesalius—The Reformer of Anatomy. St Louis: Medical Science, 1910.
10. Garrison D, Hast M. Andreas Vesalius's *De Humani Corporis Fabrica*. Evanston, IL: Northwestern University, 2003.
11. Paré A. Les Oeuvres de M. Ambroise Paré. Paris: Gabriel Buon, 1575.
12. Packard FR. Life and Times of Ambroise Paré. New York: Paul B. Hoeber, 1921.
13. Paget S. Ambroise Paré and His Times, 1510–1590. New York: G. P. Putnam's Sons, 1897.
14. Malgaigne JF. Surgery and Ambroise Paré. Norman, OK: University of Oklahoma, 1965.
15. Fay M. L'Art Dentaire dans les Oeuvres D'Ambroise Paré. Revue Odontologique 1932;53:315–334.
16. Eustachi B. Tabulae Anatomicae. Rome: Francisci Gonzagae, 1714.
17. Scultetus AH. The life and work of the German physician Johannes Scultetus (1595–1645). J Am Coll Surg 2003;196:130–139.
18. Finlayson J. An Account of the Life and Works of Maister Peter Lowe. Glasgow: James Maclehose and Sons, 1889.
19. Jones E. The life and works of Guilhelmus Fabricius Hildanus. Med Hist 1960;4:112–134.

20. Weinberger BW. Dental literature: Its origin and development. J Dent Res 1924;5:305–388.
21. Endelman J. A dental book of the sixteenth century. Dent Cosmos 1903; 45:39–43.
22. Hemard U. Recherche de la vraye anathomie des dents, nature et propriete d'Icelles. Lyon: Rigaud, 1582.

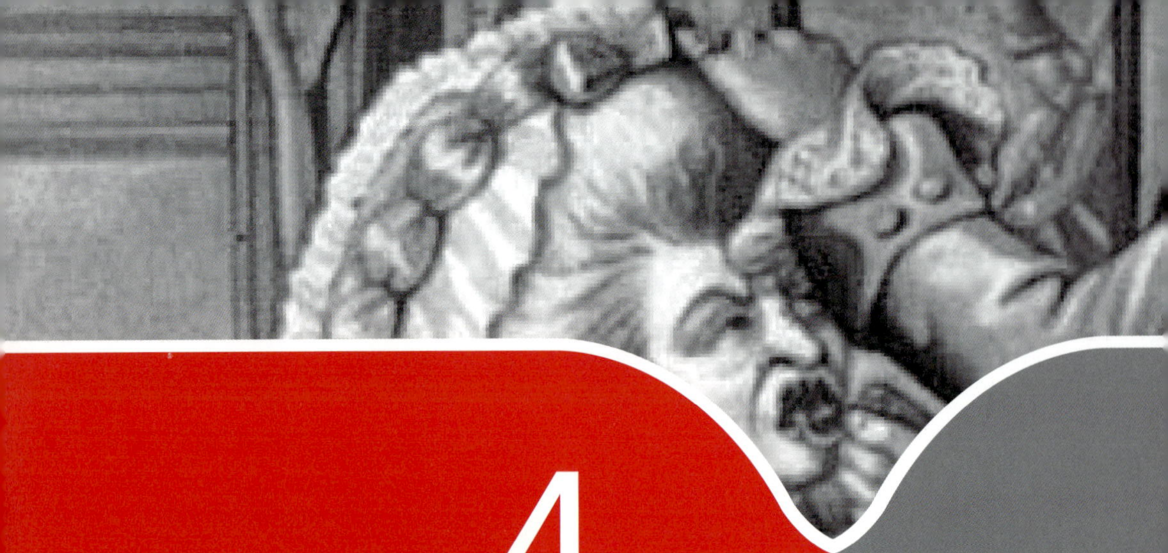

4

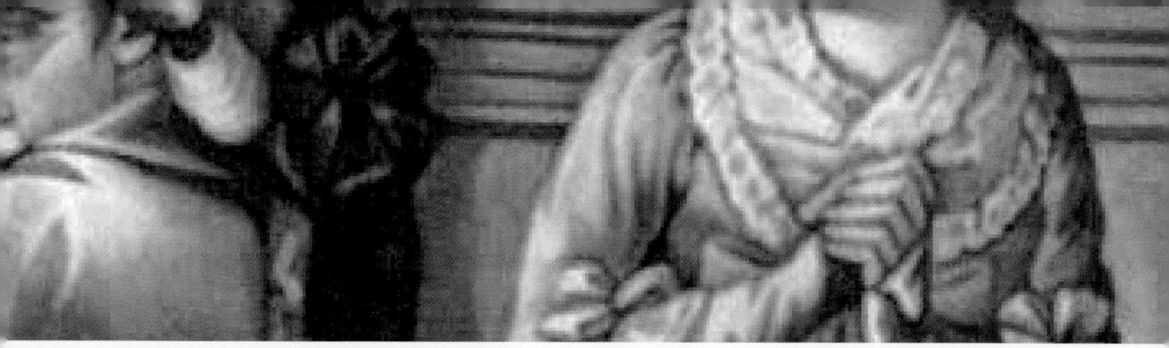

Birth of a Profession

From the end of the Renaissance to the 17th century, there evolved out of the ranks of the barber-surgeons a new class of practitioner specializing in dentistry. Formal recognition of a dental branch of barber-surgeons came in 17th-century England and France when dental surgeons were appointed to the staff of royal households. Dental surgeons were under the supervision of the First Physician and First Surgeon to the King. They were called upon to care for the teeth of the king, members of the royal family, and other members of the aristocracy. Through such appointments, some surgeon-dentists developed large practices at court. During the reign of Charles V of France, Thomas de Pisan, a surgeon-dentist, was permitted to set up shop in the Louvre Castle, where he held a large practice serving the courtiers. The ennoblement of dental surgeons, begun during the reign of Louis XIII, gave the profession of dentistry its royal approval and in so doing made the care of the teeth and the mouth a sign of higher status, a practice of the better educated or informed members of society.[1]

Dental Surgery in Royal Families

Some of the earliest records of the practice of dental surgery are found in the memoirs of the French royal families and from those of other members of the court at Versailles. Philip I, Charles VII, Francis I, Henry III, Henry IV, Louis IX, Louis XIV, and Louis XVI of France suffered from bad teeth, all in need of the attention of dental surgeons.[2] Louis IX (1215–1270) is reported to have died with only one remaining tooth, a consequence attributed to having been exposed to scurvy while on his Crusade to the Holy Land.[2] The expertise of his dentist, Pierre de la Brosse, must be questioned, because although he treated Queen Blanche "with dexterity," Marie of Brabant was less fortunate in that she received "clumsy and painful operations."[2] Catherine de Medici, the Italian mother of Henry III, is said to have set the standard for proper toiletry at court by introducing cosmetics, perfumes, rouges, wigs, and artificial teeth. A common treatment for toothache at that time was to wear a small black plaster applied to the skin of the cheek nearest to the affected tooth. The black plaster, set off by the whiteness of the skin, came to be viewed as an embellishment and was the forerunner of the fashionable beauty spot. Joubert, physician to Henry III (1551–1589), wrote on the virtues of mouthwash:

> *One must not forget the mouth in order to preserve the teeth, gums, and good breath, which is of great importance to health, because the air which one inspires and expires through the mouth comes in contact with the dirty teeth and gums, thus infecting the air which gives its bad qualities to the lungs and heart.*[2]

Henry III may have worn some artificial teeth, and Henry IV is believed to have had gold fillings.[2] Charles VII not only had bad teeth, but he also developed a buccal cancer incited by the jagged edges of a carious tooth. At the time of his death, an official report to the dauphin stated "some time since a certain disease attacked the King... which commenced at first as a toothache, following which the cheek and a large part of his face was much changed and a great amount of matter discharged."[2]

The most dramatic case involving dental surgery at court was the treatment of Louis XIV's maxillary fistula. In 1685, a part of Louis XIV's maxillary bone, along with a portion of the floor of the maxillary sinus, was torn away during the extraction of an infected and decayed maxillary left molar. The King (Fig 4-1) was left with a large fistula through which food and drink escaped from his mouth into his nasal cavity. After a consultation by D'Aquin (the First Physician), Felix de Tassy (the First Surgeon), and Dubois (a surgeon-dentist), it

Fig 4-1 Louis XIV, King of France.

was determined that cauterization of the wound's edges was the best treatment likely to induce a healing response. Special cauterization instruments were shaped by Dubois so as to contact all borders of the fistula to its very end. Cauterization was applied 14 times to the King by Dubois. According to the King's physicians, Dubois appeared to suffer more than the King, no doubt from fear of imprisonment in the Bastille if the treatment should fail. Three weeks later, a second series of cauterizations was applied; after several months, the entire wound was closed by bone regeneration and soft tissue formation.[2] Fagon, who replaced D'Aquin as First Physician to Louis XIV, was no model of dental hygiene; according to Charlotte-Elisabeth de Baviere, the King's sister-in-law, all of Fagon's maxillary teeth were black and rotten.[3]

The official appointment of dentists as members of the medical faculty at the French Court was begun under Louis XIV. Appointment to the royal household brought with it ennoblement, and as a member of the nobility (no doubt the lesser nobility) the royal dentist enjoyed certain privileges, including the right to bear a coat-of-arms. The king's daily oral hygiene was performed by his barbers and valets. The royal dentist was called to perform more thorough dental cleanings with special instrumentation and to carry out filings, fillings, and cautery as directed by the First Physician.[4]

In the histories of the royal families of England, there is similar evidence of dental and oral diseases. As early as the 13th century, the physician John of Gaddesden is reported to have extirpated a salivary stone from King Edward I. John of Arderne, surgeon to Edward III, used henbane and mustard seed as toothache remedies. Henry VIII's physician, Andrew Boorde, attributed tooth decay to worms. His treatment was to smoke them out with burning candles of wax and henbane. Beginning in the 16th century, dentists (or *operators for the teeth*) were appointed to the royal households. The first to receive that title was Peter Hemet in 1727 in the reign of King George II. Peter's grandson, Jacob Hemet, while serving as Operator for the Teeth to Queen Charlotte, profited from the sale of his "Essence of Pearl and Pearl Dentifrice." Thomas Berdmore, author of the 1768 *Treatise on the Disorders and Deformities of the Teeth and Gums* is said to have amassed a fortune in practice while serving as dentist to George III.[5]

Attention given to the oral health of the aristocracy gave impetus to the notion that good teeth were an element of respectability. Concern for how one appeared in public was especially important at the Court of Versailles. One could not afford to be seen at Versailles in anything less than the most glamorous attire. A pleasant smile revealing clean teeth, without gaps from previous tooth extractions, was essential to anyone aspiring to win at the game of social advancement.[6] The upper bourgeoisie of Paris were not far behind in their pursuit of vanity. Cosmetics, extravagant hairpieces, and fine clothes were used to cover up the ravages of time. Mme de Cornuel, when asked why the aging Mme de Lyonne continued to use makeup and to load herself up with jewelry, replied that "it's the cheese in the mouse trap." Pearly white teeth revealed in a pleasant smile were just as important then as they are today. To be seen in public with rotten or missing teeth was to be avoided. The demand for dental care, especially for the replacement of missing teeth, created a stimulus for the development of dental prosthetics. The main function of false teeth ("dents de parade") was cosmetic, seeing as how they were useless for mastication. It is said that Mlle de Gournay kept hers by her plate, inserting them adroitly whenever she was going to speak and removing them to continue her meal. But for the peasants in the country and the less fortunate citizens of Paris, missing teeth were all too common, and their only "treatment" was extraction, usually at the hands of a toothdrawer or charlatan.

When a new manufacturing process made mirrors more affordable, it became easy to judge one's shortcomings and to commit to improving the image one presented in public. Newspaper announcements of services by both qualified practitioners and charlatans increased public awareness of the availability of an increasing number of remedies for dental and oral problems, as well as the location of practicing dental surgeons. The increased demand for dental care is reflected in the growing respectability of the surgeon-dentist and the increased number of practitioners in Paris.[7]

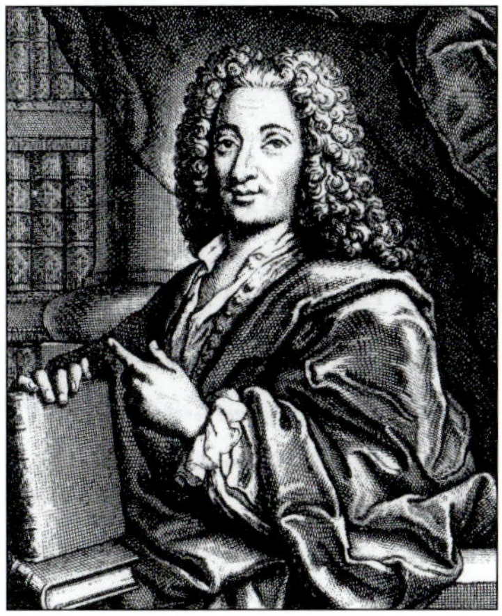

Fig 4-2 Pierre Fauchard with the second edition of his two-volume treatise on dentistry.

Pierre Fauchard

Pierre Fauchard (Fig 4-2) represents the crowning example of the successful dental surgeon of the early 18th century. Pierre Fauchard lived from 1678 to 1761, at the height of the Enlightenment, a period of enormous intellectual and political ferment in France. In Paris, books on all subjects were being printed and circulated at rates that were previously unimaginable. It is no surprise that during this surge of new knowledge someone would come forward with a synthesis of all that was known in dental practice. In 1728, at age 50 years, Fauchard published his famous treatise on dentistry, *Le chirurgien dentiste, ou traite des dents (The Surgeon Dentist; Or, Treatise on the Teeth)*. It was the first true textbook of dentistry, a treatise in which the full spectrum of 18th-century dental practice was laid out in a lucid and comprehensive manner. It was also an equally important guide to a professional ethic.[8] Fauchard's treatise was based on actual personal experience. Fauchard spent his early years in practice in Angers, France, following his discharge from the Royal Navy. In 1719, he settled in Paris, where he set up practice on the Rue de la Comedie Francaise in the heart of the University of Paris. His reputation attracted eminent physicians and surgeons of the faculty, such as Helvétius, La Peyronie, Hecquet, and Winslow as patients.[7]

Fauchard's book was not translated into English until 1969 by Lilian Lindsay. His treatise contained 42 full-page engravings, making it the best-illustrated book on dentistry in its time. The fact that Fauchard set down in writing what he had learned from experience and study, and thus was able to share it with fellow practitioners, testifies his desire to promote education among fellow dental practitioners. In that time period, it was customary to protect one's methods from competitors. He deplored the lack of formal schooling in the newly developing science and art of dentistry in 18th-century France:

> *For the rest there is no record of any public or special course in surgery where the theory of diseases of the teeth could be fully taught, and where thorough instruction in the practice of this art which is so necessary for the cure of these diseases and those which attack those parts by which the teeth are surrounded. The most famous surgeons having abandoned this part of the art, or at least having paid little attention to it, have caused by this negligence, the rise of people who without theory or experience, have degraded it, and practiced haphazard, without principles or method.*[9]

Fauchard accused the untrained and unprincipled charlatans of having brought disdain for what otherwise should have been recognized as an honorable endeavor:

> *It is with regret that I have to decide to remove teeth, not because of the violence of the operation, which is never so excessive as the toothache, nor the annoying sequelae, I hesitate, I elude and I defer to draw them because of the stress I lay upon their important function. If everyone else had the same respect for them, the teeth would be as much conserved as they are recklessly drawn, and there would not be so much contempt for tooth drawers, of whom some only in truth deserve such a title, while many more deserve that of tooth conservators, since they conserve not only as many teeth as the rules of the art permit, but more, they use their genius in imitating Nature in repairing defects in a mouth when the work of that artist is lacking. To these last the title of surgeon dentists should not be refused, since they practice in its entirety a part of surgery which is not only estimable in itself but which would never have become despised if certain people had not brought it into contempt by practicing without ever having acquired the necessary and sufficient knowledge, and who have deceived and shocked the public. As a result the public, not being always capable of making a just estimation of merit, have confounded the honest man with the fraud, the qualified with the ignorant, and finally the dentist has been despised, and his profession, which without such drawbacks, would always have been considered as useful and as important for the preservation of mankind as other parts of surgery.*[9]

Fauchard also identified dishonest methods among some dentists who practiced restorative dentistry. A common fraud was the use of fake gold leaf for plugging teeth. This was accomplished with the use of thin leaves of lead or tin stained to look like gold or beaten lead covered with gold leaf. Another form of dishonesty was to promote oneself as having special expertise, as by use of an inordinate number of unnecessary instruments: "Some of those who clean teeth have as a rule an assortment of instruments of all kinds and try to persuade by this that they cannot be properly cleaned without all these instruments which are useless for operating but necessary to impress the public."[9]

Fauchard endorsed the need for qualifying examinations before a panel of experts as a prerequisite to practice.[8] He urged the authorities that in the case of candidates for the title of surgeon-dentist, the panel of examiners from the College of St Come (surgeons) and the medical faculty of Paris should contain an eminent and experienced surgeon-dentist as well as physicians and general surgeons. This measure would further assure the competency of certified candidates. More than 250 years later, it is difficult to find more concise and forceful endorsements of dental education as the vehicle for the advancement and preservation of dentistry as a respected profession.

Fauchard deplored the fact that most dental care was being provided by unskilled amateurs. He rightly pointed out that the public neglected to obtain dental care because they feared dental surgeons. He attempted to educate patients that regular dental care, provided in a humane and intelligent fashion, could preserve a dentition. Fauchard had received most of his practical training while in the health service of the French Navy.[7] His mentor, surgeon general M. Alexander Poteleret, was especially knowledgeable in scorbutic disorders, because this was the most common ailment affecting seamen. Fauchard devoted an entire chapter of his textbook to the effects of scurvy on the teeth and gums:

> *Scurvy occasions considerable swelling, lividity, yellow color, importunate and intolerable irritation, sordid ulcers, serous exudation which is putrid, it oozes at the slightest touch, bleeding is sometimes considerable...This cruel evil loosens the teeth, exposes their roots and makes them very loose.*[10]

Fauchard's book contains evidence that he continued to learn and study throughout his life. He notes that he has made direct observations on tooth development with Mr Winslow, professor and demonstrator of anatomy in the Faculty of Medicine at Paris: "It is he who has made me see on a new born subject the order which I have just reported of the layers of the tooth." He describes the tissues of the dental germ, its high vascularity, and the manner in which enamel is believed to be formed. It is significant that Winslow, a distinguished anatomist of the medical faculty, shared his knowledge and research interests with a surgeon-dentist, considering that there existed a long tradition of animosity between the very conservative members of the medical faculty of the University of Paris and the surgeons of the College of St Come. Fauchard had not only gained the respect of master surgeons at St Come but was also held in high esteem by the medical faculty of the University of Paris. In the preface to his treatise, Fauchard urges the study of anatomy:

> *As the diversity of diseases of the teeth, the causes which they produce and their symptoms are infinite, the operations which surgery has devised for their cure demand as much variety of knowledge, and practice alone does not suffice to carry these operations to perfection, at least when it is not governed by an exact study of the anatomy of the mouth.*[10]

Perhaps the most valuable parts of Fauchard's book are his numerous case reports. These accounts give insight to the way he practiced and the way he consulted with his dental and medical colleagues, and they demonstrate his keen powers of observation and his common sense. The scope of his practice included operative dentistry, prosthodontics, oral surgery, periodontics, and orthodontics. In each of these areas, he provides the details of his methods so that others may profit from his experience. From 58 case reports, it is clear that the public he treated was a cross section of the upper middle classes of Paris: M. Octavien, a painter; M. Duchemin, comedian; Claude Cussant, wine merchant; Abbé Cherier of the faculty of Paris; M. Bretonnier, attorney to Parliament, etc. These case reports also reveal the names of referring surgeons and physicians who were among the most respected members of the professions: Winslow, professor of anatomy at the Jardin du Roy in Paris; Jussieu, naturalist at the Jardin du Roy; and Helvétius, the elder, First Physician to Marie Leszczynska, Queen of France, are just a few who sent him patients or who sought his advice.

The case of the wine merchant, Claude Cussant, illustrates Fauchard's skill and the best level of care available at that time:

> *The renowned Claude Cussant, wine merchant at Saint Bri near Auxerre, aged forty-six years, in 1725 had the two last large molars of the right side of the lower jaw so carious that there only remained a small part of their roots. An overgrowth of the flesh of the gums was*

caused by this caries and in less than a year it grew to the size of a pullet's egg. The tumour was quite hard and prevented the mouth from shutting closely enough to chew food, because the molars of the upper jaw on the same side bit on a portion of the growth. The patient was in a sad state, consulted M. de Lisle his surgeon who advised him to seek surgeons of the Hotel Dieu at Auxerre and to consult them about it. These gentlemen finding the tumour considerable advised the patient to come to the hospital of the Brothers of Charity of Paris. The monks to whom he applied and the surgeons of the hospital found the disease extraordinary and believing it contagious and incurable refused to take him in. Then one of the surgeons at the hospital said that it might be a good thing to extirpate the tumour. This patient then sought M. Fremont sworn surgeon of Paris who feeling the need of good advice sent him to the St. Come to consult with him and several of his confreres. These gentlemen after expressing their opinion resolved to send the patient to me. I examined him and found that it was indeed of consequence and that nothing should be neglected. I told the patient that if these gentlemen wished to abandon the treatment to me I would hope to guarantee a cure. M. Fremont had the goodness to tell him that he could put himself in my hands with the utmost confidence. The next day at the appointed time the patient came, where Messieurs Du Lessis, Saure and Verdier, Master Surgeons whom I had invited, were there already. When we examined the patient we agreed that the growth should be removed. To proceed with this operation, the patient being seated in an arm-chair his head leaning on the back, I took several lengths of waxed silk with which I encircled the tumour by the back and two sides in order to draw it forwards. Holding the two ends of the silk in my left hand I held a curved bistoury in my right, with which I began to cut this growth on its posterior part and its sides. Then I took a hook with which I held these growths already divided, and I continued to cut with the curved scissors. In this way I removed the greater part of the carcinomatous tumour. The state of the patient and the effusion of blood caused me to pause from complete extirpation. I stopped the hemorrhage with styptics.

The operation started at ten o'clock in the morning, at eleven the patient returned to his inn in Isle St. Louis. He returned to me the same day at four in the afternoon after having drunk some beer and wine, very frightened at seeing that his blood flowed abundantly; I reassured him with good encouragements and at the same time I worked to stop the bleeding. This day a surgeon came to me and assisted me with advice and here we were in agreement. After applying several times different styptics in vain, I used tampons, compression and alternately the actual cautery, the bleeding always started afresh. At eight o'clock we decided to keep the patient in my house, I gave him a room and a bed, on which we made him sit propped up with cushions after which we were only occupied in finding something more efficacious to help. We renewed the applications of the actual cautery, as much with the idea of stopping the hemorrhage as to consume at the same time the remains of the carcinomatous growth. On this flesh and these vessels so many times cauterised we applied tampons and pledgets steeped in

> *my styptic of which I have given the prescription in Chapter XII, Vol. II, and we took great care to hold this adjusted and compressed. At last in this way we mastered the hemorrhage. Later it began again with more violence than before which decided us to use Cyprus vitriol in powder, we made balls and pledgets of it and powdered them—this was applied with order and circumspection and covered over with little compresses doubled and soaked in my styptic water. This was held and compressed with the fingers for a long quarter of an hour. Seeing that this hemorrhage was arrested we abandoned the compression to the pressure of the jaws and we advised the patient to keep them shut continually and firmly to hold the compression equal and sufficient. This hemorrhage stopped an hour after midnight. We did not leave the patient until two o'clock, nor did we take any repose until we were sure of his condition. We advised him to remain seated for the whole night and not to go to sleep nor open his mouth. His wife and the servant of the house watched over him to perform those things we had ordered for him. We saw him at seven o'clock in the morning and found him as we had left him, without hemorrhage, fever or pain only having a longing for sleep. We examined the mouth, we made him rinse it, there was not a single drop of blood, the dressing was like a lump of putty. We gave him milk to drink, as much for nourishment as to take away the bad influence which the vitriol, swallowed with the saliva, had had on his mouth and on the primae viae. After all these precautions we were easy in our minds and we allowed him to lie down and not to be troubled about anything and to rest quietly. I kept him two days in my house, on the third he was able to return to his inn without any fear. I expected the dressing would come away by itself. The scars made by the caustic came away on the fifteenth day without any trouble. There remained some part of the tumour which I consumed with the actual cautery. As the patient had not suffered much pain by the preceding applications of the actual cautery which gave less trouble than cutting instruments this decided me to consume the growth by several applications of the actual cautery. When the scars came away I drew the roots of the carious teeth which were the cause of this disease. I applied the actual cautery once more and for the last time on several growths which needed it and when the scars had fallen the bone of the jaw was exposed and without caries. I only applied several compresses steeped in the balsam of the Commander and the scar was perfect in three weeks. After this the surgeons who had been present at the operation saw the patient and found him completely cured. During the treatment the patient had some fever, he was bled and purged, and the fever was cured without return. Since then he has returned to Paris several times, I examined his mouth and have always found it in good condition.*[9]

Throughout his book, Fauchard is seen as a practitioner who enjoys the challenge of successfully treating difficult cases and, when necessary, developing new instruments and techniques to achieve an optimal result. He developed a new double pelican that facilitated the extraction of teeth. An entire chapter is devoted to describing its design and method of application. Further, Fauchard claims that dental caries is a "most baleful affliction which can attack the teeth." For caries that have not reached the pulp, he recommends four remedies: "the first is that by filing and rasping; the second the application of lead, the third by oils or essences of cinnamon and cloves mixed or separate and the fourth by the actual cautery." If a tooth is only slightly carious, "it is enough to remove the caries by instruments...and to fill the cavity with lead." Deeper cavities are treated with cotton dipped in oil of cinnamon or cloves. After several days, when the pain has subsided, the cavity should be filled. Cautery is used when the above treatments fail. During these operations "the dental patient must be seated in an arm chair, which is steady and firm...The dentist will be sometimes on the right side and sometimes on the left, sometimes in front but seldom behind the patient." Fauchard rejected the old idea that for extractions the patient should be seated on the ground. He gives ample space to attacking charlatans who "abuse the credulity of the public" by promoting all types of liquors and plasters for alleviating toothache: "The ease with which they find dupes in credulous persons and with which they amass money is a bait too strong not to increase the breed; they are found of all kinds, sexes, and professions."[9]

A study of Fauchard's case reports shows that nearly 50% of his practice centered on extractions of teeth and the extirpations of tumors and other growths. Orthodontic alignment of teeth also forms a good part of his practice: 13 of the 58 case reports deal with minor tooth movement. Periodontal treatment and operative dentistry are less prominently described. Prior to the development of techniques to achieve peripheral seal, maxillary dentures were difficult to retain in place, supported only by the mandibular teeth and pressure from the cheeks. Dentures were used primarily for ornament and pronunciation. It was a rare individual who could become sufficiently accustomed and adept to use these "dents de parade" for masticating food. Fauchard achieved limited success in solving this problem by joining full maxillary dentures to full or partial mandibular dentures via posterior springs (Fig 4-3). Fauchard illustrates such a case:

> *In 1737 a lady, of the highest circle, about sixty years of age, who had not lost a single tooth in the lower jaw, came to M. Caperon, a very skilful dentist to the king, in the hope that he would be able to provide her mouth with an upper denture. He told her, as the lady repeated to me, that as she had no teeth in this jaw to which to attach it, it would be as easy to build in the air: he advised her to come and see me and that if I could not do what she desired there was no hope for her. This lady followed his advice, and when I had examined her mouth I begged her to give me a few days to reflect on the means to carry out her wish. After*

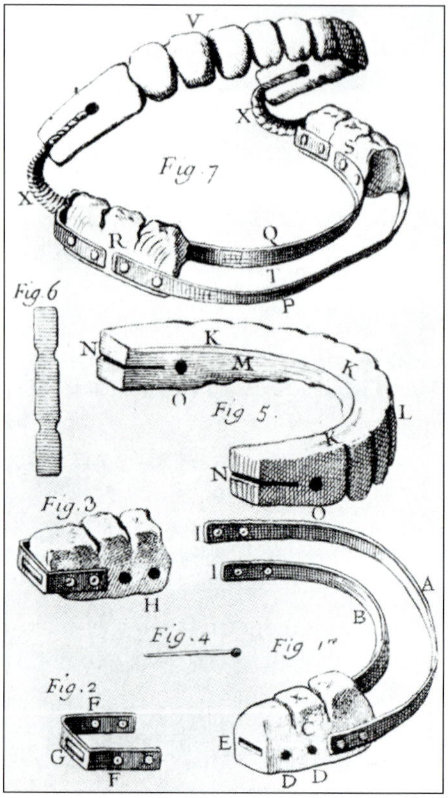

Fig 4-3 Full maxillary denture held over the mandibular natural dentition by a framework linked to the maxilla by springs. (From Fauchard,[10] 1728.)

having thought over it well, I invented a machine like that shown in plate 41, being connected with the teeth of the lower jaw, which would be capable of fastening and keeping in the upper jaw a row of teeth almost entire. This lady wishing only to have teeth in the front of the mouth for ornament and a more perfect pronunciation, I made the denture less extensive with which she could eat easily and which she would hardly notice. For greater cleanliness she has two similar ones, which she wears alternately. I shall tell willingly how I came to make this machine.[10]

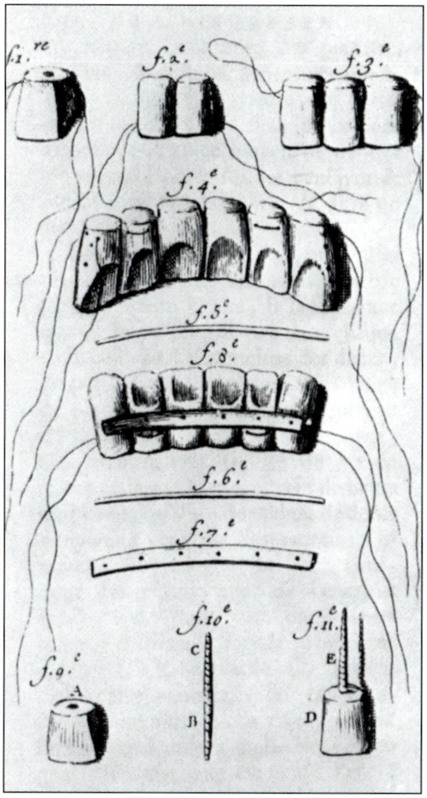

Fig 4-4 Partial dentures made of artificial teeth drilled to accommodate threads by which they are attached to abutment teeth. Silver bars are used to join the pontics. (From Fauchard,[10] 1728.)

The idea of using springs for retention was not new, but his designs and materials were improvements (Figs 4-4 to 4-6). His use of the term *machine* to describe this prosthesis is perhaps a reflection of his sympathy for the contemporary philosophy of life held by many medical men of that time, in which man was described in mechanical terms.

Fauchard rightly deserves to be called the "father of modern dentistry," because his treatise was the first comprehensive description of dental practice. The book received the approbation of many members of the Faculty of Medicine of the University of Paris, including M. Finot:

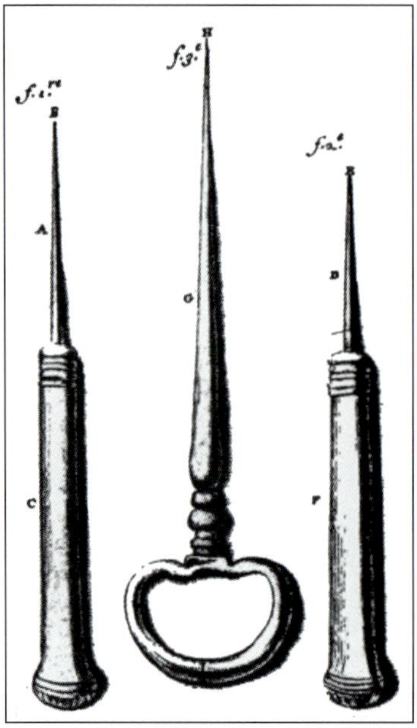

Fig 4-5 Instruments used to enlarge pulp canals prior to insertion of pivot teeth. (From Fauchard,[10] 1728.)

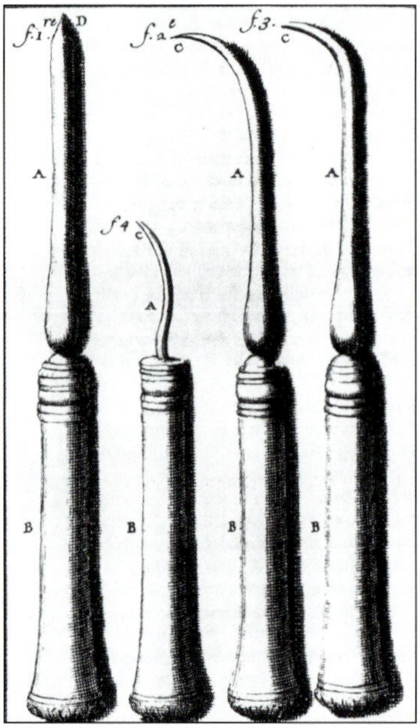

Fig 4-6 Instruments for packing and filling teeth. (From Fauchard,[10] 1728.)

> *I have read M. Fauchard's book with much pleasure, from this book the public will derive very solid advantage. It contains many facts exactly recounted, judicious reflections on diseases of the teeth and the means of curing them. These reflections, founded on assiduous work and drawn from confirmed experiment to which nothing may be added, have given him a perfect knowledge of these different diseases of which no other dentist has attained up to the present. It is by this exact knowledge that he has improved even invented successfully a very large number of instruments, fitted for operations on the teeth and for their preservation in many seemingly doubtful cases. There is nothing but praise for a work which has cost him so many pains; a work which he has produced with so much clarity and precision from the obscurity which has enveloped it and the superficiality with which it has been treated hitherto.*[9]

In breaking new ground, Fauchard had set high standards for those who would follow. He turned the craft of dentistry into a profession deserving a place among the specialties in medicine and surgery. Others in France, England, and Germany would soon follow his lead.

Other Noteworthy French Dentists

Pierre Baron has provided an exhaustive study of dental practitioners in Paris at the end of the 18th century. Three categories are described: *(1)* surgeon dentists who had qualified by completing studies at the surgical college of St Come, *(2)* dentists skilled by apprenticeship, and *(3)* the untrained charlatans who performed mainly tooth extractions. Baron's study reveals that at the end of the 18th century, Paris had no shortage of dentists.[11]

Claude Gerauldy

Claude Gerauldy, surgeon-dentist to the Duc d'Orleans, published his methods of practice in *L'art de conserver les dents* in 1737. He characterized dentistry as widely practiced but little understood. Gerauldy noted that most men who engage in dental practice, especially in the provinces, apply themselves to the mechanical aspects, while but a few pursue the theory or science of dentistry. Thus, it should be no surprise that they are unable to cure or prevent a whole host of maladies or the sequelae resulting from dental disease.[12] In general, Gerauldy's book echoes many of the methods previously described by Fauchard, but they lack the extensive case reports provided in Fauchard's work.

Gerauldy described dental decay as a corrosion of dental tissues arising from both external and internal sources. Early external lesions are treated by filing away the diseased enamel, such as that caused by retention of food debris on interdental surfaces. Gerauldy notes that most caries begins internally as a result of the transmission of acidic and corrosive substances that escape from the tooth's internal blood vessels. Often these lesions are only detected by probing the tooth surface or from pain originating in the tooth. Caries lesions are not reversible, and the only recourse is the excavation of the decayed substance and plugging of the cavity with lead. If the tooth is too painful to be plugged, it may benefit from a temporary dressing consisting of cotton pellets soaked in a concoction made from wine, cloves, cinnamon, and powdered chamomile roots.[12] When the nerve (pulp) is exposed, it is best to cauterize the tissue with a hot probe before plugging the cavity. Teeth that have been restored in this manner serve equally well as normal teeth in mastication and can be retained for the life of the patient.[12]

Gerauldy taught that when the crown has been entirely destroyed by caries, the root may be left in its alveolus if it is asymptomatic; otherwise, it must be extracted. For extractions, he recommended that the patient be seated lower than the dentist and that the patient's head be secured between the left arm and body of the operator. With the fingers of the operator's left hand, the patient's lips are parted, and the cloth-covered head of the pelican is positioned adjacent to the tooth. With the claw engaged on the opposite side of the tooth at the cervical margin, the tooth is then extracted by applying leverage with the pelican. Extraction should not be performed when the surrounding tissues are swollen and inflamed, nor when the patient is pregnant. However, if an abscess has formed, the extraction need not be postponed. To prevent the loss of loose and unsteady teeth, they should be tied together with gold thread after the removal of all tartar.

Gerauldy described four varieties of gingival lesions: inflammatory tumors, gingival outgrowths, ulcerations, and fistulas. Inflammatory tumors were characterized by swelling with engorged and dilated blood vessels. Because these tumors were believed to arise from accumulations of stagnant blood, they were treated by bloodletting, gingival scarification, and the use of a variety of herbal mouthwashes. Gingival abscesses were covered with a roasted fig and herbal plaster to induce rupture. If this failed, Gerauldy recommended that the abscess be incised to fully drain it of all fluid. These lesions must be closely watched to avoid penetration of the suppuration into the jawbone. Other outgrowths from the gingiva that are soft and whitish in appearance were thought to arise from stagnation of the lymphatic vessels. Gerauldy notes that these may attain a large size, interfering with speech and swallowing, so they must be cut away before they ulcerate or invade the jaws.[12]

Etienne Bourdet

Etienne Bourdet, one generation after Fauchard, was equally effective in describing the practice of dentistry in an excellent treatise published in 1757. The fame of Fauchard continues to overshadow the merit of Bourdet's original contributions, especially in the area of periodontal disease.[13] Bourdet must be viewed as the second most important dentist of the 18th century. Bourdet was appointed surgeon-dentist to the Queen of France in 1759 and to King Louis XV in 1760. He is best noted for his treatise *Recherches et observations sur toutes les parties de l'art du dentiste (Research and Observations on All Aspects of Dentistry)*, published in Paris in 1757. In the preface, Bourdet notes that written works on dentistry are abundant and outnumber those for any other branch of surgery, a sign of the growing demand for dental care.

Although there was much that was new in both technique and theory in the works of Bourdet (Fig 4-7), there remained many

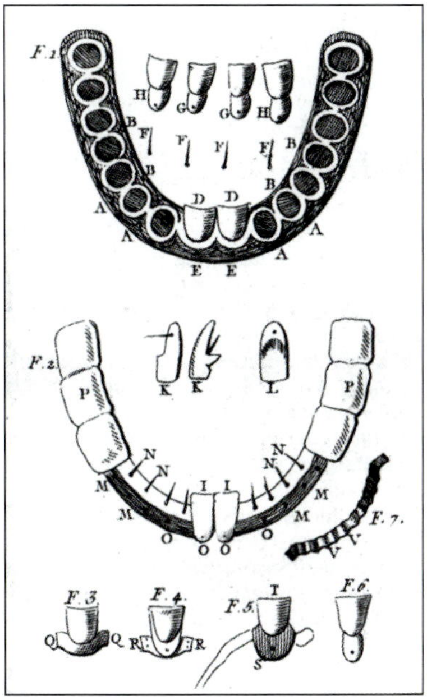

Fig 4-7 Methods of attaching artificial teeth to carved denture bases and to metal bars. (From Bourdet.[14])

ideas that simply repeated old humoral theories of dental caries and tartar formation. Bourdet continued to make the false assumption that exhaled air carried noxious vapors from the stomach and lungs, which upon contact with the teeth formed a corroding deposit. Like his contemporaries, he was right in recommending sobriety, healthy foods, and vigilance in performing oral hygiene to preserve healthy teeth. He viewed sugary foods as being particularly destructive to the teeth. Bourdet also warned that exposure to certain metals, such as arsenicals, as in metal workers, could damage the teeth and surrounding tissues.[14]

Bourdet diagnosed and treated bruxism, the nocturnal grinding of the teeth. For this condition, he adjusted the occlusion with files and fabricated gold shell crowns to protect the occlusal surfaces of the molars. A technique he advocated for the remedy of a painful tooth was luxation of its nerve supply. By use of the pelican, the offending tooth was partially elevated from its alveolus and quickly returned to its original position. The loosened tooth was stabilized by ligating it to its neighbors until firmness was reestablished. Bourdet claimed to have much success with this method. Dupont, dentist to Louis XIII of France, had previously published a small pamphlet in 1633 describing subluxation of teeth as a sure and easy method to cure toothache.[15] Another controversial technique was replantation of extracted

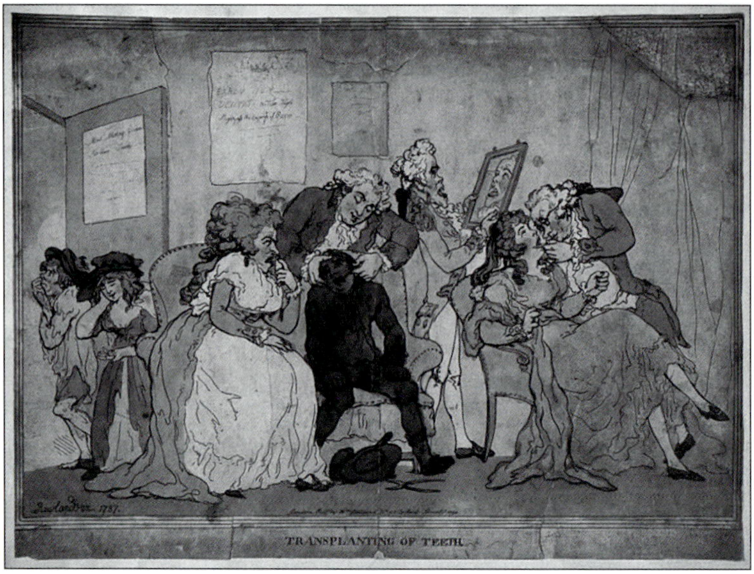

Fig 4-8 Thomas Rowlandson's 1787 etching mocking the practice of tooth transplantation.

teeth that were first cleaned of carious tissue and all cavities and pulp canals plugged with lead or gold. This method was recommended for incisors and premolars.[14]

Bourdet, like many of his contemporaries, also carried out transplantation of teeth, a procedure introduced as far back as the early 17th century by Dupont.[15] The implanted teeth could be obtained from cadavers; a common practice was to collect teeth from dead soldiers on the battlefield, hence their being called *Waterloo teeth*. But it was just as common to buy one or more teeth from a younger person of the poorer class at the scheduled day of implantation. The dentist often had several donors waiting in his dental parlor ready to have their teeth matched to the recipient, in the hope that one might obtain a donor tooth of the right dimension for the recipient's alveolus. Bourdet suggested that because of the variations in size and shape of the roots, "one should make sure you have several donors, Savoyard boys or others, so that if the tooth of one does not fit, it can be put back in (replanted), so that the donor be not deprived of it, and several others can be tried." Many poorer individuals sold their anterior teeth in this trade. Some dentists spoke out against this practice as an unethical exploitation of the poor. Charles Allen of York, England, who produced the first dental textbook in the English language in 1685, regarded it as commonplace (Fig 4-8) but objected to the practice on moral grounds. He claimed that it was inhumane, attended by difficulties, and not a true restorative procedure because the repair of one dentition was at the expense of another. Thomas Berdmore, surgeon-dentist to King George III of England, strictly rejected tooth transplantation. However, it was not until symptoms of syphilis began to appear in patients following tooth transplantation, and the development of porcelain teeth, that the practice was gradually eliminated.

A study of Fauchard's and Bourdet's concepts of gingival and periodontal pathology, and their methods of managing these diseases, reveals their many similarities but also their significant differences. Bourdet linked gingival inflammation to local alveolar bone loss with much insight.[13] For Bourdet, the health of the alveolus was clearly dependent on the health of the gingival tissues: "The gingivae in their natural state must be rose colored and of a firm texture. They should not cover the enamel but terminate exactly at the cervical neck of the crown." He noted that gingival disease could originate from scurvy or from venereal disease, but the most common damaging agent was the accumulation of tartar. His treatment included the removal of tartar, lancing of the gums to express the blood and fluids, and excision of the most highly swollen parts, such as the interdental papillae. In cases involving spontaneous bleeding from the gums, it was necessary to decrease the volume of the blood by bloodletting and to purge the patient.[14]

Bourdet noted that suppuration of the gingiva was as common as dental caries and just as likely to cause tooth loss.[13] He suggested that men were more likely to be affected by this condition because they did not have monthly menstruations, which served to cleanse the blood, because he believed the contemporary medical dogma, which held that most pathology was traceable to disturbances and imbalances in body humors, especially the blood. He also made the observation that suppuration of the gingiva was not likely to occur prior to the age of 30 years and that it became more common in 40- to 50-year-old individuals. Furthermore, he stated that "this disease causes the loss of otherwise perfectly good teeth, without ordinarily causing anything but very minor pain."

His writings display the origin of the concept of the gingival pocket and of an ulcerated pocket epithelium. Furthermore, his treatment rationale, based on a clearly defined concept of the local pathology, was developed through personal observation:

> *I have always noted that gingival suppuration developed in areas devoid of alveolar bone, and that this suppuration came precisely at the spot where the bone was destroyed. Why it is produced, is due to*

> *the failure of the gingiva to recede, and it, being now deprived of alveolar support can no longer attach itself to the root, itself as well as the gingiva having been denuded of periosteal tissue. Thus, this gingiva which naturally seeks to reunite and reattach, finds in the denuded root a foreign body, whose presence induces an infinite number of small ulcers, the source of this suppuration. These tiny ulcers, having formed on the surface of the gingiva which corresponds to the root, produce an incessant yet beneficial flow of viscous, white pus. As to the external surface of the gingiva, no ulcers are to be found: it is but more or less firm, often flaccid, spongy, swollen, or thin, depending on the duration of the problem. The color of the gingiva in this condition is almost always brown to lead-like; and in pressing the gingiva with the finger one can express material such as I have described above. To convince oneself that there no longer is any alveolar bone at the site from which this exudate originates, one has only to introduce a probe between the gingiva and the root; the instrument will soon measure the depth of the void produced by the absence of bone, and will also give the sense that the root has been denuded, which is confirmed when one opens the gingiva to stop the suppuration.*[14]

He described his method for treating this condition—the use of thin, flat instruments to cauterize the inside of the pocket and the excision of unattached gingiva, with care to preserve the gingival contours. Bourdet noted that when the affected tooth was extracted, the gingiva was restored to health within 24 hours. When the disease was not too far advanced, one could stop the suppuration by excision of the unattached gingiva, thereby removing the ulcerated area. Teeth treated in this manner would become firm.[14]

Charlatans

While Fauchard, Gerauldy, and Bourdet represented the new professionals of the dental art, the average man in the street was unlikely to be the recipient of their services. They were more likely to fall into the hands of a toothdrawer or charlatan. Fauchard and Bourdet had the courage to attack charlatans and to identify malpractice. They lived at a time when most people suffered from dental caries and periodontal disease and whose only recourse was to wait until the pain was unbearable before placing themselves at the mercy of an unskilled ambulant dentist. These fellows made their living by extracting teeth and selling mouthwash or other medications, usually with extravagant claims and false testimony.[11]

The most notorious of the charlatans who practiced in 18th-century Paris was Le Grand Thomas (Fig 4-9), who set up "shop" on the Pont Neuf, near the Louvre and the Île de la Cité.[1] He was

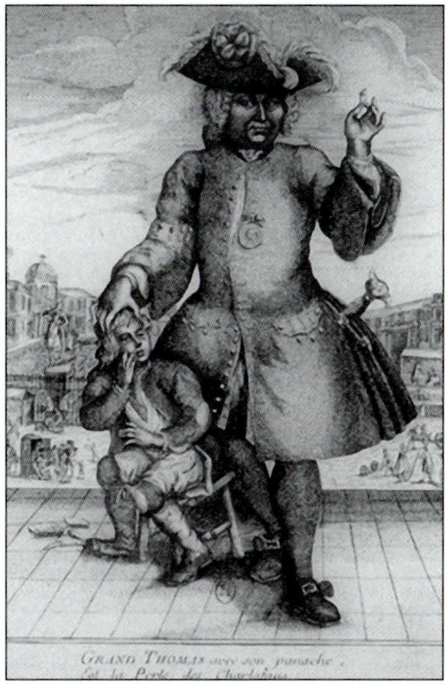

Fig 4-9 Grand Thomas, the notorious dental charlatan of Paris.

a gargantuan man who possessed the strength of a brute. Dressed in a scarlet military coat and a tricorn hat over his wig, "fat Thomas" attracted attention among the many charlatans and tradesmen who stationed themselves on the Pont Neuf. He extracted teeth to the sound of trumpets and drums and sold secret medicines for all types of diseases. He claimed his Orvietan could cure venereal disease.

In his book, Fauchard describes how these charlatans operated:

> *The knowledge that I have of the teeth and the diseases which attack them has always convinced me that these kinds of people have only one method, by throwing dust in people's eyes. The trouble I have taken to discover the mystery of these impostors has shown me and put me in possession of their cheat. All their cleverness consists in getting hold of some unfortunates, who push themselves among the people listening to the promises of the empiric. These pretended paid sufferers come up from time-to-time to the operator who holds in his hand a tooth all ready wrapped in a very fine skin with blood of a chicken or some other animal, introduces his hand in the mouth of the pretended sufferer, drops into it the tooth hidden in his hand. Then he has only to touch the tooth or do something of the sort with a powder or a straw or the point of his sword, he has only if he wishes to ring a bell in the ear of the pretended patient, who spits during this time that which he has*

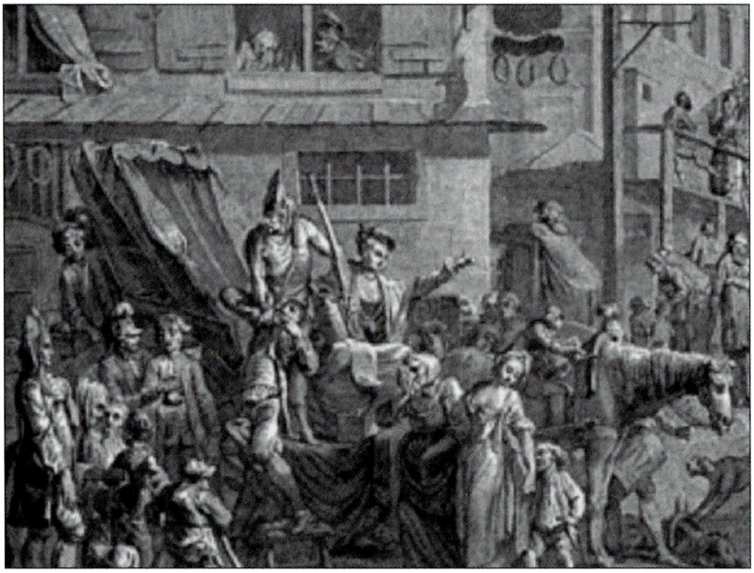

Fig 4-10 French street scene depicting a charlatan about to extract a tooth while his assistant sells a concoction to cure all ailments. Painting by Jacques Louis François Touzé (1747–1809).

in his mouth. One sees him spit out blood and his bloody tooth...If in the crowd anyone is deceived by this stratagem and presents himself to have a tooth drawn, the powder, the straw not being any longer any use, the operator soon finds a shift, he finds that the fluxion is too great, that he must have patience for a few days, or that his tooth is an eye tooth which must not be drawn, because these teeth, etc., as the empirics pretend are connected with the eye, which they say would be lost if the teeth are drawn.[10]

Fauchard goes on to point out that charlatans only remove very loose teeth and that they have no knowledge whatsoever of anatomy and the art of conserving teeth. In fact, they were not above telling prospective clients that it was useless to spend their money with practitioners who would attempt to clean, file, and plug teeth. Charlatans and toothdrawers hoped to sell tinctures and mouthwashes (Fig 4-10). They inculcated a fear of dentistry in the general public, which led to neglect. When business fell off or too many unfulfilled promises had been made, it was time to hit the road and head for the next village or fairground.

In parallel with the rapid developments in dentistry in France, similar events were taking place across the channel in England. Here guilds of barber-surgeons and colleges of the physicians were formed in part to protect themselves from encroachment from irregular practitioners and charlatans. They petitioned Parliament and obtained charters to restrict outsiders from practice. Henry VIII, in granting charters, had defined the scope of practice for physicians, surgeons, and barber-surgeons. But the resulting efforts to curb illegal practice in London led to an outcry of the public for the continued practice of irregulars who charged less to tend to their mundane ills, even if such irregulars were quacks.[16] In response to the mounting public resentment toward the regular members of the guild for their high prices and their persecutions of local irregulars, Henry VIII modified his previous law by instituting the following Act, which stated the following:

> *Mindful only of their own lucres, and nothing the profit or ease of the diseased or patient, have sued, troubled, and vexed divers honest persons, as well men as women, whom God hath endued with the knowledge of the nature, kind, and operation of certain herbs, roots, and waters, and the using and ministering of them to such as be pained with customable diseases, as women's breasts being sore, a pin and a web in the eye, uncomes of hands, scaldings, burnings, sore mouths, the stone, strangury, saucelin, and morphew, and such other like diseases, &c. &c. Therefore it shall be lawful for any person to cure outward sores, notwithstanding the statute of the 3rd of Henry VIII.*

Therefore, anyone who ministered to oral sores and dental diseases could practice without regulation.[16]

In 1685, Sir William Petty calculated that the number of people residing in the 124 parishes of London was about 696,000, a population much larger than that of any other European city and 10 times as large as that of London at the end of the 14th century.[17] The incidence of dental disease in London (Fig 4-11) at that time can be estimated by referencing the bills of mortality. For the year 1661, when 19,771 deaths were registered by the parish clerks, teeth and worms accounted for 1,195 deaths.[16] Thus, there was a need for individuals who had developed skills in tooth extraction and the treatment of minor oral diseases and who were available to the public locally and at relatively low cost.

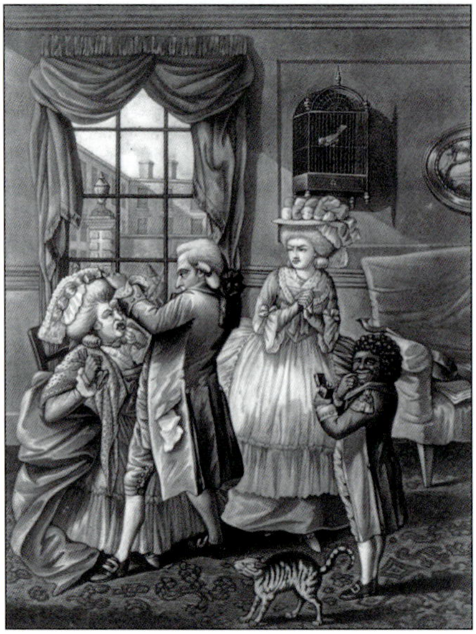

Fig 4-11 *The London Dentist* by watercolorist Robert Dighton (1762–1814).

Dentistry in England

Through the publication of Charles Allen's *Operator for the Teeth* in 1685, dentistry made progress in England, albeit at a slower pace than in France. The dental books of Fauchard and those of his French colleagues were not translated into English until the 20th century. A significant advance in English dentistry was made by Thomas Berdmore, surgeon-dentist to King George III, who published his *Treatise on the Disorders and Deformities of the Teeth and Gums* in 1768. Demonstrating the age-old competition with the French, Berdmore claimed that he owed nothing to French dentists, because they had only published to increase their fame.[18] Despite his claim to originality, however, there was little of merit or anything new in his work. England's most renowned contributor to the advancement of dental science was John Hunter. His books *The Natural History of the Human Teeth* (1771) and *Practical Treatise on the Diseases of the Teeth* (1778) are landmarks in the history of dentistry and are discussed in chapter 6.

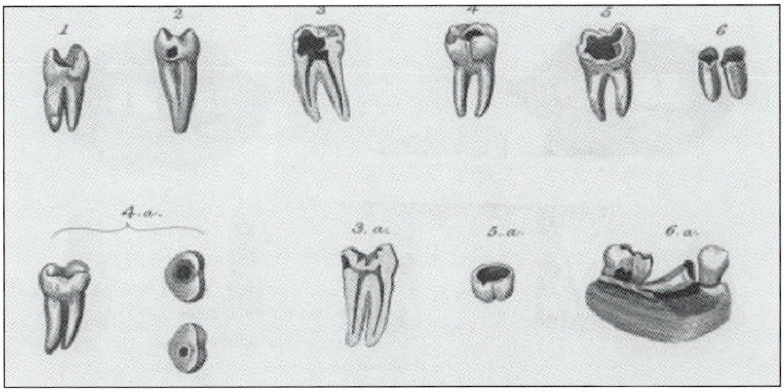

Fig 4-12 Figures representing the progress of dental decay. (From Fox.[19])

Joseph Fox

Joseph Fox (1775–1816), one of the most highly regarded dentists of his time, was the author of two key textbooks, *The Natural History and Diseases of the Human Teeth* (1803) and *The History and Treatment of the Diseases of the Teeth, the Gums, and the Alveolar Processes, with the Operations Which They Respectively Require* (1806). Both were seminal works that proved particularly influential in training the next generation of dentists. Fox, a pupil of John Hunter, was a lecturer in dentistry at London's Guy's Hospital. Fox's descriptions of dental and gingival diseases have a ring of modernity when compared with earlier works of a similar nature. His descriptions, illustrated by a large number of excellent engravings, reveal an underlying inquiring spirit, one who examined the pathologic gums and teeth with a view to understanding the etiologies of the various diseases. In this regard, he is an equal to Bourdet and Fauchard.

In beginning his treatise, he sets out to explain dental decay (Fig 4-12) and the methods to deal with this most common ailment:

> *Caries, or as it is commonly called, decay, is the disease with which the teeth are most frequently affected. It has at first its origin in the bony part (dentin) of the crown of the tooth, the structure of which becomes gradually destroyed, and the disease proceeds until the whole*

of the crown of the tooth, both enamel, and bone (dentin), is entirely removed. When caries has made some progress internally, a small, opaque spot appears upon the enamel, where it covers that part of the tooth which is diseased and the bony part of the tooth situated underneath this spot will be found of a dark brown color; when the decay has advanced so far as to destroy the texture of part of the bone (dentin) of the tooth, the enamel loses its support, then breaks away, and a cavity is discovered in the tooth. It is in this way that, in the first instance, caries originates; and it is by no means uncommon for a person, in a very short space of time, to discover cavities in several teeth which had been supposed perfectly sound. In the mastication of hard substances, pieces of the enamel are broken off, on account of the texture of the bony part being destroyed by the caries which had previously gone on for some time internally. There is no one part of a tooth more particularly liable to become diseased than another. In some the caries appears in the irregularities of the grinding surfaces of the molares, and resembles a crack filled with a black substance, which at length breaks into a cavity in the center of the tooth; in others it commences in the side of the tooth next the cheek; and sometimes at the neck of the tooth, the decay extending into the body of the tooth underneath the enamel. The decay very often commences on those sides of the teeth which are placed in apposition to each other; this is the worst possible situation for the disease, because it often makes considerable progress without being discovered, and is much less conveniently placed for the performance of any operation to arrest its progress. In the incisors, the caries most commonly begins at the sides, between the teeth; in some, it appears near the neck, the cavity extending across the tooth, and the disease proceeds until the tooth is nearly divided in two; in this case, whilst biting something hard, the lower part of the tooth usually breaks off, leaving the fang in the socket, and a small portion of the body of the tooth. The molares seem to be more subject to this disease than any of the other teeth: the incisors of the upper jaw are very frequently affected by it, whilst the incisors of the lower jaw very seldom become decayed. When a decayed tooth is examined, the carious part appears to be disposed in strata, the external is the most decayed, is black and so soft that it may be easily picked away. Underneath this, it will be found of a harder texture, and not so black in colour, and the substance of the tooth is less decayed and becomes more dense, until we arrive at the sound part. Whenever a decay has taken place in a tooth, and the enamel, by becoming opaque, begins to exhibit the appearances of this disease as having gone on underneath, if the tooth be sawn through, a brown mark will be found extending into the natural cavity of the tooth. It is in this direction the decay always proceeds, and, when the cavity is exposed, the membrane which lines it, and upon which the nerve and the blood vessels ramify, most commonly becomes inflamed, and produces pain. During the progress of caries in a tooth, it is the internal part of the crown which is the soonest removed, causing the tooth to appear as if the inside had been scooped out.[19]

Fox speculated from his clinical observations that some teeth were more susceptible to decay by virtue of a diminished content of "earthly matter" (mineral). Furthermore, this condition or disposition to decay might be constitutional, or in modern terms, systemic, because it often appeared to be bilateral in its occurrence:

> *The teeth of many persons are formed with a less quantity of earthy matter than of animal substance, on which account they do not acquire such a density as is necessary to make them durable, and resist those various causes of decay to which the teeth are constantly exposed. Teeth thus formed are at first very white, and have a certain transparency; but they soon begin to decay, and frequently, in a very few years, the disease extends through the greater part of them…This original defect in the structure of the teeth must depend upon a want of healthy action in the pulps, during the time of the formation of the teeth. It is impossible to conjecture what can be the cause of this imperfection, but it is very singular, and also very certain, that the same kind of structure may be observed in the teeth of many individuals in the same family, who, in all other respects, are very healthy. That the teeth acquire this disposition to decay from some want of healthy action, during their formation, seems to be proved by the common observation, that they become decayed in pairs; that is, those teeth which are formed at the same time being in a similar state of imperfection, have not the power to resist the causes of disease, and, therefore, nearly about the same period, they exhibit signs of decay, while those teeth which have been formed at another time, when a more healthy action has existed, have remained perfectly sound to the end of life. Decay of the teeth is often the consequence of certain states of the constitution, in which the functions of the body are performed irregularly, inducing various dyspeptic symptoms. In these cases, the caries affects many teeth at the same time, and often proceeds so quickly as, in a short period, to destroy the crowns of the teeth, leaving only the fangs. It is remarkable that the caries, arising from these constitutional affections, has often a whitish appearance, and the bone of the tooth is then much softer than when it proceeds from a simple inflammation.*[19]

Following his description of the pain of toothache, Fox advises the removal of the decayed tissue and the stopping (filling) of the cavity:

> *More commonly, at first, the pain of tooth-ache is slight, and occurs at intervals, being occasioned by exposure to cold, or the accidental pressure of some adventitious substance, such as a piece of crust, the seed of some fruit, or anything sweet: either of these getting into a tooth, partially decayed, generally causes some uneasiness. This kind of pain may almost always be relieved by a little tinctura opii, or it may subside of itself. In either case a recurrence may generally be prevented, by filling up the cavity of the tooth with some substance sufficiently hard and durable to keep out particles of food, and not liable to be acted upon by the*

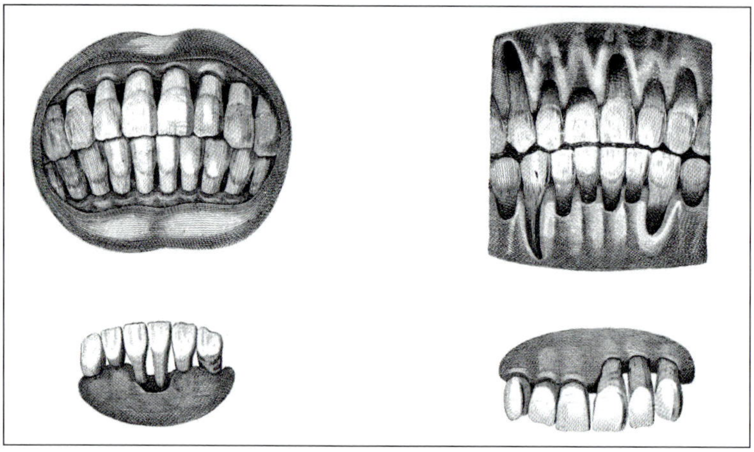

Fig 4-13 Drawings depicting "absorption of the gums and sockets, leaving the fangs of the teeth uncovered and black," considered to be the first illustration of periodontal disease. (From Fox.[19])

moisture or heat of the mouth. For this purpose wax, gum mastic, etc. have been employed, but they are soon dissolved and destroyed, therefore are improper. Formerly it was very much the practice to stop teeth with lead leaf, but the use of this substance ought to be forbidden, as it becomes corroded by the saliva, and the introduction of a very small quantity of this metal into the body is found to be productive of deliterious consequences: there is indeed reason to believe that, being dissolved by the menstrua contained in the saliva, it may occasion pains in the stomach, or other uneasy sensations. On this account, nothing ought to be used but what is insoluble or, if soluble, innoxious. Gold leaf is the most proper substance: also pure tin, beaten into leaves, may be used with nearly equal advantage: it is not so durable as the gold, as the saliva gradually acts upon it, but it cannot do any injury to the constitution. By thus excluding the air, and preventing any particles of food from lodging in the cavity, the progress of decay may be greatly retarded, the pain prevented, and the teeth preserved for many years.[19]

Fox recognized a disease of the alveoli characterized by resorption of bone, loss of attachment, inflammation and recession of the gingiva, and tooth loss (Fig 4-13):

The alveolar processes have certain diseases peculiar to themselves, independent of affections arising from the teeth and gums. The most common disease to which they are subject, is a gradual absorption of their substance, whereby the teeth lose their support, become weak, and

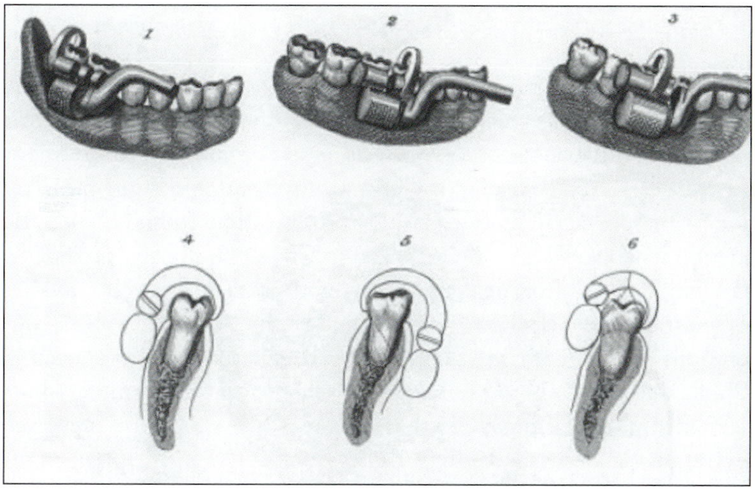

Fig 4-14 Fox's depiction of the proper use of the key for extraction of posterior teeth. (From Fox.[19])

> *at length are so loosened as to drop out. This disease usually begins to show itself between forty and fifty years of age; and, from its frequent occurrence without any evident cause, it would seem to be a consequence of having passed the middle period of life. The gums, being supported by the alveolar processes, partake also of the disease; for, as the absorption of the bony matter advances, they lose their attachment to the teeth, and recede in proportion to the wasting of the sockets. Hence, when an absorption of the sockets is taking place, the necks of the teeth being exposed, the teeth appear to become longer.*[19]

Fox preferred the use of the key for extraction of premolars and molars. Forceps were used on anterior teeth. Fox illustrated the use of an improved key enabling the placement of the claw anterior or posterior to the bolster (Fig 4-14). He also illustrated the proper positioning of the bolster on the gums to minimize fracturing of the crown.

By the end of the 18th century, Londoners could avail themselves of dental services if they had the means to do so. From an analysis of city trade directories and newspaper advertisements, it is estimated that there were at least 43 individuals practicing dentistry during the 1790s.[20] The great majority had no formal training, often combining hairdressing, corn cutting, and the sale of toothpowders and other elixirs to make a living.

Dentistry in Germany

The evolution of dentistry as a separate profession occurred in Germany around the same time as in France and England. The first book on dentistry, the *Artzney Buchlein*, was published in Germany in 1530.[18] Lorenz Heister, a German physician and surgeon, is remembered for his pioneering study of mastication. In his "Dissertatio anatomico-physiologica de masticatione" of 1711, Heister provided a thorough description of the anatomy and physiology of the muscles of mastication.[17] In his *Chirurgie* of 1718, he described various operations on the teeth and gingiva. Excerpts have been reproduced in Shklar and Chernin's *A Sourcebook of Dental Medicine*.[21] Among Heister's recommendations were that carious teeth should be preserved by removing decay and filling the cavity with wax. Incipient decay should be removed with a rasp. Deep caries that does not respond to anodyne fillings must be cauterized. Extractions should be avoided if the patient's gums are inflamed.[18] Heister also described cancer of the lip and its surgical removal.[21]

The Berlin surgeon Philipp Pfaff published a treatise on teeth and their disorders in 1756 in which he criticized Fauchard's book for its lack of brevity and order.[18] As court dentist to King Frederick of Prussia, Pfaff achieved clinical fame and respect among his peers. His contributions to clinical practice included his admonitions against the use of acids for cleaning teeth and caution in tooth transplantation as a potential source of cross infection. He was the first to recommend the use of sealing wax for taking impressions of the mouth for subsequent production of a plaster model.[18]

Porcelain Teeth

Prior to the invention of porcelain teeth, artificial teeth were carved from animal bones or from elephant and hippopotamus ivory. The teeth were fastened by a variety of methods to baseplates, also carved from the same substance. Because these teeth and plates were made of organic material (bone or ivory) and were exposed to saliva, they underwent decomposition over time. Accordingly, they were a source of an "insufferably offensive odor which cannot be corrected or prevented. They may be washed half dozen times a day, and taken out and cleansed at night, but it will still be grossly perceptible."[22] Individual teeth were often repaired by removing the decayed crown and attaching the crown of an extracted human tooth to the retained root by means of a screw of gold or silver. A less permanent option was to attach the crowns of extracted teeth by wire to adjacent teeth.

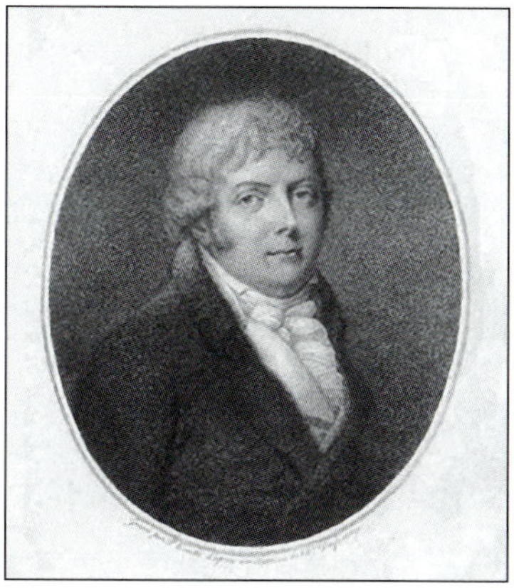

Fig 4-15 Nicholas Dubois de Chemant.

Porcelain teeth were first invented in Paris by chemist Alexis Duchateau with the aid of M. Guerhard, a porcelain manufacturer.[18] However, Nicholas Dubois de Chemant (Fig 4-15) perfected the invention and made it public in 1788. He characterized his newly invented teeth as incorruptible, imperishable, and odorless.[18] Initially the teeth and gums were baked as a single block; in 1808, however, Fonzi (a notable Italian dentist) introduced individual porcelain teeth with baked-in platinum pins (or staples). Dubois de Chemant's method received the approbation and formal endorsement from the Faculty of Medicine of Paris. Committee members reported that Dubois de Chemant's teeth and dentures were not altered by acid and were not broken when thrown to the floor (the supreme test of a good set! [Fig 4-16]). They also noted that the dentures weighed less than the fine porcelain from Sevres.[23] The French Royal Academy of Sciences in 1789 confirmed the report of the Faculty of Medicine, noting among the many advantages that the teeth and the gingival parts of the dentures were of a natural color and well adapted to the contours of the underlying tissue. Patients that had worn the dentures attested to the superior quality of the porcelain dentures before the Academy.[23] Because of controversy over priority rights of invention and the turmoil of the upcoming French Revolution, Dubois de Chemant moved to England, where he was well received. He claimed to have had success in 12,000 cases. The English translation of his book, *A Dissertation on Artificial Teeth*, was published in 1804.

Dubois de Chemant extolled the benefits of his artificial teeth in numerous case reports:

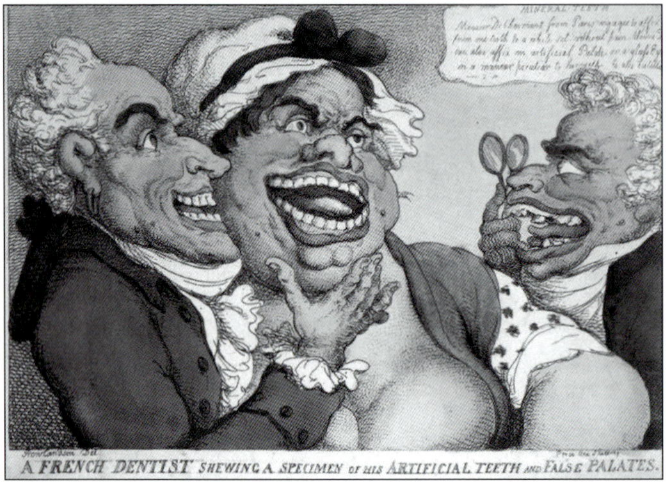
A FRENCH DENTIST SHEWING A SPECIMEN OF HIS ARTIFICIAL TEETH AND FALSE PALATES.

Fig 4-16 Thomas Rowlandson's caricature of the use of porcelain teeth.

> *I extracted in the presence of Sir Walter Farquhar, twenty-eight stumps and bad teeth, from a lady of quality, whose thinness, livid and yellow complexion, frequent complaints of the stomach and continual uneasiness, seemed to presage her approaching end. Her teeth were so decayed that the crowns of them were entirely destroyed, and there proceeded from them an insupportable odour; the discharge had corroded the internal parts of the sockets so that the teeth had all become loose. The desire to get rid of this distressing malady produced sufficient courage in this lady to submit, though contrary to my advice, to the extraction of 26 stumps at one sitting, and two the next day. Some weeks after, the fetid smell of the mouth and the symptoms of disease went off, and in two months more she had acquired the embonpoint and complexion which were natural to her before the decay of her teeth; because I made for her a complete set, with which she could eat as if she had preserved her natural ones.*[23]

In promoting his new product, Dubois de Chemant was quick to point out the corruptible nature of teeth carved from animal bone. A patient referred to him by the celebrated Mr John Hunter is said to have

> *experienced violent pains in the stomach, his breath was so offensive that it was impossible to remain near him. He wore two partial rows of teeth, made of sea horse tooth (hippo), placed between some natural ones which remained; having attentively examined them, I perceived that they were the cause of his indisposition: two days after they had been laid aside, his mouth exhaled no offensive smell, and his health which had suffered, began to improve.*[23]

Dubois de Chemant also condemned the use of cadaver teeth and the practice of transplantation of living teeth as a source of infection and transmission of disease, such as syphilis.

Fonzi (1768–1840) created individual porcelain teeth (indestructible "terro-metallic" teeth) that were subsequently bound to a metallic denture base by a platinum stud.[18] Fonzi experimented with various paste compositions and was able to develop 26 different tones resembling those found in natural teeth. The internal or opaque part was composed of Limoges clay, and the outer transparent part was fired from Limoges silica. Before firing, a platinum pin was inserted into the back of each tooth, later soldered to the silver or gold denture baseplate. His invention led to the industrial fabrication of individual porcelain teeth, thereby eliminating the use of human natural teeth (cadaver teeth). Porcelain teeth were not introduced in America until Dr A. A. Plantou, arriving in Philadelphia from Paris in 1817, carried with him a supply of porcelain teeth.[18]

Voltaire

While Fauchard, Bourdet, and other notable dentists in England and Germany were perfecting the practice of dentistry, the most prominent citizen of the Enlightenment—Voltaire—was suffering from advanced periodontal disease and tooth loss.[24] His case is included here because it illustrates the difficulties facing even the wealthiest and most famous people of that time. Voltaire, the leading French intellectual of the 18th century, was a notorious hypochondriac. His numerous letters contain hundreds of references to his medical and dental disorders, as well as to those of his close friends. Voltaire lived to be 84 years old, but not without suffering from several systemic medical disorders and periodontal disease, diagnosed as a scorbutic condition, that left him nearly edentulous by middle age[24] (Fig 4-17). As a result of neglect and from possible mercury intoxication, his periodontal disease worsened. He lost most of his teeth and suffered facial collapse because he chose not to wear a dental prosthesis (Fig 4-18).

The first mention of dental problems is found in a letter Voltaire addressed to the King of Prussia, Frederick II, dated January 1, 1749: "I have had a sickness which rendered me deaf in one ear and causes me to lose my teeth." Two years later, in a letter written at Berlin to Claude Darget, Voltaire writes that "The sickness which sequesters me from society is killing me." He most likely was afflicted by a dental or oral disorder, because he goes on in this letter to add that

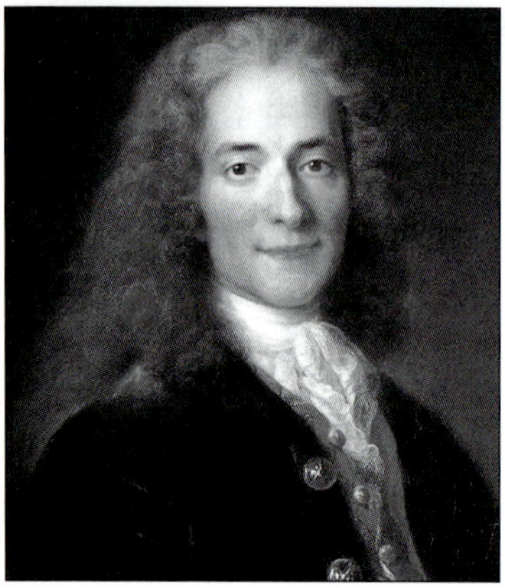

Fig 4-17 Voltaire in early middle age.

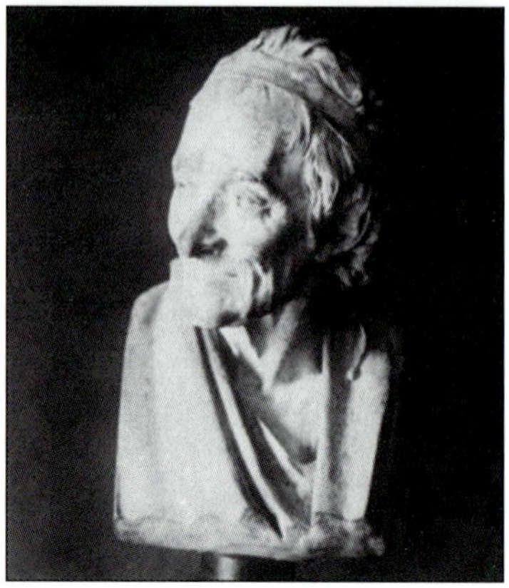

Fig 4-18 Houdon's sculpture of Voltaire in old age.

both La Mettrie and Codenius, physicians at Frederick's court, were prescribing antiscorbutiques. One month later, on February 20, 1751, writing again to Darget, Voltaire complains that "this cruel sickness which knaws at me does not permit me to eat suppers." The key statement comes one week later, again to Darget: "my gums are not any better." In the same letter, with his usual sarcasm, he says that he has great faith in La Mettrie: "Show me a better student of Boerhaave, and one who has written better of his profession." In August of that year, Voltaire wrote the following to his niece: "After having passed through the hands of physicians, charlatans and cooks...I have lived comfortably for six months with my King, eating like a devil, and taking like him, a little rhubarb and powder (laxative) every third day." In October of the same year, he revealed what had been suspected: "The king makes me as happy as a man could be who has been attacked for six months by a cruel sickness that has caused me to lose nearly all my teeth. One can hardly hear me when I speak."[24] It is reasonable to assume that Voltaire's reference to having been put into the hands of a charlatan indicates a visit to a toothdrawer, after having been prescribed useless antiscorbutic medications by La Mettrie and Codenius and special diets following tooth extraction.

In December of 1752, Voltaire wrote the following to a Parisian surgeon, Bagieux: "I came to Berlin with about 20 teeth, I have about six left." From this information, it can be concluded that Voltaire lost 12 teeth prior to going to Berlin, assuming that at one point he had a full dentition of 32 teeth. He probably lost most of those 12 teeth in 1749 at Cirey (see letter to Frederick II, dated 1/1/1749, quoted above). Although there is no proof that Bagieux was the surgeon that may have treated Voltaire in France, it is easy to suspect such a connection, because Bagieux is the recipient of several letters containing news of Voltaire's dental problems. There is no evidence that Voltaire was treated, other than for tooth extraction, by a surgeon-dentist prior to or even after his exile in Berlin. The dentist L'Ecluse, known to have been acquainted with Voltaire, does not enter the picture until 1761, when Voltaire was well established at Ferney and by then almost completely edentulous. While at Ferney, L'Ecluse made dentures for Voltaire's niece, but there is no record to suggest that he treated Voltaire. Although there is no evidence that Voltaire used dentures, it is evident that he was self-conscious of his edentulousness, because he spoke of it on several occasions. Writing to the duchess of Brunswick to decline an invitation, he notes that "For your royal dinner parties one needs teeth." And to countess Bentinck: "Will my doctors give me back my teeth and will God give me back my Madame du Chatelet." In October of 1752, he wrote that "It has been eight months since I have been out of my apartment. I lost my teeth—I am dying bit-by-bit."[24]

What might have been the outcome of Voltaire's dental problems had he been so fortunate as to have been a patient of Fauchard or of Bourdet? Might he have preserved his teeth longer and enjoyed life a bit more?

Summary

By the end of the 18th century, a subspecialty of surgery dealing with dental diseases had been established in the major cities of the West. This new practice was largely a craft learned by apprenticeship without a scientific basis and devoid of formal educational criteria. The works of Fauchard and other prominent surgeon-dentists of the 18th century demonstrated a perfection of practices begun at an earlier age that now encompassed the basis for the formation of a self-standing profession. From this baseline, rapid advances in both the mechanical arts and the science of dentistry would flourish; during the next century and a half, dentists would establish associations and rules of practice to set themselves apart from untrained charlatans. The science of the oral cavity would develop alongside the rapid growth of the basic medical sciences and, before long, the groundwork would be in place for the birth of dental schools.

References

1. King R. The Making of the Dentiste, c. 1650–1760. Aldershot, UK: Ashgate, 1998.
2. Stein JB. The teeth and dentists of some monarchs of France. Dent Cosmos 1914;56:578–587.
3. Coignerai-Devillers L. Medecine, dietetique et sante a la cour de Louis XIV d'apres les lettres de la princess Palatine. Revue D'Histoire De La Pharmacie 1983;30:265–274.
4. Dagen G. The dentists of the kings of France from Louis XIV to Louis Philippe. Dent Cosmos 1928;70:60–63.
5. Dobson J. The royal dentists. Ann Royal Coll Surg England 1970;46:277–291.
6. Garant PR. Dental health in the reign of Louis XIV: Anecdotes in the memoirs of Saint-Simon. Bull Hist Dent 1992;40:67–71.
7. Viau G. The life of Pierre Fauchard (1678–1761). Dent Cosmos 1923;65:797–808.
8. Garant PR. Lessons to be learned from Pierre Fauchard. J Am Coll Dent 1990;57:32–36.
9. Lindsay L. The Surgeon Dentist; Or, Treatise on the Teeth by Pierre Fauchard (as translated from the French). Pound Ridge, NY: Milford House, 1969.
10. Fauchard P. The Surgeon Dentist; Or, Treatise on the Teeth, ed 2. Paris: P. J. Mariette, 1746.
11. Baron P. Dental practice in Paris. In: Hillam C. Dental Practice in Europe at the End of the 18th Century. The Wellcome Series in the History of Medicine. Amsterdam: Rodopi, 2003.
12. Gerauldy C. L'art de conserver les dents. Paris: Le Mercier, 1737.
13. Garant PR. The contribution of Etienne Bourdet (1722–1789) to the diagnosis and treatment of periodontal disease. Bull Hist Dent 1993;41:69–72.
14. Bourdet M. Recherche et observations sur toutes les parties de l'art du dentiste. Paris: J. T. Herissant, 1757.
15. David T. Les dentistes de la cour de France. L'Odontologie 1887;7:472–583.

16. Poore GV. London: From the Sanitary and Medical Point of View. London: Cassell, 1889.
17. Unwin G. The Guilds and Companies of London. London: Methuen, 1908.
18. Hoffmann-Axthelm W. History of Dentistry. Chicago: Quintessence, 1981.
19. Fox J. The History and Treatment of the Diseases of the Teeth, the Gums, and the Alveolar Processes, with the Operations Which They Respectively Require. London: Thomas Cox, 1806.
20. Hargreaves A. Dentistry in the British Isles. In: Hillam C. Dental Practice in Europe at the End of the 18th Century. The Wellcome Series in the History of Medicine. Amsterdam: Rodopi, 2003.
21. Shklar G, Chernin DA. A Sourcebook of Dental Medicine. Waban, MA: Maro, 2002.
22. Dexter JE. A History of Dental and Oral Science in America. Philadelphia: S. S. White, 1876.
23. Dubois de Chemant N. Dissertation sur les avantages des nouvelles dents et rateliers artificiels, incorruptibles et sans odeur. Paris: Gattey, 1789.
24. Garant PR. Voltaire, medicine, and dentistry. Quintessence Int 1991;22:405–411.

5

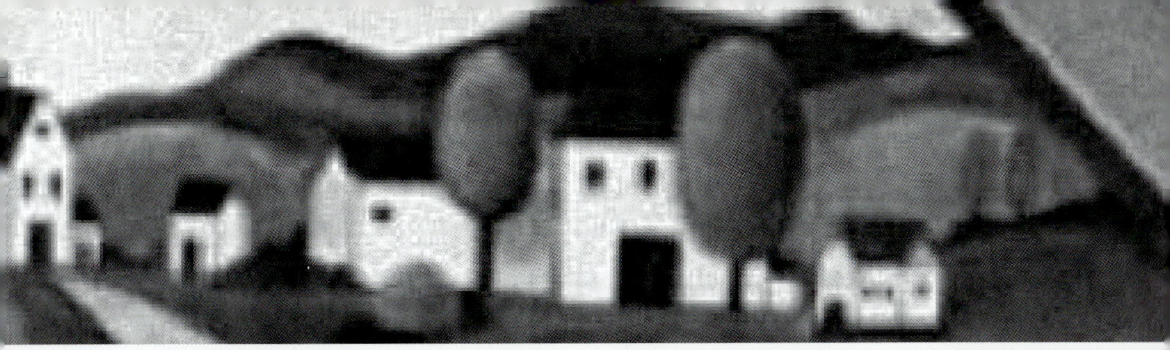

Dentistry in Colonial America

American colonists, out of necessity, managed every aspect of their daily lives, including dealing with injury and sickness. Pain was to be borne with stoic acceptance as retribution for one's sins, according to the Reverend Cotton Mather.[1] Dental caries and periodontal disease went mostly untreated, until the pain of toothache became intolerable and was only then relieved by tooth extraction. Because there were few trained dental practitioners, tooth extractions were often performed by local physicians who kept dental forceps in their instrument bag for such occasions. But if the local physician was unavailable, the butcher, the schoolmaster, or the blacksmith could fill in.[2] Joseph Sewall, a student at Harvard College in the early 1700s, informed his father, the famous Massachusetts Chief Justice Charles Sewall, that he had "a tooth pulled out by Madam Oliver's maid."[3] William Byrd, an aristocrat of Virginia, when attacked by toothache in the wilderness of the Carolinas, dealt with his problem in the following manner:

> *I had an impertinent Tooth in My upper jaw, that had been loose for some time, and made me chew with great caution. Particularly I cou'd not grind a Biscuit but with much deliberation and presence of mind. Tooth-Drawers we had none amongst us, nor any of the Instruments they make use of. However, Invention supply'd this want very happily, and I contriv'd to get rid of this troublesome Companion by cutting a Caper. I caused a Twine to be fasten'd roune the Root of my Tooth,*

> *about a Fathom in Length, and then ty'd the other End to the Snag of a Log that lay upon the ground, in such a Manner that I cou'd just stand upright. Having adjusted my String in this manner, I bent my Knees enough to enable me to spring vigorously off the ground, as perpendicularly as I cou'd. The force of the Leap drew out the Tooth with so much ease that I felt nothing of it, nor should have believ'd it was come away, unless I had seen it dangling at the End of the String.*[4]

Almanacs and Home Remedies

Colonials who could read sought relief of pain in almanacs and home remedy books. These books had a long history, having evolved from the 13th-century *Thesaurus pauperum* of Petrus Hispanus, a compendium of herbal remedies copied from Dioscorides's *De materia medica.*[5] The *Thesaurus pauperum* was used by mendicant monks to treat the poor. With the invention of moveable type in the 15th century, the *Thesaurus pauperum* was printed in numerous editions. In 1612, the first English home remedy book, *A Rich Storehouse or Treasury for the Diseased*, presumed to have been written by George Whetstone, a poet and contemporary of Shakespeare, was very popular.[5] In it are recipes for making various herbal concoctions and mouth rinses to cure toothache and gum diseases. It is likely that such a book would have been among the possessions of the Pilgrims at Plymouth Plantation.

Almanacs first appeared in printed form in Germany in 1448 following Gutenberg's invention of the printing press.[6,7] These printed pamphlets contained calendars, the positions of the heavenly bodies, weather forecasts, planting guides, and medical and dietary advice. For the early settlers of New England, the almanacs were essential (Fig 5-1). Rural families probably owned a Bible and an almanac, their only sources of information for regulating their lives. From the early 1700s, almanacs included practical information such as food recipes, currency conversion, interest tables, and medical advice. Advertisements also appeared in almanacs; in the 1698 edition of *Tully's Almanac*, there was an advertisement that a barber-surgeon's shop had opened next to the post house in Boston.[6]

In a survey of 1,685 colonial almanacs, 506 contained medical advice, and 56 contained specific advice on dental problems.[6] Remedies for toothache, gum infections, and teething problems were given along with preparations for cleaning teeth.[8] Folk remedies contained in Varlo's *A New System of Husbandry*, published in Philadelphia in 1789, were mostly prepared from common household goods and were probably beneficial, but other remedies, such as the advice to "rub the

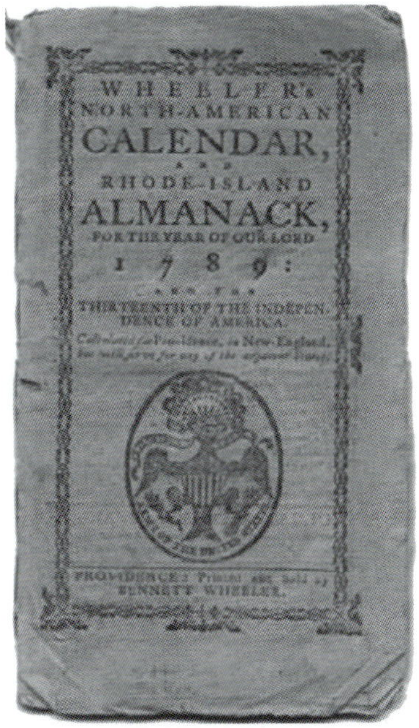

Fig 5-1 Almanac from Rhode Island.

gums with gun-powder till they bleed" for relief of toothache, were rather excessive.[6] In general, the medical content found in almanacs continued to reflect the old humoral theory of disease as taught by Hippocrates and Galen.[7]

Development of Dentistry

Because there were no legal restrictions to medical practice, anyone could establish himself as a physician. Medical training for those who did not have the means to go to Europe was through apprenticeship. David Harris has stated that in the colonies at the end of the American Revolution, there were over 3,000 medical practitioners, of which only 400 had earned medical degrees, mostly from Edinburgh or London.[9] Some physicians included dentistry in their practice, as did Charles Walker of Northampton, Massachusetts.[2] While physicians would extract teeth and lance infected tissues, they were unlikely to practice tooth replacement. For those individuals who lived in major cities and had the financial resources, they might seek out the local ivory turner or silversmith for the fabrication of artificial teeth.

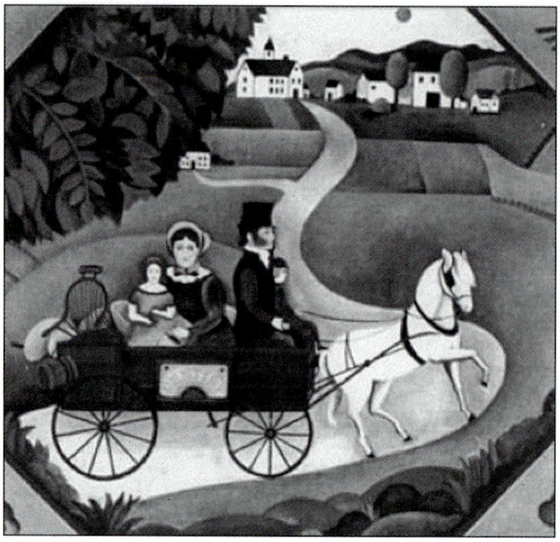

Fig 5-2 Primitive painting of an itinerant dentist. (Adapted from Ring ME. Dentistry: An Illustrated History. New York: Abradale, 1985.)

Among the first settlers of the Plymouth Colony in Massachusetts were a company of physicians, an apothecary, and three barber-surgeons. Only one of these three barber-surgeons is known—William Dinly, who froze to death in a violent snowstorm in the winter of 1638 while on his way to relieve a man of toothache.[10,11] Nearly 100 years would elapse before new information about dental practice in America would surface in early newspaper announcements and other sources. Weinberger compiled a list of 71 individuals who practiced as toothdrawers, operators for the teeth, surgeon-dentists, and dentists in the major cities of the American colonies from 1733 to 1799. According to Weinberger, the list is incomplete, "for there were many more men who practiced in this country during the period."[11] Although little is known about many of these men, several placed lengthy public advertisements, thereby providing a view of dentistry in that time period.

Boston, New York City, and Philadelphia, the three largest ports along the eastern coast, were first to see the development of dentistry (Fig 5-2). Newspaper advertisements appearing in these cities are a valuable source of information on early development of dentistry in America.[11,12] The *Independent Advertiser of Boston* announced in 1749 that Sieur Roquet, a dentist from Paris, had established a dental practice in town. Roquet claimed to "cure stinking breath by extracting teeth and broken stumps painlessly" and to burn (cauterize) gums down to the bone, also without pain: "Sets of African Ivory Teeth... will be nicely fitted to the jaws, that people of the first fashion, may eat, drink, swear, talk, scandal, quarrel, and show their teeth, without the least indecency, inconvenience, or hesitation whatever."[12]

In 1767, on arriving to New York City, Robert Woofendale, an Englishman apprenticed in dentistry to Thomas Berdmore, dentist to King George III, announced that he practiced "all operations on the teeth, gums, and sockets; and likewise fixes in artificial teeth so as to escape discernment, and without the least inconvenience."[10,12] After 1 year of practice in Philadelphia and New York City, Woofendale returned to London after failing to establish a financially profitable practice in the colonies.[11,13]

John Baker

John Baker was one of the first dentists to practice dentistry in America. Weinberger's research suggests that Baker was trained in medicine in Cork, Ireland, and practiced dentistry on the Continent from 1752 to 1762 before establishing himself in Boston around 1763.[11] While building a successful practice in Boston, Baker provided the seed for the development of dentistry in America by giving instruction in dentistry to Paul Revere, Josiah Flagg, and Isaac Greenwood. In 1768, Baker left Boston to practice in major cities of the Eastern seaboard. Weinberger traced his moves through New York, Philadelphia, Williamsburg, Baltimore, Annapolis, and Rhode Island from newspaper announcements and advertising circulars. From such documents, it is also possible to gain an idea of the scope of Baker's services and conclude that "Baker must have been a dentist of more than average ability, well grounded in the fundamentals of his profession, and deeply and sincerely concerned with the health and the proper care of the teeth of the community."[11]

From a circular for the proper use of his mouthwash and dentifrice, printed in Philadelphia around 1779, Baker described his practice:

> *The Doctor may be consulted on all disorders of teeth, gums, sockets, ulcers, cancers, abscesses, fistulas, suppurations, inflammations, fungi excrescenses, exposure of the roots of the teeth, recess of the gums, formation of the different kinds of tartar, change of positions, loosenesses, luxation, caries, and exostosis of the bones which form the sockets, caries of the teeth, loss of enamel, matter collected in the maxillary sinuses, sometimes in the cancellated substance of the lower jaw; fractures, obstructions of nerves and vesicular parts of the teeth,*

> *softness and bleeding of the gums, compression of tartar that obstructs the regular course of the fluids, which will be liable to putrify and destroy, in a short time, the gum, the socket, and the periosteum of the root, etc.... He also may be consulted in all disorders incident to children in teething... Those who have had the misfortune of losing their teeth, may have natural teeth transplanted, or grafted on the old stumps. Also artificial teeth, from a single tooth, to a complete set.... The Dentifrice and Essence (with proper brushes) may also be had.*[11]

It should also be noted that Baker filled teeth with lead and gold. If Baker is to be believed, his scope of practice was not unlike Fauchard's.

During his time in Virginia, Baker was consulted by George Washington. Washington's account books between 1772 and 1774 contain entries for toothbrushes, dentifrice, and services of John Baker, surgeon-dentist. In 1791, John Baker returned to New York City, where he purchased a 46-acre farm for the price of £3,600, which at present would be located between 76th and 81st streets. Upon his death, the proceeds from his estate were used to support the Trinity School of New York City.[11,12]

Dentistry as a second profession

In 1766, James Daniel, a wigmaker, informed the public that he operated on teeth in New York City.[10] Wigmakers/barbers, many who served as toothdrawers, were common at the time.[14] In the colonies, as in Europe, the wearing of wigs was a custom among the wealthy aristocrats and gentlemen of the professions. Williamsburg, Virginia, listed 30 wigmakers who practiced during the 18th century. Andrew Anderson, a Williamsburg wigmaker, submitted a bill for services rendered to the Jones family from 1741 to 1743 that included drawing teeth and bleedings, both of which earned him less than a tenth of what he received for making and bobbing wigs.[14]

Paul Revere (Fig 5-3) was a skilled ivory turner and outstanding gold- and silversmith. Although not considered a dentist, he did fabricate artificial dentures for practitioners in Boston. Revere advertised this service in the *Boston Gazette* for December 19, 1768:

> *Whereas many persons are so unfortunate as to lose their foreteeth by accident and other ways, to their great detriment, not only in looks, but speaking, both in public and private: This is to inform such that they may have them replaced by artificial ones that look as well as the natural and answer the end of speaking to all intents. 'By Paul Revere, Goldsmith, Near the head of Dr. Clarke's wharf.'*[15]

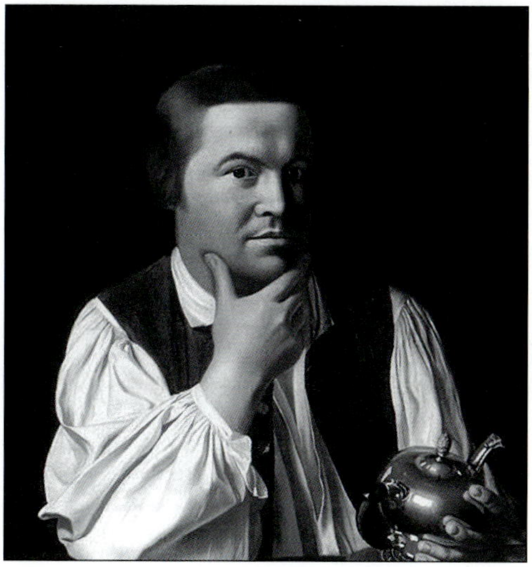

Fig 5-3 Paul Revere.

Revere is said to have identified the body of Dr Joseph Warren at the Battle of Bunker Hill from the dental prosthesis he had made for Warren.[15;1]

The persecution of Huguenots in France led to the emigration of numerous professionals to England and the American colonies. The American Revolution, supported by French naval forces, also contributed to the arrival of French-trained dentists on American shores. In Philadelphia in 1800, there were 30 dentists of whom 15 had arrived from England or France. Asbell named Michael Poree, M. Glabeau, Le Mayeur, Jacques Gardette, M. Leger, Le Breton, Chauvet, and Duvivier as of French origin.[16] By 1800, people with means in the major cities along the Eastern seaboard had access to dentists, but out in the country, dental care, if at all available, was still provided by the country doctor.

[1] This forensic dental identification preceded by about 100 years Dr Keep's identification of the denture of Dr Parkman in the famous murder trial of Harvard professor Webster.

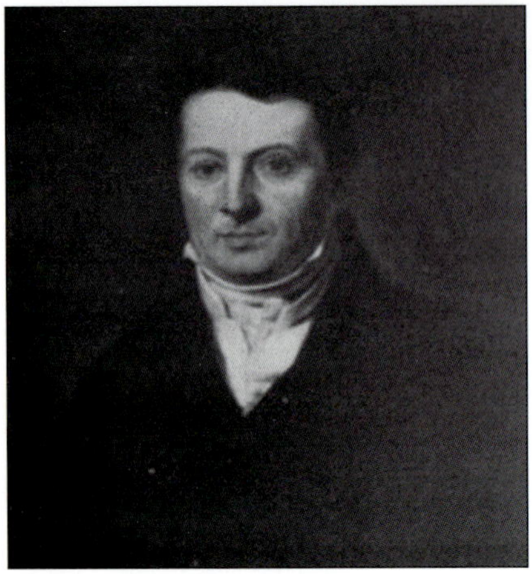

Fig 5-4 James Gardette.

James Gardette

James (Jacques) Gardette (Fig 5-4), who sailed from France with General Lafayette, arrived in Plymouth, Massachusetts, in 1778. A naval surgeon with training in dentistry, he treated men in Rochambeau's army in Rhode Island.[12] Gardette established his practice as a surgeon-dentist in Philadelphia in 1784, advertising that he

> *begs to inform the ladies and gentlemen that he makes artificial teeth (which imitate the natural) from a single tooth to whole set, and places them, without the least pain, so regular, that it is impossible to distinguish them from the natural ones, and in such a manner, that the persons may take them out and fix them again themselves with the greatest ease; he can place them over stumps, if the person don't chuse to have them drawn. He also takes the scales or tartar from the teeth without pain, and renders them (by help of a powder that he composes) as clean and white as ever.*[11]

Gardette is credited with fabricating the first maxillary denture that was supported by suction rather than by springs.[13] As one of the early dentists who adopted gold foil instead of lead or tin as the best material for filling teeth, Gardette related that he prepared gold foil for his own use from Dutch ducats.[17] In 1791 while in practice in Philadelphia, Gardette invited his brother, an engraver working in Paris, to come to America, where Gardette would train him as a dentist. Gardette suggested that he could earn in 1 hour of dental practice what he was presently making in 1 week "scratching copper in France."[18] Gardette also asked his brother to bring with him Fauchard's, Bunon's, and Bourdet's new textbooks.[18]

Weinberger shed new light on Gardette's observations on transplantation of teeth by reproducing an article that appeared in the *Medical Recorder* of Philadelphia for January 1827. In that paper, Gardette expressed his opposition to transplantation:

> *I shall preface this paper, by informing my readers that I arrived in Philadelphia in June, 1784, and began to practice my profession; and that Mr. Lemayeur, with the reputation of an eminent dentist, had transplanted one hundred and seventy teeth in this city, in the course of the winter of the years 1785 and 1786, as he told me himself, at Baltimore, in the fall of the last mentioned year; and that, of all those transplanted teeth, not one succeeded! Some became firm, and lasted, more or less so, for one or two years, in the sockets in which they had been inserted; but those cases were very rare. In the course of my practice, after that time, I had occasion to extract at least fifty of these transplanted teeth—most of them without an instrument, with my fingers only—and to replace them by artificial teeth.*[11]

Although Gardette viewed the transplantation of a tooth from one person to another to be contraindicated, he did practice the replantation of teeth within the same individual. He reported cases where he had "extracted the tooth with a straight forceps, cleared the cavity of its carious parts, filled it with gold, washed it in warm water, and inserted it in its alveola; all this was done in the space of five minutes... that tooth rendered service to the lady for nearly eighteen years."[11]

Gardette holds the distinction of having been a dentist to George Washington in 1789. When Washington sat for his portrait by Stuart in 1795–1796, he was wearing a set of teeth made by Gardette.[11] Washington's bulging lips do not speak well of Gardette's skills as a fabricator of dentures.

Gardette retired to France after 45 years of practice in Philadelphia, during which time he formed friendships with Drs Benjamin Rush, Caspar Wistar, and William Shippen, among the elite of American medical practitioners.[11]

Jean Pierre Le Mayeur

Jean Pierre Le Mayeur came from London in 1781 to settle family business in America. He had been trained in dental surgery in Paris at a time when dental transplantation was popular. Bernard Weinberger's research on Le Mayeur has refuted the idea that Le Mayeur arrived in America with French forces under Rochambeau at Newport and that he had instructed Josiah Flagg in the art of dentistry.[19] Le Mayeur is of special interest to American dentistry on two counts: *(1)* as dentist and friend to George Washington and *(2)* for practicing transplantation of teeth in New York, Philadelphia, and Virginia. Weinberger's study of Washington's diary and letters revealed that Le Mayeur treated Washington at his headquarters in Newburg, New York, in 1783 and at Mount Vernon, Virginia, in 1784.[11,19] General Washington, writing from his headquarters in Newburg to Lieutenant-Colonel William Smith, inquiring about Le Mayeur's skills, revealed his own dental condition:

> *Having some teeth which are very troublesome to me at times, and of which I wish to be eased, provided I could substitute others (not by transplantation, for of this I have no idea, even with young people, and sure I am it cannot succeed with old) and gums which might be relieved by a man of skill. I would thank you for making a private investigation of this man's character—knowledge in his profession, and if you find them such as I can derive any benefit from, encourage him to come out, and to take this on his way to whatever Port, or place he may be bound. At any rate, if he is really skillful, I should be glad to see him with his apparatus. I would not wish that this matter should be made a parade of, and therefore give you the trouble of arranging it.*[19]

Colonel Smith confirmed that Le Mayeur was "a man of polished manners, strict integrity, at the head of his profession, and a friend to this Country." General Washington was treated at Newburg and in the following year at Mount Vernon, where Le Mayeur was received as a dinner guest on several occasions.[19] Le Mayeur settled for a time in New York City, where he practiced and advertised transplantation of teeth. While in Virginia (1785–1788), it is reported that he accepted teeth from slaves for transplantation. Later in Philadelphia, he boasted having transplanted 123 teeth in 6 months.[10] Weinberger's research of the correspondence between Le Mayeur and George Washington revealed that Le Mayeur had accumulated substantial wealth and liked to breed horses.

Other colonial dentists

Edward Hudson was born in Ireland in 1772 and educated at Trinity College, Dublin, before coming to Philadelphia in 1803. Hudson had learned his dental skills in Ireland, where he perfected the use of gold for dental restorations. He was one of the first to fill root canals with gold foil, an operation for which he charged $20.[20] Hudson was regarded as a leading figure among Philadelphia's nascent dental profession.

One of the more colorful dentists was Charles Whitlock; while maintaining a dental practice, he achieved fame as an actor. Whitlock performed on stage in Boston, Baltimore, New York, Charleston, and Philadelphia from 1794 to 1802, at which point he retired to his home in England. The *Baltimore Daily Gazette* in 1795 announced that he performed all aspects of dentistry, including scaling and cleaning teeth, filling teeth with gold, placing artificial teeth, and regulating teeth.[11]

Richard C. Skinner was another dentist to arrive in the colonies from England. Skinner began practice in Philadelphia in 1789 and later moved to New York City. He had been trained in London by the Italian dentist Bartolomeo Ruspini.[2] Skinner announced his services in the *Federal Gazette* of Philadelphia as follows:

> *Mr. Skinner, Dentist,—Two doors below Dock in Second-street—Transplants natural as artificial teeth, from a single tooth to a complete set; those transplanted grow as firm in the jaw, and are equally as useful as the original teeth—The artificial are of a peculiar kind, the enamel of which is as beautiful as they upon the human teeth; they do not change their color, neither can they be distinguished by strict inspection from natural teeth. Mr. Skinner being perfectly acquainted with the practice and remedies of one of the most eminent and skillful dentists in London, engages to cure, in a few moments, that excruciating pain proceeding from carious teeth, without extracting them. He demands no compensation for any operation that does not equal the most sanguine expectations.*[11]

For his transplantation practice, Skinner advertised that he paid one guinea for live front teeth and a lesser but "generous" price for dead front teeth. The crowns of the dead teeth were used as pivot teeth for mounting in artificial dentures.[11]

Skinner, like contemporary dentists in Europe, was especially concerned with cleaning teeth from deposits of tartar to ensure healthy gums:

> *He cleanses and restores the teeth to their original whiteness and the breath to its natural sweetness, by removing tartar, which by negligence and inattention collects upon the teeth, insinuates itself under the gums, separates them from the teeth, eventually occasions their loosening and falling out of the jaw, and is the first cause of introducing those vitiated juices or scorbutic humors commonly called the scurvy, evils that ought to be early noticed and remedied by all classes of people.*[11]

---

[2] Ruspini was the author of *A Treatise on the Teeth, Their Structure and Various Diseases*, published in London in 1768. He emphasized treatment of the gingiva for alleviating scurvy.

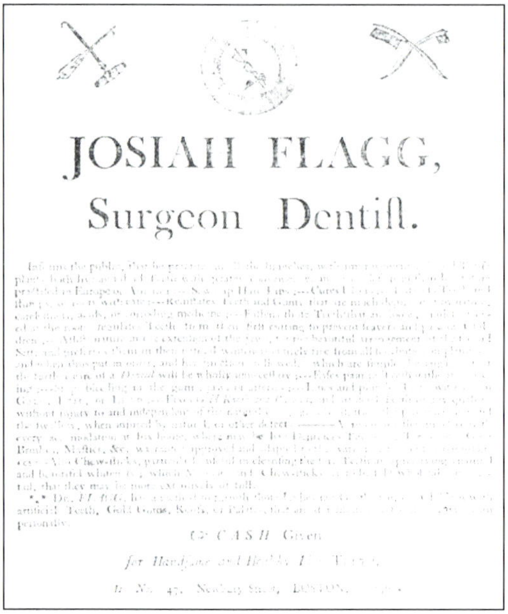

Fig 5-5 Announcement of Josiah Flagg's dental practice.

Like most colonial dentists, Skinner made periodic visits from his main base of practice in New York City[3] to nearby cities, where he would conduct practice for a week or more. From newspaper notices, Skinner is known to have spent time in Hartford, Connecticut; Hudson, New York; and Baltimore, Maryland.[11] Skinner holds the distinction of having been the first dentist to serve in a hospital setting (the Dispensary of New York). He is also credited with producing the first printed dental book in America, a small, 26-page treatise on dental practice and oral hygiene, which he offered free to his patients.[11]

Josiah Flagg has often been said be the first dentist native to America. It has also been said that he served in the Continental Army and may have received training in dentistry from Le Mayeur or Gardette while in Newport, Rhode Island, during the encampment of Rochambeau's army.[10,15,17] However, Weinberger's research disputed all of these claims.[11] Flagg, who practiced in Boston and in surrounding towns, may have been trained by Revere. Flagg boasted of an ambitious list of services (Fig 5-5), as judged in his handbill:

---

[3] Weinberger's *An Introduction to the History of Dentistry*[11] contains a map of colonial New York with the location of 19 dental practices.

> *Dr. Flagg transplants teeth; cures ulcers and eases them from pain without drawing; fastens those that are loose; mends teeth with foil or gold to be as lasting and useful as sound teeth, and without pain in the operation; makes artificial teeth, and secures them in an independent, lasting, and serviceable manner. Sews up harelips, and fixes gold roofs and palates, greatly assisting the pronunciation and the swallow... Cuts the defect from teeth and restores them to whiteness and soundness, without saws, files, acids, and such abusives as have shamefully crept into the profession, and which have destroyed the confidence of the publick.*[17]

In the service of the American resistance in the war of 1812, Flagg was captured by the British and for a brief time was incarcerated in England.[11] Upon his release from prison, he became acquainted with several English surgeons from whom he gained additional expertise before returning to the States.[10]

Noteworthy Dental Families

A characteristic of a craft learned by apprenticeship was its passage within members of a family, father to son or brother to brother. Two dental families of the colonial period famous for their skills and leadership qualities were the Greenwoods and the Parmlys.

The Greenwood family

In just two generations, the Greenwood family produced seven dentists.[11;4] Isaac John Greenwood is considered America's first native-born dentist.[11] Originally a craftsman in the business of wood and ivory turning, umbrella manufacturing, and the import of items for ladies, he would later take up tooth cleaning, the sale of toothbrushes, and the replacement of teeth on plates of gold or silver around 1778 in Boston.[11] Descendants of Isaac John Greenwood achieved fame as colonial dentists. Isaac Greenwood, Jr, extended his practice beyond toothdrawing, tooth replacing, and tooth filling to treatment of the gums and regulation of the teeth (orthodontics). Judging from his advertisement in New York City's *Rivington Gazette* and the *Independent Journal* of 1784, his practice was all-inclusive.

[4] A chart of the genealogy of the Greenwood family is contained in Weinberger's *An Introduction to the History of Dentistry*.[11]

Greenwood announced that he

> *begs leave to acquaint the publick that he preserves the Teeth and Gums by removing an infectious tartar, that destroys them and renders the natural purity of the breath offensive. He cures the Scurvy in the Gums; also fastens the teeth by causing the gums to grow up and adhere to them. He extracts and replaces the Teeth, regulates, gives them proper vacancies, cleanses the Teeth, and makes them white. He substitutes Artificial Teeth in so neat a manner as not to be perceived from natural ones, without drawing the stumps or causing the least pain. They give a youthful air to the countenance, and render pronunciation more agreeable and distinct; in a word, both Natural and Artificial are of much real service—it is a folly to neglect them. And as he would ever have his work recommended him, he requires no pay from those that are not completely satisfied with his performances. He has Pills for the Tooth Ache, that seldom fail to give relief; likewise boxes of Teeth Powder and Brushes that will recommend themselves.*[2]

John Greenwood

The most celebrated of the Greenwood family was John Greenwood (Fig 5-6), the second son of Isaac Greenwood, Sr. He achieved special fame as a friend and dentist to George Washington. Although he was apprenticed as a cabinetmaker at the age of 13 years, his training was interrupted by the Revolutionary War. As a volunteer in the colonial army, he served in Canada and New Jersey. Following capture and escape from imprisonment, he settled in New York City in 1875.[15]

Up until this time, John Greenwood had no prior experience or training in dentistry. The story of how he became a competent and respected dentist, as recounted by Weinberger from his extensive research of original family documents, illustrates the ease with which one could establish oneself as a "dentist" when there was a total lack of professional regulations or standards: One day as he was employed in woodcarving and instrument repair, "out of fun…by the desire of Dr. Gamage,[5] I attempted to draw a tooth for him. I had never seen one drawn before in all my life. It came out well and encouraged me to attempt others…then I thought I would undertake to make teeth."[11] Just 1 year later in 1786, he placed a notice in the *New York Advertiser*:

---

[5] Dr Gamage was a respected physician who had been instrumental in forming the Medical Society of the State of New York. Greenwood, through his friendship with Gamage, may have been introduced to medical books and encouraged to pursue his interest in dentistry. Greenwood is known to have owned and thoroughly read and annotated a copy of Hunter's *Natural History of the Teeth*.

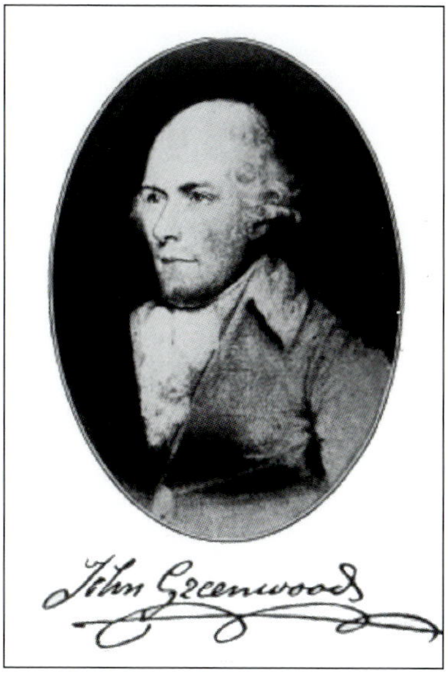

Fig 5-6 John Greenwood.

> *Encouraged by the success of his practice, [he] begs leave to acquaint the public, that he preserves the teeth and gums, by removing an infectious tartar, that destroys them, and renders the natural purity of the breath offensive; cures the scurvy in the gums; fastens the teeth by causing the gums to adhere to them, he cleanses the teeth, makes them white; substitutes artificial teeth in so neat a manner as not to be perceived from the natural; they give a youthful air to the countenance, and render the pronunciation more agreeable and distinct; in a word both natural and artificial are of such real service as are worthy the attention of every one.*[11]

By 1787, John Greenwood was devoting his full-time attention to dental practice. Soon he was using the title of surgeon-dentist and operator for the teeth when announcing that he transplanted teeth and that he had invented a method of fixing artificial teeth with springs. He advertised that he was employed by "the first families in the United States, as well as foreigners."[11] In 1800, John Greenwood ran an advertisement in the *New York City Directory* in which he labeled himself as "Dentist to the Late President George Washington," including the following excerpt from one of President Washington's letters: "I shall always prefer your services to that of any other in the line of your present profession."[11]

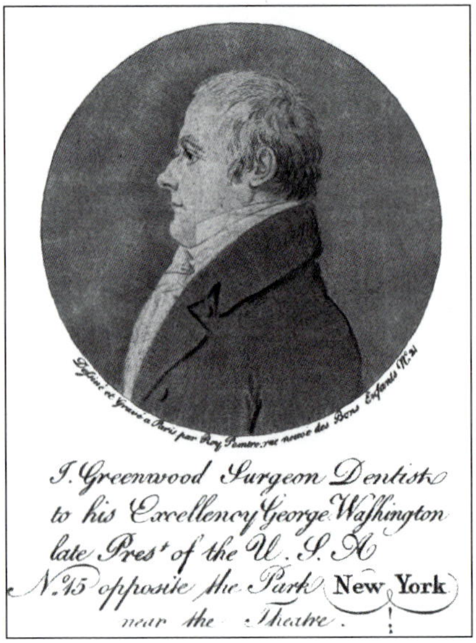
I. Greenwood Surgeon Dentist
to his Excellency George Washington
late Prest of the U. S. A
N.o 15 opposite the Park New York
near the Theatre.

Fig 5-7 Business card of John Greenwood.

John Greenwood traveled to Paris in 1806, where he met the elite of the dental profession. While there, he had his portrait painted by Roy, which he later reproduced on his engraved business cards[11] (Fig 5-7). It is said that he returned to the United States with a keg of natural human teeth.[12] He did have an active practice in transplantation and fabrication of artificial plates, as noted by the 1792 advertisement in the *New York Weekly Museum*:

> *Possessing a perfect knowledge of Mr. John Hunter's practice of the human teeth (Surgeon Extraordinary to the King), with the general approbation of the first families of the United States as well as foreigners, he transplants and grafts natural teeth; those transplanted grow as firm in the jaw as the original teeth. Mr. Greenwood makes and fixes artificial teeth of a peculiar kind, the enamel of which is as beautiful as that upon the human teeth; they neither change their colour nor can they be distinguished from the natural.*[21]

John Greenwood achieved lasting fame as the dentist of George Washington.[11,12] Throughout his life, George Washington suffered from bad teeth and gums. He was the patient of John Baker, Le Mayeur, Gardette, and John Greenwood. John Greenwood fabricated a gold plate denture for George Washington in 1789. The teeth were

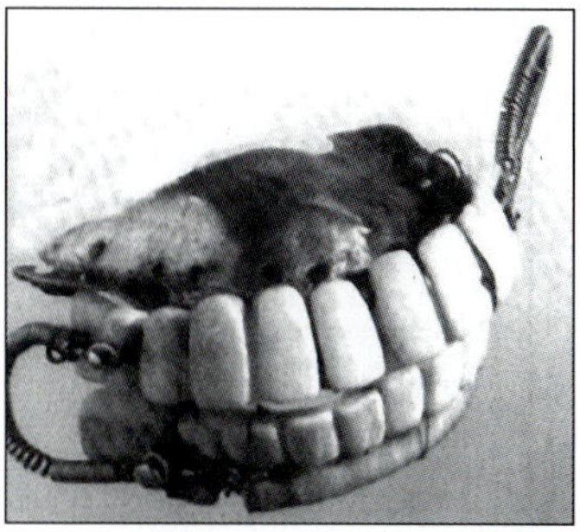

Fig 5-8 President Washington's denture.

carved from hippopotamus ivory and were held in place by springs (Fig 5-8). Washington had had several sets of dentures made for him, none of which was ever comfortable or useful. Greenwood instructed George Washington on how to take good care of his dentures, including making repairs to holes caused by acid and avoiding soaking them in port wine:

> *Sir: I send you enclosed two sets of teeth, one fixed on the old bars in part, and the sett you sent me from Philadelphia, which, when I received, was very black, occasioned either by your soaking them in port wine, or by your drinking it. Port wine being sour takes off all polish and all acid has a tendency to soften every kind of teeth and bone. Acid is used in coloring every kind of ivory, therefore it is very pernicious to the teeth. I advise you to either take them out after dinner and put them in clean water and put in another sett, or clean them with a brush and some chalk scraped fine.*[10]

Greenwood goes on to advise Washington on how to repair holes created by acid in the ivory teeth:

> *First observe and dry the teeth, then take a piece of wax and cut into small pieces as you think will fill up the whole; then take a large nail or any other piece of iron and heat it hot into the fire, then put your piece of wax into the hole and melt it by means of introducing the point of the nail to it.*[10]

By 1789, Washington had only a single tooth left, the mandibular left second premolar. When it was so loose that it could be extracted, Washington presented it to John Greenwood, who had it encased in a gold locket that is now displayed at the New York Academy of Medicine.

The Parmly family

The Parmly family had 13 practicing dentists over two generations.[12] The two most famous members of the family were Levi S. Parmly and Eleazar Parmly of New England. Levi Spear Parmly was a Vermont-born and Boston-trained dentist. He was one of five brothers, four of whom became dentists. In Boston, Levi received dental instruction from the English dentist S. Petrie and Dr John Randall.[22] After a brief period of practice in Montreal and Quebec City, Levi sailed for Europe, where, from 1817 to 1820, he studied and practiced in London, meeting Bell, Tomes, Nasmyth, and others among the leaders of the profession in England.[22] He also went to Paris to study dentistry in 1819. Levi Parmly returned to practice in New York City in 1820 before moving to New Orleans, where he conducted a highly successful practice for over 30 years. In his practice, he gave free dental care to many children in schools and orphanages, work that earned him the title of "father of dental hygiene and children's dentistry."[23] President James Monroe and his family were among his patients.[23] As a leading maker of gold foil restorations, he soon joined those who crusaded against the use of amalgam.

He collected thousands of teeth from dead soldiers to examine the stages of dental caries. While on a trip to Niagara Falls, he ventured into Canada to collect teeth from the skulls of soldiers who had perished in the 1814 Battle of Bridgewater. From his examination of carious teeth, he concluded that caries started externally from decomposition of food and penetrated into the tooth through minute openings in the enamel.[23] This notion was at odds with the generally held theory that decay originated inside the tooth and progressed outward from the dentin. His ideas on the origin and progress of dental caries led him to advocate oral hygiene as the best defense against caries, as described in two books. In 1816, he published a book on dental care titled *Practical Guide to the Management of the Teeth*, in which he promoted oral hygiene as the best preventive measure to combat caries.[22] The second edition of this book was dedicated to his friend Benjamin West, the American artist. In 1820, while in London, he published his second major book, *Lectures on the Natural History and Management of the Teeth; the Cause of Their Decay; the Art of Preventing its Accession; and Various Operations, Never Hitherto Suggested, for the Preservation of Diseased Teeth*, in which he gave his account of the progress of dental decay.[23]

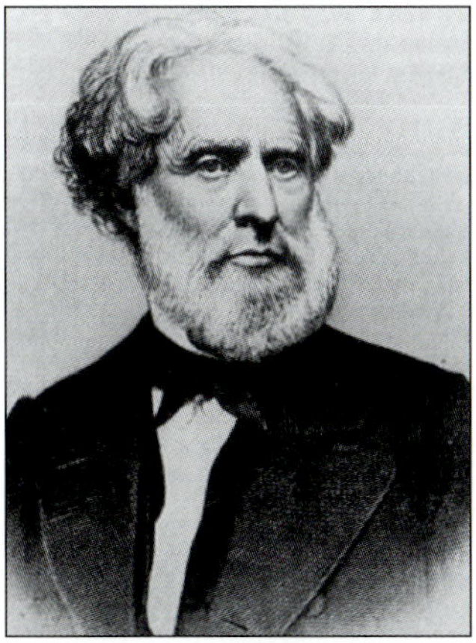

Fig 5-9 Eleazar Parmly.

Eleazar Parmly

Eleazar Parmly (Fig 5-9), younger brother of Levi, was one of the major figures in the history of American dentistry. Born in Vermont in 1797, he pursued his dental apprenticeship in Montreal with his elder brother, Levi. From 1817 to 1820, he traveled south to New Orleans, practicing in Pittsburgh and Cincinnati along the way. He recorded his travels in verse as he floated down the Ohio and Mississippi Rivers. In 1820, he sailed for England, where he studied and practiced dentistry in London. While in London, he published the first edition of *Natural History of the Teeth* (1820).[22] After 3 years, he returned to New York City, where he enjoyed an extensive practice. The Parmly practice included extractions using the turn-key, cleaning with scrapers, separating teeth and removing caries with files, filling cavities with tin and gold foil, carving dentures from ivory and bone, and attaching false teeth with gold or silver wires.[22] In perfecting the gold foil technique, he helped to establish it as the standard of good care for that time.

Eleazar Parmly was, to a large extent, responsible for establishing American dentistry as a respected profession, with national societies, ethical principles, dental degrees, national journals, and the development of dental colleges. In addition to being a successful dentist, Eleazar Parmly was a gifted poet who set down his autobiography in verse. In 1839, He joined Solyman Brown, Horace Hayden, and Chapin Harris to form the *American Journal of Dental Science*, the first dental periodical in the world. He was also instrumental in convincing Harris and Hayden to start the first dental school in Baltimore, Maryland (see Fig 5-10).

A distinguishing characteristic of Eleazar Parmly was a scrupulous attention to details, which, joined to integrity and cultivated taste, laid the foundation for both his large fortune and his popularity. Parmly served as the first president of the New York College of Dentistry. He retired from active practice in 1861 after accumulating the fortune of $3 million.

In 1834, the Crawcour brothers arrived in New York City from London to promote the use of amalgam through blatant newspaper advertisements, in which they extolled amalgam as the "Royal Mineral Succedaneum." Eleazar Parmly and other better dentists in the city opposed its use as injurious. The campaign against the Crawcours led to the formation of the world's first dental association, The Society of Surgeon-Dentists of the City and State of New York, in 1834.

Opening the First Dental School

Solyman Brown

Solyman Brown, born in Litchfield, Connecticut, in 1790, graduated from Yale in 1812 and was ordained a Congregational minister in 1814. He preached and taught school until 1822, when he moved to New York, where he preached Swedenborgianism. Although Solyman Brown was in demand as a minister, in 1832 he gave up preaching because of trouble with his throat and began a new career when his close friend Eleazar Parmly offered to teach him dentistry. Parmly not only taught him the basics of dentistry, but the two also worked together to perfect porcelain teeth for dentures. Brown settled in New York City, where he began a dental practice in conjunction with Dr Samuel Avery. They advertised in the *Evening Post* that Solyman Brown was doing mechanical dentistry (ie, dentures and bridgework) exclusively and that Samuel Avery was doing all necessary surgery. It was through his friendship with Parmly that Brown had become acquainted with all the leading figures of the dental profession at the time. Dr Brown was also recognized as a poet of merit, contributing *Dental Hygeia* and *Dentologia* to the approval of his colleagues as well as the public.[10]

Brown and Parmly, along with other dentists of equal merit, recognized that in order to establish dentistry as a profession on a par with medicine, they needed to establish three things: *(1)* develop formal schooling, *(2)* create an organization, and *(3)* build a literature. Until 1839, these things did not exist in dentistry. In May 1839, several dentists—including Parmly, Elisha Baker, and Chapin Harris—met at Brown's home and founded the first dental periodical in the world, the *American Journal of Dental Science*. The first issue appeared a month later on June 1, 1839, with Brown as the editor.

American dentistry in the first third of the 19th century was in chaos. There were no legal requirements for treating patients; one could do so even if one had no schooling. Quacks and charlatans abounded, and the public was at their mercy. No regulations existed as to the type of training a practitioner must have. Because there was not a single school of dentistry anywhere in the world, practitioners of the trade were taught through apprenticeship, and what was taught was left to the discretion of the established dentist or physician tutor. Brown, Harris, Hayden, and Parmly, working together in 1839, founded the world's first dental school, the Baltimore College of Dental Surgery (see Fig 5-10). The state legislature of Maryland empowered them to grant the Doctor of Dental Surgery (DDS) degree. Because Brown lived and practiced in New York City, it was impossible for him to teach at the new school. However, he helped shape the curriculum and the school's goals.

Horace Hayden

Horace Hayden, a native of Connecticut, after a brief period of involvement with architecture and geology, turned to the study of dentistry under the tutelage of John Greenwood in 1793.[12] He also studied anatomy and medicine, with a focus on glandular function. In 1810, Hayden obtained a license to practice dentistry issued by the Medical and Chirurgical Faculty of Maryland.[24] This is believed to be the first license issued in America to practice dentistry. In 1819, he was invited to give lectures on dentistry at the University of Maryland Medical School.[12] He joined with Chapin Harris in an unsuccessful attempt to form a dental school in the University of Maryland Medical School. As noted above, they subsequently founded the Baltimore College of Dental Surgery in 1839, the first such institution in the world.

Dr Hayden, at the advanced age of 70 years, serving as the chair of dental physiology and pathology in the new school, entered into his work with high zeal and energy. His lectures, reflecting his long experience, were both interesting and instructive. As far back as 1817, Dr Hayden had broached the idea of a national convention of dentists, but as it was said, "the pear was not ripe." After more than 20 years, on

August 18, 1840, the best dentists then in the profession assembled in New York City for the purpose of forming the American Society of Dental Surgeons, the first regularly organized dental association in America.[15]

Chapin Harris

Chapin Harris studied medicine and dentistry under the tutelage of his older brother, John Harris, a physician with expertise in dental matters.[12] John Harris was also preceptor to his other brother, James, as well as to James Taylor and John Allen, the latter two achieving national prominence along with Chapin Harris as leaders in the newly developing dental profession.[25] It was suggested that Bainbridge, Ohio, the site of John Harris's teachings, should be considered the "Cradle of Dental Education."[26] Chapin Harris later settled in Baltimore, Maryland, to practice dentistry. As an early student of dentistry, he is said to have studied the works of Hunter, Fox, and Delabarre. In 1839, he published his first book, *The Dental Art, a Practical Treatise on Dental Surgery*.[10] Harris served as editor of the first dental journal, *The American Journal of Dental Science*, established in 1839. Among his many contributions to dental literature were his *Monograph on the Physical Characteristics of the Teeth* (1840) and *Dissertation on the Diseases of the Maxillary Sinus* (1841).[15] Harris revised his *Principles and Practice* through several editions and compiled a *Dictionary of Dental Science and Biography*. He also translated the works of Delabarre from French into English.

Baltimore College of Dental Surgery

The world's first dental school, the Baltimore College of Dental Surgery (Fig 5-10), was chartered in March 1840 by the state of Maryland. Horace Hayden was professor of dental physiology and pathology and president of the college. Chapin Harris was professor of practical dentistry and dean. Thomas Bond, MD, was professor of special pathology and therapeutics, and H. Willis Baxley, MD, served as professor of anatomy and physiology. Harris recognized that the development and expansion of dentistry as a learned profession could only be accomplished by creating facilities for instruction comparable to those provided in medical schools.[25] Harris suggested that medical schools might set up departments for teaching dentistry, as he believed dentists needed to master medical science as well as the mechanical aspects of dentistry. When Hayden and Harris first approached the medical faculty of the University of Maryland with a

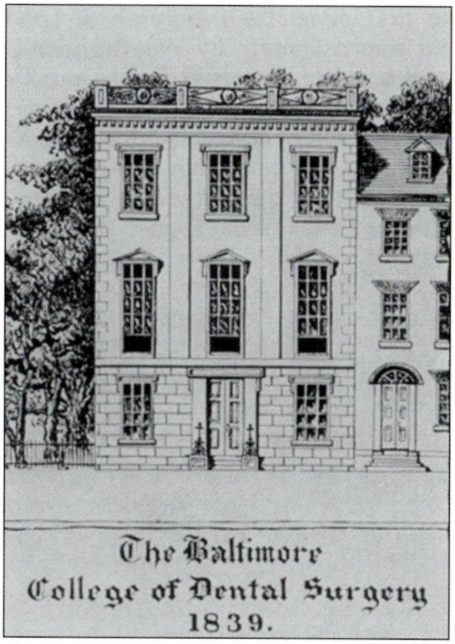

Fig 5-10 The Baltimore College of Dental Surgery.

proposal to establish dentistry as part of the medical program, they were turned down, being told that "the subject of dentistry was of little consequence and thus justified their unfavorable action."[10] After being denied space in the Medical College of Baltimore, they petitioned the state for a license to form an independent college. The State of Maryland empowered them to establish an independent school and to grant the DDS degree. Five students were enrolled in the first class. The course of study consisted of 2 years, each including a 4-month series of lectures and demonstrations and the remaining time spent in a dental office. Harris, in his address to the first graduating class of the Baltimore College of Dental Surgery stated the following:

> *Elevate the standard of the qualifications of the dental surgeon to a level with those of the medical practitioner, and the results of his practice will always be beneficial, which at present are frequently the reverse. Require of the practitioner of dental surgery to be educated in*

the collateral sciences of anatomy and physiology, surgery, pathology, and therapeutics, and the sphere of his usefulness and his respectability will be increased. Require of him to be thus qualified, and he will be able to contribute to the advancement and dignity of his calling, and by a zealous devotion to it he will soon arrive at an excellence to which heretofore but few, comparatively, have attained, and enjoy the high gratification of knowing that he is a benefactor of his fellows.[17]

At a meeting of dentists in New York City held on October 8, 1860, to establish the Harris Testimonial Fund, Dr Eleazar Parmly, longtime friend of Dr Harris, opened the meeting with the following remarks:

> *My long acquaintance with Dr. Harris, in the societies to which we belonged, and my more intimate acquaintance with him in the Baltimore College of Dental Surgery, while I held the office of Provost in that institution, enable me to say, with truth, that I have never known a man of more generous impulses, or more genial feelings, than he whose death has awakened our sympathies, and brought so many of his professional brethren together to express their high respect for his professional character, their admiration of his attainments, and their esteem for his moral, social, and personal worth. As one to whom he was long known and endeared by the many virtues that adorned his character, I trust it will not be deemed unbecoming in me to give this testimony concerning one who has labored more arduously as a practitioner, more untiringly as a writer, and more devotedly as a teacher of the principles and practice of dental surgery than any person who had, in any way, or in any country, ever been connected with our professional art.*[27]

Summary

The seeds of a dental profession had been planted in the American colonies by a small number of immigrant surgeon-dentists and physicians who recognized the need to treat dental and oral diseases. Through an apprenticeship system, they imparted their knowledge to succeeding generations, until the rapid development of dental schools, beginning with the Baltimore College of Dental Surgery in 1839. Throughout most of the 18th and 19th centuries, the preponderance of dental care in America was provided by unlicensed, unregulated practitioners of widely different standards. The challenge was to reign in and regulate, and eventually to replace, this corpus of amateurs with graduates of accredited dental schools, educated in basic and medical science and proficient in all aspects of dental care. This goal was achieved through the efforts of a relatively small number of dentists who organized dental associations, petitioned for the establishment of laws regulating practice, and spearheaded educational reforms. Their story is told in the following chapters.

References

1. Beinfield MS. The early New England doctor: An adaptation to a provincial environment. Yale J Biol Med 1942;15:99–132.
2. Trueman WH. The advent of dental science in the United States. Dent Cosmos 1896;37:713–723.
3. Graham JS. Puritan Family Life: The Diary of Samuel Sewall. Boston: Northeastern University, 2000.
4. Cairns WB. Selections from Early American Writers 1607–1800. New York: Macmillan, 1922.
5. Geshwind M. A rich storehouse of medicines for diverse and sundry diseases, an Elizabethan "treasurie for the poorer sort of people." J Hist Dent 1997;45:17–22.
6. Geshwind M. Early American almanacs and dental history. Bull Hist Dent 1994;42:5–39.
7. Curth LH. The medical content of English almanacs. J Hist Med Allied Sci 2005;60:255–282.
8. Geshwind M. Dental remedies in early American husbandry books. J Hist Dent 1998;46:67–69.
9. Harris D. Medicine in colonial America (part I). California West Med 1939;50:355–358.
10. Taylor JA. History of Dentistry. Philadelphia: Lea and Febiger, 1922.
11. Weinberger BW. An Introduction to the History of Dentistry. St Louis: Mosby, 1948.
12. Lufkin AW. A History of Dentistry. Philadelphia: Lea & Febiger, 1948.
13. Hoffmann-Axthelm W. History of Dentistry. Chicago: Quintessence, 1981.
14. Chermin D. Wig-maker, barber, bleeder and tooth-drawer. J Hist Dent 1996;44:125–127.
15. McManus C. The makers of dentistry. Dent Cosmos 1902;44:1105–1128.
16. Asbell MB. A Century of Dentistry: A History of the University of Pennsylvania School of Dental Medicine. Philadelphia: University of Pennsylvania, 1977.
17. Dexter JE. A History of Dental and Oral Science in America. Philadelphia: S. S. White, 1876.
18. Viau G. The life of Pierre Fauchard (1678–1761). Dent Cosmos 1923;65:797–808.
19. Weinberger BW. Jean Pierre Le Mayeur in America—No longer the man of mystery (1781–1789 in America). Dent Cosmos 1934;76:569–578.
20. Thorpe BL. A brief review of the prominent pioneer manipulators of gold foil. Dent Cosmos 1906;48:389–399.
21. Kirk EC. Pioneer dentistry in New York: An historical study. Dent Cosmos 1906;48:981–997.
22. Brown LP. The greatest dental family. Dent Cosmos 1923;65:251–260.
23. Chermin D, Shklar G. Levi Spear Parmly: Father of dental hygiene and children's dentistry in America. J Hist Dent 2003;51:15–18.
24. Robinson JB. Dr. Horace H. Hayden and his influence on dental education. Dent Cosmos 1932;74:783–787.
25. Ward ML. Landmarks in dental education. Dent Cosmos 1934;76:3–23.
26. Mills EC. Bainbridge, Ross County, Ohio, the cradle of dental education. J Am Dent Assoc 1932;19:361.
27. Parmly E. Harris testimonial fund. Dent Cosmos 1860;2:220–223.

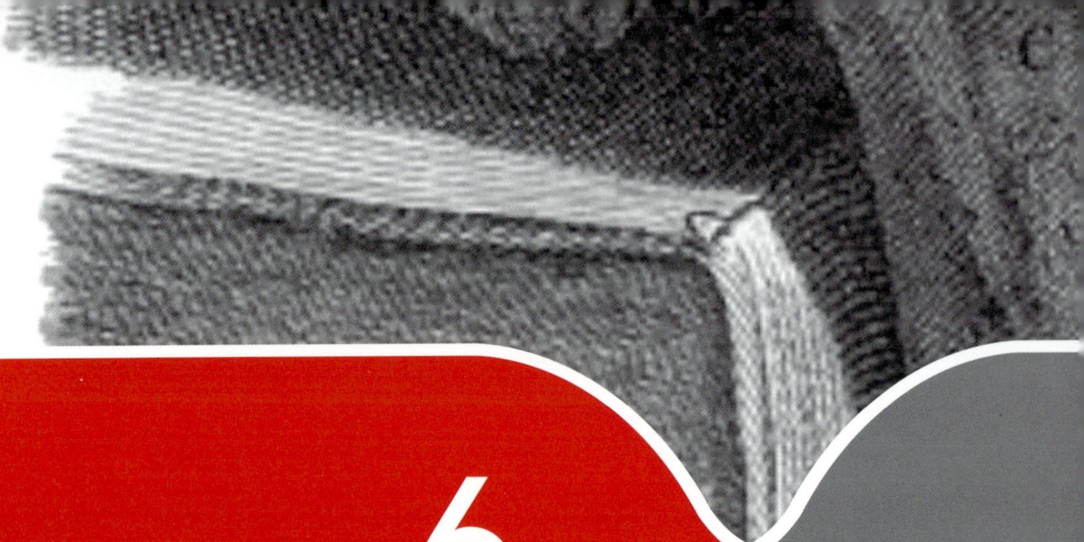

6

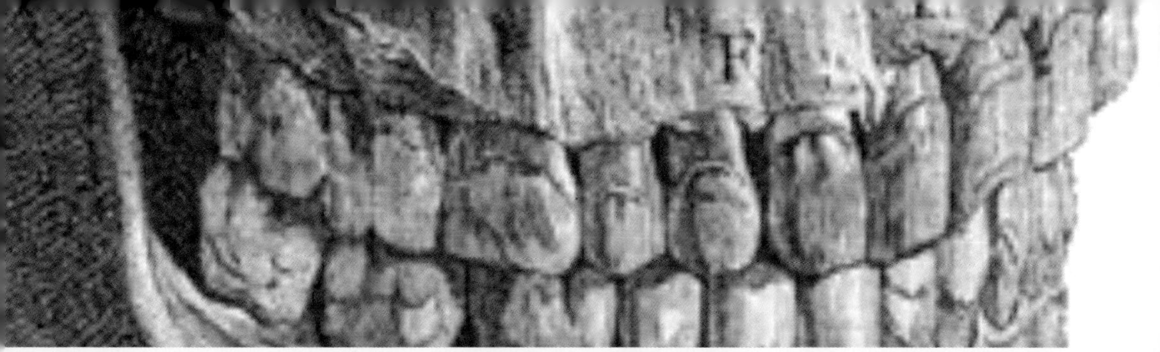

The Birth of Dental Science

The birth of dental science as a separate discipline may be said to have started with the description of the gross anatomical features of the jaws and individual teeth in Vesalius's *De Humani Corporis Fabrica*. But Bartolomeo Eustachi holds the title of first dental anatomist, because in 1563 he described the macroscopic anatomy, physiology, and development of the teeth in his Libellus de dentibus, the first book dedicated solely to the teeth.[1] Eustachi described the number of roots, their variations in length and form, and the periodontal ligament. He noted the penetration of blood vessels and nerve fibers into the apex of the roots, differentiated the enamel from the dentin, and described tooth buds.

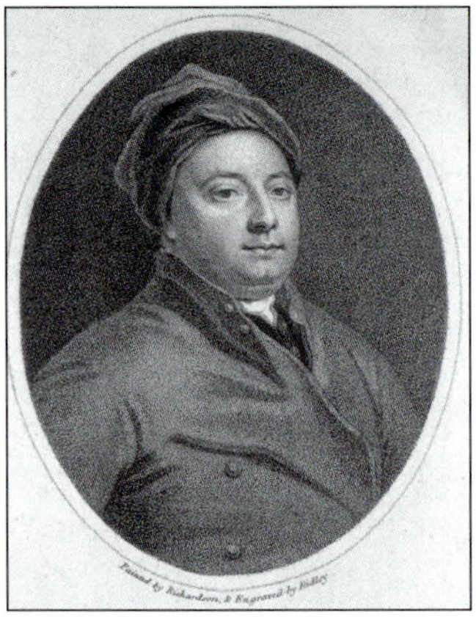

Fig 6-1 William Cheselden.

It took nearly 100 years before deeper insights into tissue architecture and function began to appear. William Cheselden (1688–1752) (Fig 6-1) was an English anatomist and surgeon who published *The Anatomy of the Human Body* in 1713 and *Osteographia, or the Anatomy of Bones* (Figs 6-2 and 6-3) in 1733, two beautifully illustrated books with outstanding engravings made with the camera obscura technique. Cheselden, a member of the London Company of Barber-Surgeons, had studied anatomy in London under William Cowper (1666–1709) and began lecturing on anatomy in 1710. In 1718, he was appointed surgeon at St Thomas' Hospital, London.

In describing his observations of the nervous system, particularly of the brain and the major nerves emanating from its base, Cheselden wrote:

> *From undeniable evident experiments, all anatomists are now convinced that to the nerves we owe all our sensation and motion, of which they are the proper organs; and sensations in the minutest parts being very distinct, therefore the instruments of such sensations must have distinct origins and course to each part. Though all are agreed as to the effect, yet a hot dispute has arisen about the manner how it is produced, viz. whether sensation and motion are occasioned by a vibration communicated to the nerves, which these gentlemen suppose entirely solid and tense, or by a liquid contained and moved in them. The last of these opinions I rather incline to, for these reasons, because the nerves proceeding from the brain bear a great analogy to the excretory ducts of other glands.*[2]

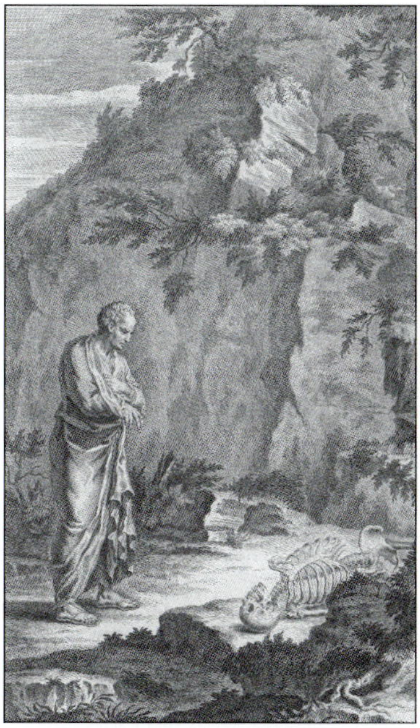

Fig 6-2 Frontispiece from Cheselden's *Osteographia.*

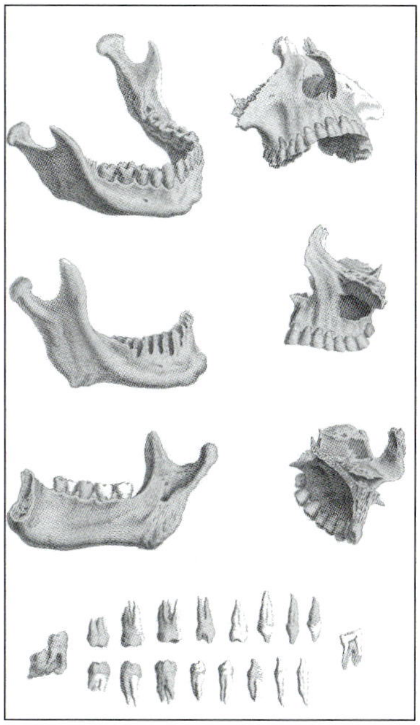

Fig 6-3 Plate depicting the jaws and dentition from Cheselden's *Osteographia.*

Cheselden conjectured that neural ganglia might serve as reservoirs of a nervous liquid. He summarized his concept of neural activity as follows:

> *That the nerves are instruments of sensation is clearly proved from experiments, but how they convey those sensations to the brain, is a matter of dispute. The most general opinion is; that they are tubes to contain animal spirits, by whose motion these sensations are conveyed: and diligent enquiry has been made to discover their cavities, but hitherto in vain; and if each nerve is distinct from its origin, as I have endeavored to show, and too small to be the object of the best microscope, I do not see how such cavities are likely to be discovered. Nevertheless nerves may be tubes, and possibly a fluid, whose cohesion is very little, and whose parts, no finer than light, may move freely in them.*[2]

While advancing the science of gross anatomy to a new peak, Cheselden correlated his observations to clinical applications relevant to dental practice. He correlated clinical findings of toothache to the distribution of the second and third branches of the fifth cranial nerve:

> *The second branch of the fifth pair, which may be called maxillaris superior, passes out through the foramen rotundum ossis sphenoidis, and immediately gives nerves to the fat under the crotaphite muscle, and to the palate, sinus sphenoidalis, and nostrils. The remaining trunk insinuating itself into the channel on the top of the antrum highmorianum, to which cavity and to the teeth of the upper jaw it gives small twigs, at last comes out at the orbiter externus hole, and is spent on the musculus orbicularis palpebrabrum, nose, and upper lip, where some branches of the seventh pair seem to unite themselves to the twigs of this. The third branch, or maxillaris inferior, goes out at the foramen ovale, or fourth hole of the wedge-like bone, and soon splitting into a great many branches, is distributed to the musculus crotaphites, masseter, pterygoides, digastricus, buccinator, mylohyoideus, geniohyoideus, genioglosius, and basioglossus, glandusa sublingualis maxillaris inferior, and parotis, to the external ear, where it seems to join the portio-dura to the substance of the tongue, in which it is pretty much confounded with the ninth pair: from the root of this last branch the chorda tympani is reflected. The last ramification of this branch which I shall mention is that which enters the canal of the lower jaw, furnishing the teeth there, and comes out at the chin, on which and the lower lip it is bestowed; at this place it is again conjoined to the seventh pair. From this short sketch of the large fifth pair of nerves, and by offering several phaenomena, which happen to these parts to which they are distributed, we might have a much farther confirmation of the general doctrine of nerves delivered, and see, at least, the way pathed to a rational account of these phaenomena, for reasoning on which we should not otherwise have the least ground. We can for example, from the chorda tympani and the nerves of the teeth, being derived from the same common trunk, understand how the sound of any vibrating body held between our teeth is sensible to us, when another cannot possibly hear the least of it. By the like rule we know why in a violent toothache the muscles of the face are sometimes convulsed; nor shall we be surprised to hear one plagued with the ach in his upper teeth, complain of a gnawing pain deep seated in the bones of his face, or to see his eyelids much swelled, or the tears trickling down in great abundance; whereas the lower teeth aching, the ear is pained, and the saliva flows in great quantities.*[2]

The Microscope

Although the camera obscura had made it easier to produce very accurate representations of the human body and its various organs, it was not until the invention of the microscope that the development of the new science of histology, or the study of the minute structure of the internal architecture of the body, was born.

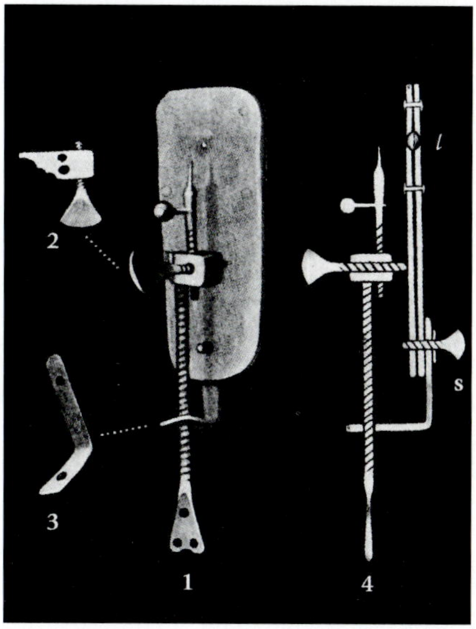

Fig 6-4 Leeuwenhoek's simple microscope.

Antoni van Leeuwenhoek

Antoni van Leeuwenhoek (1632–1723), using simple microscopes, gets credit for providing the first glimpses of the microscopic structure of dentin and the discovery of bacteria in saliva. The spirit of inquiry and individual ingenuity so characteristic of the Renaissance is illustrated by the investigations of Leeuwenhoek. He was born on October 24, 1632, in Delft, Holland, and at the age of 16 years was apprenticed in a shop that sold cloth. Leeuwenhoek may have been introduced to the microscopic world when using magnifying glasses to determine the quality of cloth. He discovered that simple microscopes constructed of a single lens could produce hundred-fold magnifications with minimal distortion. Soon he began to design and build his own simple microscopes as a hobby. His convex lenses were very small (about the size of a pinhead) and mounted over a hole on a brass plate. When the lens was held close to the eye, one could observe a magnified image of a specimen secured on the end of a movable pin[3] (Fig 6-4). Leeuwenhoek constructed a separate microscope for each item to be examined, because the technique of using transparent glass plates to hold the specimens had yet to be developed. Leeuwenhoek's microscopes, which were considered by many to be of the highest quality, provided extraordinarily clear images. After Leeuwenhoek's death, 26 of his microscopes were obtained by the Royal Society and subjected to examination by Henry Baker. His analysis showed that the best magnification achieved with these microscopes was 160×.[3]

More recent investigations using one of Leewenhoek's instruments indicated that a magnification of at least 266×, with a resolution of 1.3 mm, was attained.[4] By illuminating the specimen with indirect light, Leeuwenhoek may have created a similar effect to dark-field illumination, a method best suited to observation of bacteria and other microscopic forms.[3,5] Leeuwenhoek pursued his hobby of making microscopes for over 40 years, during which time he made original observations of bacteria, sperm cells, red blood cells, and cells of the epidermis. Over time, Leeuwenhoek made over 250 microscopes and 400 lenses, nearly all of which were kept in his possession until after his death.[6] He refused to sell his instruments and guarded the secrets of his method. Leeuwenhoek was a successful businessman who lived all his life in Delft, Holland. He was a close friend of the artist Jan Vermeer and may have served as a model for Vermeer's paintings *The Astronomer* and *The Geographer*.[5]

Leeuwenhoek's fame as an amateur microscopist began in 1677 when he reported to the Royal Society of London that rainwater contained microscopic living organisms. The Royal Society greeted this report with skepticism and appointed Nemiah Grew and Robert Hooke to procure microscopes and to investigate the matter.[7] Robert Hooke was a gifted microscopist and author of *Micrographia*, the first book dedicated to the science of microscopy. After several failed attempts, Grew and Hooke reported that no such beings were present in rainwater. Meanwhile, Leeuwenhoek had also discovered that these "animalcules" could be transmitted in air. At long last, using improved lenses, Hooke demonstrated microorganisms at a meeting of the Royal Society, at which an amazed Christopher Wren called the finding "a new world of innumerable beings." Leeuwenhoek, in a letter to the Royal Society of London dated September 17, 1683, continued to astound the Royal Society by reporting that in the soft "scurf" of his teeth there were very small organisms, which, as shown in his drawings, may have been protozoa or bacteria[8] (Fig 6-5).

In his curiosity, Leeuwenhoek examined the microscopic anatomy of the teeth of several animals and found that they consisted of exceedingly small tubules radiating outward from the innermost part of the tooth to its surface. In 1679, in a report to the Royal Society, he described channels or canaliculi (dentinal tubules) in the dentin of man, elephant, horse, and pig:

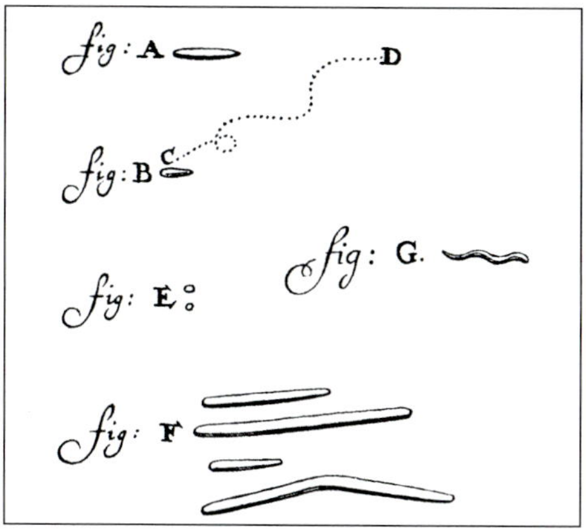

Fig 6-5 Microbes as drawn by Leeuwenhoek.

> *Having taken great pains to investigate the formation of the elephant's tooth, and examined into the nature of it by every means I could devise, I found it to consist only of a collection of tubuli, or pipes, which are exceedingly small, and all derive their origin from the inner part of the tooth, for I never could discover any of them lying longitudinally or lengthwise in it…I also examined the teeth taken from young hogs, and found them to be likewise formed of tubuli spreading from the cavity in the center, to the circumference. After this, I was desirous of examining the structure of the human teeth, and having for that purpose procured a number of the large ones, called the grinders, I found them to be formed exactly in the manner before described, namely, of tubuli, or little bony pipes, closely joined together, arising at the cavity in the middle of the tooth, and ending at the circumference or outside… the tubuli cannot be well discerned without the help of the very best microscopes.*[9]

Leeuwenhoek estimated that a molar contained 4,822,500 tubules and conjectured that they were nourished from the blood supply to the center of the tooth. Furthermore, he speculated that obstruction of the tubules might cause dental pain:

> *We may easily conceive that the boney tubuli, (being of a solid nature, and incapable of dilation or spreading) may happen to be obstructed by some gross or concreted matter, and then the small vessels contained within the cavity of the tooth must immediately by such obstruction in the circulation of their juices be defined. This distention or swelling will necessarily excite great pain, for all the vessels contained in the tooth will press closely on each other, forasmuch as they cannot swell or*

> *spread themselves as other vessels can, which are not confined within the solid substance of a bone. Again, supposing these boney tubuli to be obstructed, and the obstruction not removed, we may from thence gather the reason why our teeth partially decay, sometimes on the sides, and sometimes at the tops, the rest of the teeth remaining sound for several years after.*[9]

Here Leeuwenhoek is not merely interested in the anatomy of the tooth but is thinking of the potential consequences of the interruption of circulation within the dentinal tubules. This is the first accurate description of the structure of dentin and possibly the earliest speculation on the cause of dental decay from a physiologic perspective. Through his discovery of "animalcules," Leeuwenhoek established the origins of the field of bacteriology. From that point on, dentistry would grapple with the fact that the tissues of the mouth are exposed to and even populated by thousands of living microorganisms, raising concerns about their effects. It would be hundreds of years before Edward Miller would unravel the significance of bacteria as pathogens in dental caries.

Marcello Malpighi

Marcello Malpighi (Fig 6-6) developed the techniques for preparing tissue sections for examination in newly developed compound microscopes. Although the early compound microscopes created numerous artifacts, they served as a major impetus for the new science of microanatomy. Malpighi is regarded as the "father of histology" and is said to have initiated the fields of embryology, botany, and human microanatomy. His theories of the glandular composition of the major organs and the flow of blood corpuscles from arteries to veins through newly discovered capillaries created much controversy among medical men who were unprepared to part with past ideas. In describing the microscopic structure of the tongue, he illustrated its blood supply and innervations (Fig 6-7). Upon observing that the surface of the tongue remained dry when kept extended out of the mouth, Malpighi reasoned that the papillae of the tongue were not secretory organs and, after discovering their innervation, correctly suggested that they were involved in taste sensation.[10] Following similar observations, he proposed that the papillae of the skin were responsible for touch perception.

Malpighi is also remembered for his early description of the layers of the skin and especially for concluding that "colored cells" located at the junction between the dermis and the epidermis were responsible for skin coloration. In his studies of plant structure, he came to

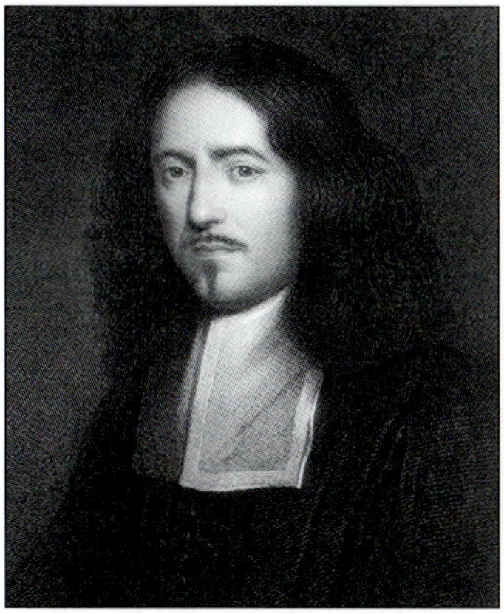

Fig 6-6 Marcello Malpighi.

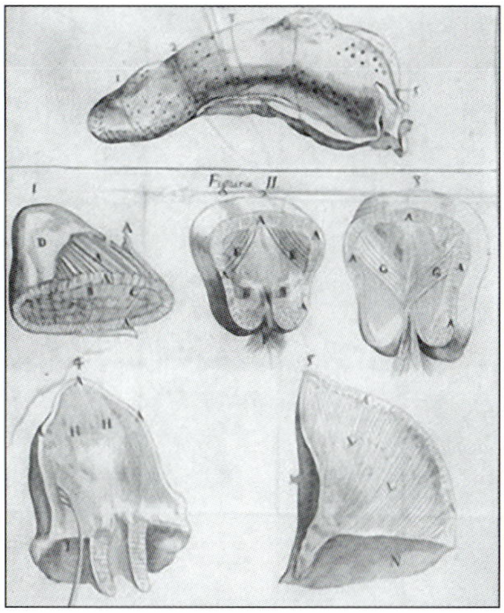

Fig 6-7 Anatomy of the tongue as drawn by Malpighi.

regard that the basic unit of tissue structure consisted of independent units called *cells*. But it would not be until 1839 that the research of Schleiden and Schwann would reveal the true cellular nature of plants and animals.[11] Important as Malpighi's studies of salivary glands were to dental science, his greatest contributions were to medicine, especially his fundamental elucidation of the microanatomy of the liver and the kidney.

Glandular Anatomy

The English physician Thomas Wharton contributed to oral science through his pioneering studies of glandular anatomy. In his *Adenographia*, published in 1656, Wharton described a rich innervation and blood supply to all glands.[10] He discovered the major duct of the submaxillary gland, which is now named for him. He hypothesized that saliva was a product of the gland and not a nonspecific "phlegm." In explaining how saliva was generated in the gland, he proposed that fluid supplied by nerves (*succus nerveus*) was filtered in glandular parenchyma before being collected in the main duct for transport to the mouth. In his view, one function of the glands was to purify the nerve fluid through removal of "excess humidity," thereby fortifying the *succus nerveus*.

In 1662, Nicolas Stensen, Danish contributor to comparative anatomy, reported the discovery of the duct of the sublingual gland as well as those of the smaller buccal glands. Unlike Wharton, Stensen recognized the primary importance of arterial blood as the source of salivary fluid.[10] Soon after these discoveries were announced, Malpighi, with the use of the microscope, uncovered the basic architecture of secretory glands, stating that they are:

> *Divided into a number of lobules, possessing not so much a spherical as a conical outline. Nor is Nature content to have made use of such a division merely; but, in a most liberal manner, has established a further division into very small parts, visible only by the aid of the microscope. For each of the lobules just described is made up of small rounded bodies, like berries (acini) crowded together after the fashion of a bunch of grapes, and connected with the whole lobule by means of "vessels."*[10]

Stensen would have been excited to learn that future research would show that these berry-like acini were made up of even smaller units, or cells.

Development of the Dentition

John Hunter

The publication of John Hunter's classic book *The Natural History of the Human Teeth* in 1741 gave prominence to the study of teeth and their diseases. The book contained an accurate description of the structure and development of the dentition. According to Sir James Paget, notable physician and biographer of John Hunter, the book may have been inspired by the works of Cheselden.[12]

John Hunter (1728–1793) (Fig 6-8), one of the world's greatest surgeons, was born in Scotland and raised on a farm as the youngest of 10 children. John's older brother, William Hunter, was a certified medical doctor who supplemented his income from the practice of medicine by conducting lectures in anatomy. He had established a private school of human anatomy in London, where lectures and dissections were given for medical students. In 1848, at the age of 17 years, John moved to London to study anatomy and surgery with his older brother. John had no prior knowledge of human anatomy or plans for a future career in medicine. His initial duties were mainly to keep the lab orderly, help secure cadavers, and collect the lecture tickets. Before long, he was participating in the preparation of anatomical dissections, a task he was soon to master. Within the space

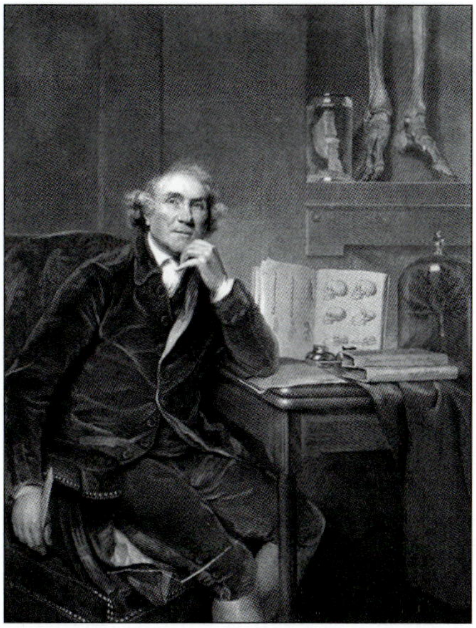

Fig 6-8 Portrait of John Hunter by Sir Joshua Reynolds.

of 3 years, he was giving presentations and had established himself as London's most gifted anatomist. John was also adept at obtaining a steady supply of cadavers for the anatomy school. He formed personal ties with some of London's best grave robbers, paid them high prices, and was not above joining in for a pint after a successful night in a church graveyard. Unlike his brother, a respected physician who moved in London's best society, John was a rough unpolished fellow, uncomfortable in genteel society.

In the hope of improving his younger brother's image, William encouraged John to attend surgical lectures at St George's and St Bartholomew's Hospitals in order to qualify him for the license to practice surgery. In 1755, again at the insistence of William, John was pushed to study classical languages and elocution at Oxford. After a short time, John dropped out because of boredom to return to full-time concentration on his anatomical investigations and the practice of surgery. When not engaged in anatomical demonstrations or in his early surgical practice, John pursued other avocations, such as collecting and raising all sorts of animals and conducting studies of their anatomy and physiology. Hunter's biographer, Stephen Paget, noted that "human anatomy was taking its place in his mind as but a part of all anatomy; he must know the whole animal world, every living structure in it; must dissect everything, noting all different forms and arrangements of the organs, each method of nature to adapt them to the necessities of life." Everard Home, John's brother-in-law, recounts how John "applied to the keeper of wild beasts in the Tower for the bodies of those which died there, and he made similar applications to the men who showed wild beasts. He purchased all rare animals which came his way."[12]

In 1759, Hunter suffered from inflammation of his lungs, possibly caused by the unwholesome air of the dissection room. After more than a decade of association with the school of anatomy and several years of hospital training under the tutelage of William Cheselden and Percivall Pott, John Hunter was compelled by ill health to make a drastic change in his life. He enlisted in the army. From 1760 to 1763, he was commissioned as a surgeon assigned to the British forces in Portugal and France. His experiences at the front increased his knowledge of inflammation and the care of gunshot wounds. Time was also made available for study and experimentation of indigenous animals and plants previously unfamiliar to John. It was here that he became intrigued with lizards, especially their ability to shed and regenerate their tails. This study led to formulation of his ideas that certain tissues contained a regenerative power or, in his words, a "living principle."

Upon returning to London in 1763, Hunter reestablished his surgical practice. Because his dominant interests resided in his study of natural history and the acquisition of new specimens for his growing collection, surgical practice was an inconvenience pressed upon him just as a means of support. With a need to increase his income, he formed a partnership with James Spence, one of London's better-known dentists. In 18th- and 19th-century Europe, dental practice was considered an abasing and unsuitable activity for one aspiring to develop a practice in general surgery. It has therefore been suggested that Hunter may have had a desperate need to raise cash while continuing his anatomical dissections and animal experimentations. Hunter's detailed knowledge of dental anatomy and advanced surgical skills were put to great use in performing dental extractions and treating gum diseases and oral infections. He also performed dental transplants for some of Spence's patients.

In his studies of comparative anatomy, Hunter focused a great deal on osteology and was one of the first to define the structure of teeth, their relationship to one another, and their position in the jaws during development and adult life. In 1771, he published the first detailed study of the human dentition, his *The Natural History of the Human Teeth* (Fig 6-9). It was the only work of his sold to booksellers. Paget notes that Hunter may have used the proceeds of his book to meet the expenses of his upcoming marriage. All of his other works were

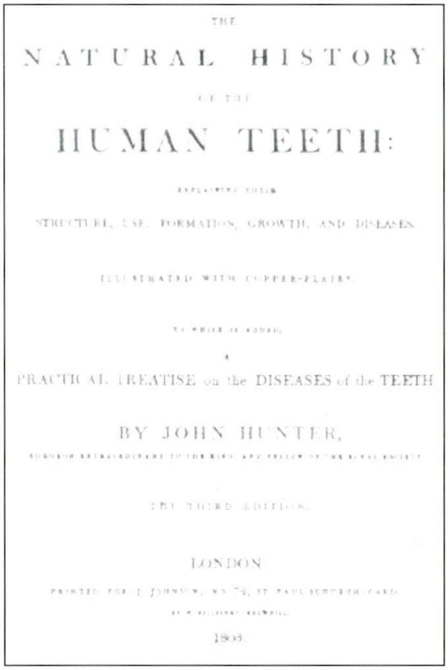
THE

NATURAL HISTORY

OF THE

HUMAN TEETH:

STRUCTURE, USE, FORMATION, GROWTH, AND DISEASES.

ILLUSTRATED WITH COPPER-PLATES.

A

PRACTICAL TREATISE on the DISEASES of the TEETH

BY JOHN HUNTER,

THE THIRD EDITION.

LONDON:

Fig 6-9 Title page of the 1808 combined edition of Hunter's *The Natural History of the Human Teeth* and the *Practical Treatise on the Diseases of the Teeth.*

published in the *Transactions of the Royal Society* or in the journals of other learned groups. The inspiration for *The Natural History of the Human Teeth* may have arisen from his former tutor, William Cheselden of Chelsea Hospital, who had previously published *Osteographia*, an atlas of the bones of the human body that was widely celebrated as the best work of its type.

In *The Natural History of the Human Teeth*, Hunter described the development and the microscopic aspects of dental tissues (Figs 6-10 and 6-11). Each tooth was described in detail, with a consideration of its role in feeding behavior. In 1773, he began offering his course of lectures on the principles and practice of surgery. Paget noted that "the labor of preparing and delivering these magnificent lectures was very heavy; there was nothing like them in London, for their comprehension of the whole circle of the sciences round surgery."[12]

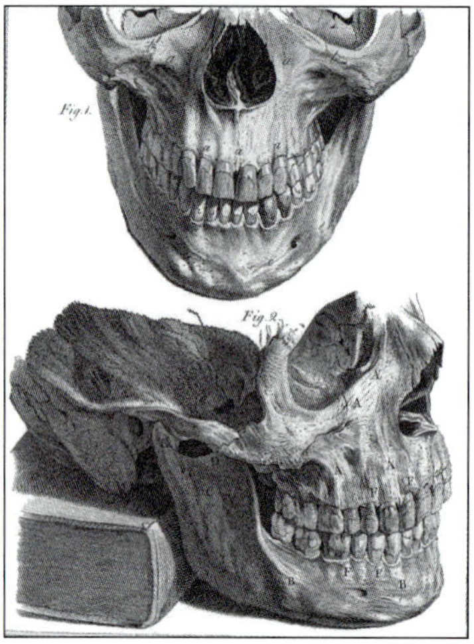

Fig 6-10 Front and side views of the jaws from Hunter's *The Natural History of the Human Teeth*. (Courtesy of Archives and Special Collections, Columbia University Health Sciences Library.)

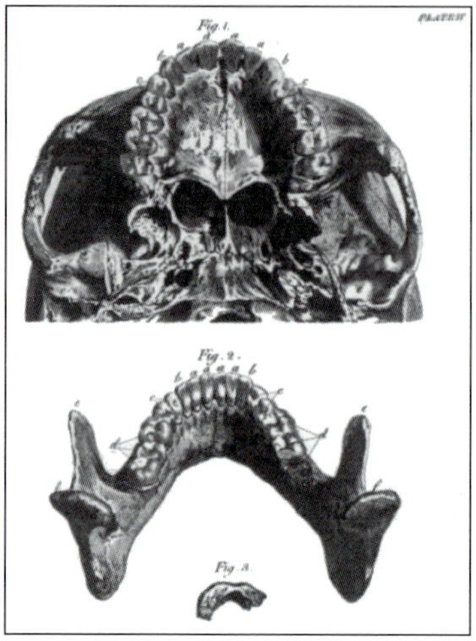

Fig 6-11 *(top)* Base of the skull and the maxilla depicting the cutting edges and grinding surfaces of the teeth. *(bottom)* Illustration of the mandibular coronoid processes and articulating condyles. (From Hunter, 1808.)

In 1778, John Hunter published *A Practical Treatise on the Diseases of the Teeth*. In this work, his experiences as a partner in William Spence's dental practice were combined with what he knew of common dental diseases, including caries, dental abscesses, inflammation of the gums, extractions, and the transplantation of teeth. He accurately described the vascularity of the pulp based on injections of the blood vessels but was less successful in tracing the distribution of nerves within the dental pulp. Hunter noted that the root was covered by a thin vascular periosteum (periodontal membrane) uniting it to the bony socket. He noted that as teeth were worn down with age, new compensatory matter was laid down in the pulp, but he dispelled the idea that teeth continued to grow in length and breadth after eruption into the mouth. In attributing dental pain to the presence of nerve fibers inside the pulp, Hunter observed that toothache was caused when the nerves became exposed to air and could be prevented by filling cavities with lead or wax. There is little evidence that Hunter actually practiced filling of teeth or had anything to do with the fabrication of artificial teeth, practices better left to mechanical dentists.

Hunter described the development of the alveoli and correctly noted their continued dependence on the presence of the teeth. He observed that the teeth and the alveolar processes were mutually dependent on each other. He described the components of the temporomandibular joint, including the articulation of the condyle against the temporal bone through an intervening "movable cartilage" (now called the *articular disc*). He described the structure of the muscles of mastication, their origins and insertions, and their mode of action during mastication. Hunter's experiments led him to conclude that enamel and dentin were avascular tissues, unlike bone. This he proved by injections of madder, a dye capable of staining both forming and mature bone but not tooth enamel and dentin, except during the formative stage. Further proof that enamel and dentin were extraneous to the circulation was the fact that once they were stained, they retained the red stain, while bone gradually lost its stain over time. Thus, Hunter concluded that the enamel and dentin of teeth, once formed, remain unchanged by age or "affections of the whole body." Hunter believed that despite their avascularity, the enamel and dentin still retained a "living principle" through which they were "capable of uniting with any part of a living body," a concept important to his explanation of the success of tooth transplantation.

Hunter is famously remembered to have been an enthusiastic proponent of tooth transplantation. He stated that "Although this operation is in itself a matter of no difficulty, yet, on the whole, it is one of the nicest of all operations, and requires more chirurgical and physiological knowledge than any that comes under the care of the dentist." He cautioned the surgeon-dentist to avoid transplanting teeth into diseased sockets or where evidence of gum disease was present. The recipient should not be taking mercury and should have several molars present in each jaw in order to stabilize the occlusion, thereby avoiding contact with the implanted tooth during mastication. He recommended having several donors on hand to ensure that a donor tooth (scion tooth) of the appropriate size (comparable in shape to but just smaller than the extracted tooth) would be available at the time of the procedure. He also advised that it was wise to have several dead (cadaver) teeth available just in case the donor tooth proved unsatisfactory.

Hunter had experimented with the transplantation of teeth, as well as with other organs, to understand the potential for tissues to unite with the body. His successful transplantation of a human tooth into the comb of a rooster (Fig 6-12), with evidence of vascular union and tissue continuity, suggested that his concept of a "living principle" in teeth was correct and that human tooth transplantation was

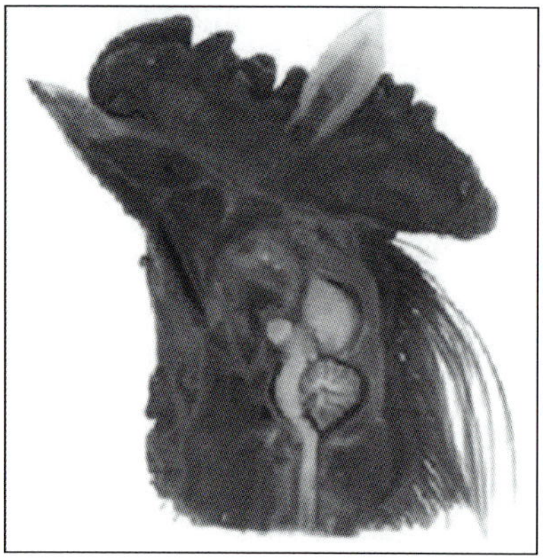

Fig 6-12 Hunter's experimental transplantation of a human tooth to a rooster's comb demonstrated the ability of the tooth to establish a patent blood supply with its host.

a biologically sound process. However, the idea of removing a sound tooth from a healthy patient (almost always younger and poorer) to provide it to a richer individual raised ethical objections among some of Hunter's contemporaries. A decline in tooth transplantation began when dentists and medical practitioners recognized that infections were spread from tooth donors to recipients.

As John Hunter's knowledge of natural science, medicine, and surgery grew, his reputation spread and his practice matured into a general surgical practice. In 1767, he was elected to fellowship in the Royal Society. He became a professor of surgery, and he soon held top posts in surgery at London's best hospitals. In 1768, he was appointed surgeon to St George's Hospital and surgeon to King George III in 1776. Wendy Moore, in her recent biography of John Hunter,[1] gives a popularized and vivid account of this greatly diverse man.

John Hunter's biographers, including Dr Stephen Paget in his 1867 account of Hunter's life, have extolled his achievements in surgery and experimental science but have not made very much of Hunter's contribution to dental science. This relative silence seems odd in light of the fact that Hunter's first major publications dealt with teeth and their diseases. From the content of these books, it is clear that John Hunter practiced dental surgery at least during his earlier years. As he matured and acquired additional experience, he appears to have restricted his practice to general surgical cases. Clearly, John Hunter intended to gain in reputation, both as a scientist and as a dental practitioner, by publication of his two treatises on dentistry. His ear-

[1] Moore W. The Knife Man: Blood, Body Snatching, and the Birth of Modern Surgery. New York: Broadway, 2005.

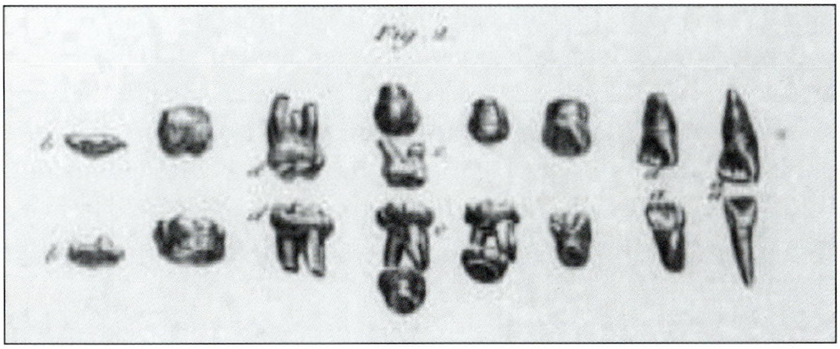

Fig 6-13 The teeth of an 8- to 9-year-old child, showing the development of the permanent teeth and beginning decay of the primary teeth. (From Hunter, 1808.)

lier work, *The Natural History of the Human Teeth*, is the first detailed description of the human dentition and a major contribution to the scientific basis of dentistry. This treatise was soon followed by *A Practical Treatise on the Diseases of the Teeth*, a publication repetitive of contemporary works by other members of the nascent dental profession but nevertheless an account of his own experiences in caring for dental diseases (Fig 6-13). Both works must have given him immediate stature in the field of dental surgery and have increased the scientific merit of dentistry, elevating it to a subject worthy of study as a science as well as a practical discipline.

Guerini agrees with the idea that Hunter initiated a new epoch in the art of dentistry in England by abandoning empiricism in favor of rigorous scientific observation. However, Guerini underlines Hunter's deficiency as a practicing dentist, noting that his *A Practical Treatise on the Diseases of the Teeth* is much inferior to his purely anatomical *The Natural History of the Human Teeth*.[13] In Sir James Paget's introduction to Stephen Paget's biography,[12] Hunter's importance to the advance of medicine and surgery is described: Hunter "introduced the exercise of the observant scientific mind into the study and practice of surgery." According to Sir James Paget, John Hunter increased our knowledge of surgery and medicine not by thinking or speculation but by experimentation and repeated careful observation. Before the mid 18th century, medicine and surgery had been based on empiric knowledge passed down almost verbatim from generation to generation. Hunter replaced empiric practice with one based on facts, established through long and careful interlocking observations of natural history, comparative anatomy, and pathophysiology. In Paget's words,

Hunter worked by the following rule: "Every thinking must be tried patiently and carefully, by experiment or repeated careful observation, before it can be safely accepted as truth."[12] Hunter brought the same scientific spirit to dentistry and thereby stimulated others to follow in his approach to the study of dental anatomy and pathophysiology.

John Hunter's contribution to dentistry can be appreciated from his own words from the introduction to *A Practical Treatise on the Diseases of the Teeth*:

> *One might, at first, imagine that the diseases of the teeth must be very simple, and like those which take place every where else in the bony parts of our body; but experience shows the contrary. The teeth being singular in their structure and some other circumstances, have diseases peculiar to themselves. These diseases, considered abstractedly, are indeed very simple; but by the relations which the teeth bear to the body in general, and to the parts with which they are immediately connected, they become extremely complicated. The diseases which may arise in consequence of those of the teeth, are various; such as abscesses, carious bones, Etc.; many of which, although proceeding originally from the teeth, are more the object of the surgeon than of the dentist, who will find himself as much at a loss in such cases, as if the abscess or carious bone were in the leg, or any other distant part. All diseases of the teeth, which are common to them with the other parts of the body, should be put under the management of the physician or surgeon; but those which are peculiar to the teeth, and their connexions, belong properly to the dentist.*[12]

Hunter went on to describe what he considered to be the proper boundaries of the practice of dentistry:

> *It is not my present purpose to enumerate every disease capable of producing such symptoms as may lead us to suspect the teeth; for the jaws may be affected by almost every kind of disorder. I shall therefore confine myself to the diseases of the teeth, gums, and alveolar processes; which parts having a peculiar connexion, their diseases fall properly within the province of the dentist.*[12]

Stephen Paget summarized John Hunter's life in the following words:

> *The whole output of his working life is fourfold—literary, surgical, anatomical, physiological and experimental; but the multiplication together of these factors does not give the whole result of his work. He brought surgery into closer touch with science. Contrast him with Ambroise Pare, a surgeon in some ways like him, shrewd, observant, ahead of his age; the achievements of Pare, side by side with those of Hunter, are like child's play in comparison with the serious affairs of*

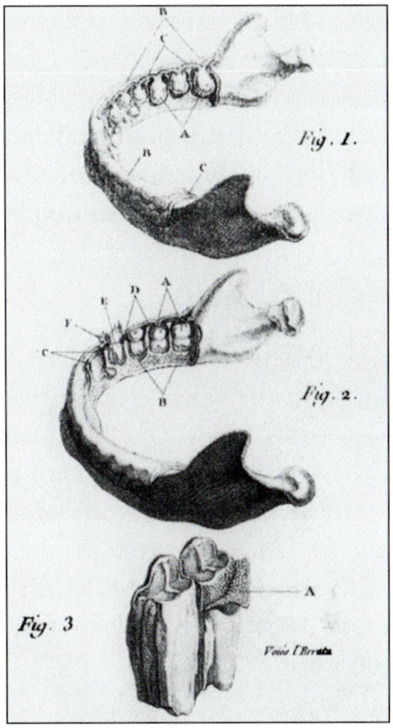

Fig 6-14 Hérissant's diagram depicting the relationship between the dental sacs and the gingiva during eruption.

> *men; Pare advanced the art of surgery, but Hunter taught the science of it.*[12]

For John Hunter, dental and oral diseases were inseparable from man's overall health and were subject to the same experimental science and pathophysiologic principles. It is the general opinion of historians that John Hunter gave the science and practice of dentistry greater respectability, launching scientific studies that would take at least 150 years to achieve full maturity.

Jean-Thomas Hérissant

In 1759, Jean-Thomas Hérissant published a short paper in the French Royal Academy describing his investigations of the formation and eruption of the primary teeth.[14] His studies led to two significant outcomes: First, each developing tooth, or, in his words, each tooth germ, was contained within a highly vascularized sac or "follicules membraneux" that was continuous with the overlying gingiva. Second, during tooth eruption, the gingiva was pierced and broken down to make way for the crown. In the process, a new gingival collar was formed from the dental sac (Fig 6-14). Hérissant called the original gingiva the "gencive passagere" or temporary gingiva and the newly formed gingiva the "gencive permanents." He speculated that the sac tissue went through an inside-out reversal during tooth eruption. In examining developing teeth of a calf with a simple hand magnifying lens, he concluded that the enamel was developed from a vesicular liquid derived from the inner surface of the dental sac.

Robert Blake

In 1801, the Irishman Robert Blake provided the first significant advance in the science of tooth development since the publication of Eustachi's *Opusculum de Dentibus* in 1563. Blake's thesis defense on the early stages of tooth formation, made before the medical faculty of the University of Edinburgh, contained information surpassing what had been written on the subject by Fauchard, Bourdet, Hérissant, and John Hunter.[15] In investigations of the earliest stages of tooth development, Blake dissected human fetuses and described the following:

> *About the fourth month after conception, I observed the rudiments or vascular membranes of twelve teeth in each jaw; specifically those of all the temporary teeth, and also those of anterior permanent grinders [Fig 6-15]. The membranes or sacs were even at this period sufficiently connected with the internal part of the gum, that they seemed derived from it, and came away with it, when torn from the groove in the jaw, leaving behind the vessels, nerves, etc. with which they had been in contact.*[15]

Blake recognized the increased vascularity associated with the developing tooth germs, noting that "the vesicles which enter the lower part of these sacs, deposit in them a substance, exactly similar to jelly in consistence and transparency; upon this the bony part (dentin) of the tooth is formed." Before the cell theory and the identification of odontoblasts had been discovered, he described the origin of a dentinal matrix from a highly vascular pulp. He noted that in the fetus, between the 8th and 9th month of gestation, "ossification had commenced on all the pulps, and at one point, even on the pulp of each of the anterior permanent grinders." The ossified matrix took the form of "elastic bony shells" over the internal membrane (pulp) of the sac. The external membrane was observed to be highly vascular and suspected to be the source for the enamel, or "cortex striates," as Blake defined it:

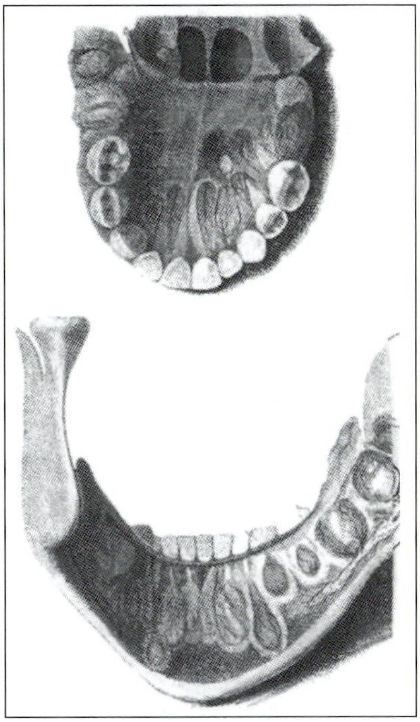

Fig 6-15 Blake's depiction of the highly vascularized dental sacs of the permanent teeth and their continuity to the primary teeth.

> *The internal part of these sacs, soon after the commencement of the bony shells, deposits on their points and sides a soft earthy matter, moistened with a mucilaginous fluid; a small quantity of which is found between the membranes and shells. This earthy matter I found even at birth so soft, that it could be scraped off with the nail of the finger. It may be proper to remark, that it is this soft earthy matter, which afterwards becomes the cortex striates.*[15]

Thus, Blake had discovered through delicate and minute dissections that dentin (bony part) ossified from a matrix derived from the pulp (internal membrane of the sac) and that enamel (cortex striatis) formed secondarily from the external membrane of the sac. Furthermore, ossification of the bony part (dentin) began earlier than the formation of the enamel.

Blake also demonstrated that in the 8th month of gestation, the sacs of the permanent incisors and canines were "not placed under the temporary teeth, nor indeed so deep in the jaw, but within side of them, that is to say, in contact with their inner surface, lying between

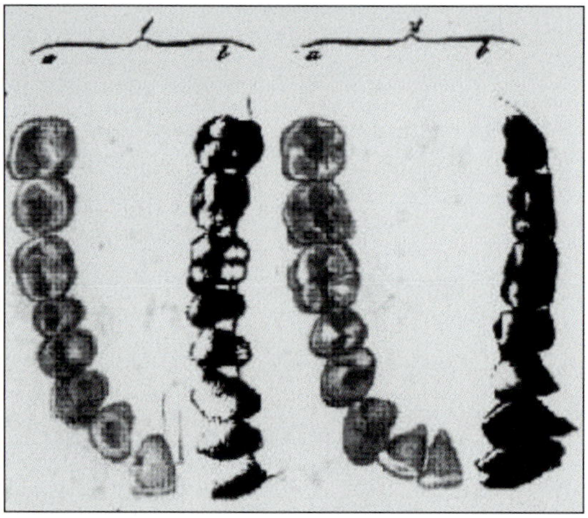

Fig 6-16 Diagram of the coronal shape of the human dentition. (From Cuvier.[16])

that and the internal plate of the alveolar process, and as Albinus remarks, they were contained in the same sockets with the temporary." Here Blake described what "had been hitherto unaccountably overlooked"—that the temporary teeth and the sacs of the permanent teeth were connected:

> *When the rudiments of the temporary teeth are tolerably advanced, the internal part of the gum, or rather the upper part of each membrane destined to form one of the temporary teeth, sends off a new sac. These sacs, situated as just now described, are each at first contained in the socket of the one to which it is to succeed; and are so intimately connected with the membranes of the temporary teeth, that they cannot be separated without tearing one or both, and may be torn along with the first sacs out of the sockets.*[15]

Blake admitted that these sacs had been observed by Hérissant and John Hunter, but he argued that the connection between the sacs of the primary and permanent teeth had not been precisely described.

Frédéric Cuvier

In the early 1800s, Frédéric Cuvier published his classic studies of the comparative anatomy of mammalian dentition. This work led to a reclassification of mammals into numerous families based on the number, shape, and occlusion of teeth (Fig 6-16). Cuvier, in the introduction to the complete edition of his work, published in 1825, described the fortuitous nature of his discovery of dental anatomy as a key to classification.[16]

Frédéric was the brother of George Cuvier, one of the most famous and productive zoologists of the 18th century. Frédéric had been assigned the study of the skeletal elements of mammals by George Cuvier, then the head of the Jardins des Plantes in Paris. At the outset of this assignment, Frédéric, struck by the similarity of the number, shape, and occlusal relationship of the teeth of members of the cat family, conceived the idea that a study of the dentinal anatomy of all mammals might lead to a better classification. He reasoned that each species of mammal had to be equipped with the organs of nutrition best able to ensure its survival; therefore, the teeth, being essential to the acquisition and preparation of raw nutrients for the digestive processes of the intestinal canal, would prove to be specific and essential characteristics, useful in sorting and classifying mammals. Furthermore, because teeth were the most indestructible part of the skeleton, they were readily obtainable for study.

Biologic Science

At the start of the 19th century, biologic science was still in its infancy but poised to grow very rapidly with the perfection of the compound microscope and the recognition that microscopic cells formed the basic units of life. The French physician and anatomist Marie François Xavier Bichat proposed that the organs of the body were composed of "membranes" or tissues, such as muscular, vascular, nervous, glandular, etc. In 1833, the English microscopist Robert Brown reported that plant cells contained an opaque spot that he called the *nucleus*. In 1838, M. J. Schleiden hypothesized that the nucleus of the plant cell was the generator of the remainder of the cell, which he called the *cytoblast*.[17] Theodore Schwann and Johannes Müller reported a similar cell-like composition for animal tissues, and when Schwann described the nucleus in animal cells in 1839, it was confirmed that both plants and animals were similarly constructed of individual units or cells.[17] Studies such as these were the cutting edge of biologic science 1 year before the establishment of the first dental school in Baltimore.

Odontology

A landmark in the science of odontology (study of structures and diseases of the teeth) occurred in 1840 with the publication of Richard Owen's *Odontography; Or, a Treatise on the Comparative Anatomy of the*

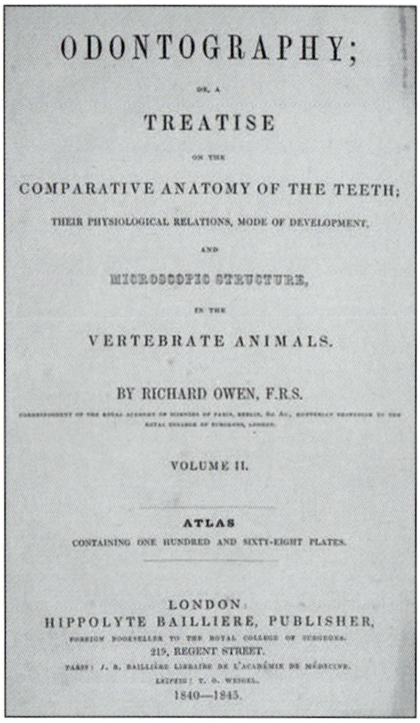

ODONTOGRAPHY;

OR, A

TREATISE

ON THE

COMPARATIVE ANATOMY OF THE TEETH;

THEIR PHYSIOLOGICAL RELATIONS, MODE OF DEVELOPMENT,

AND

MICROSCOPIC STRUCTURE,

IN THE

VERTEBRATE ANIMALS.

BY RICHARD OWEN, F.R.S.

VOLUME II.

ATLAS

CONTAINING ONE HUNDRED AND SIXTY-EIGHT PLATES.

LONDON:

HIPPOLYTE BAILLIERE, PUBLISHER,

FOREIGN BOOKSELLER TO THE ROYAL COLLEGE OF SURGEONS,

219, REGENT STREET.

PARIS: J. B. BAILLIÈRE LIBRAIRE DE L'ACADÉMIE DE MÉDECINE.

LEIPZIG: T. O. WEIGEL.

1840—1845.

Fig 6-17 Richard Owen's *Odontography*, 1840.

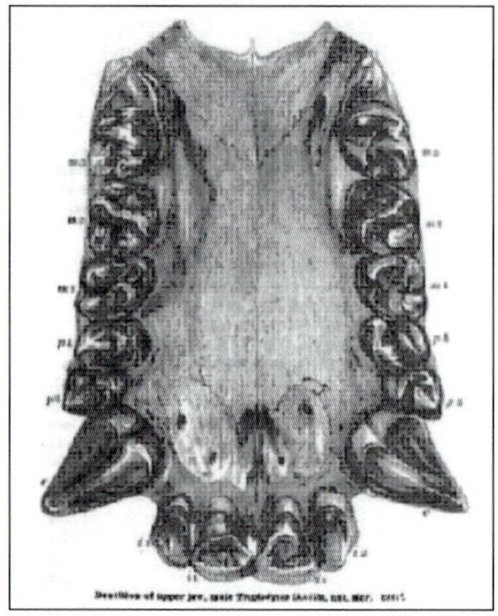

Fig 6-18 The maxilla of the gorilla. (From Owen.[18])

Teeth[18] (Fig 6-17). Based on a lifetime of research, including pioneering use of microscopy, Owen described the structure and development of teeth from fishes to mammals (Fig 6-18), including those of extinct species. He coined the word *dentine* to name the predominant substance of the tooth, replacing older terms such as *tooth-bone* and *ivory*. Owen attended Edinburgh University prior to assuming the duties of prosector for Dr John Abernathy of St Bartholomew's Hospital, London. His growth as a respected anatomist led to his appointment as assistant curator of the Hunterian Museum in 1827 and later as "superintendant" of the natural history collections of the British Museum (1856).[19] Owen's *Odontography* raised the study of tooth development and structure to a new level and thereby helped to create a scientific basis for dentistry.

Dental histology

In the middle of the 19th century, dental histology had become a field of intense investigation and controversy. Without a clear understanding of the fundamental nature of cells and their capacity to generate extracellular products, it was not possible to determine the true origin of enamel, dentin, or cementum. Early theories of the formation of dentin included the idea that pulp was transformed at its surface into mineralized substance through a coalescence of globular elements.[20] Later it was proposed that dentin arose from conversion of cellular units (ivory cells) of the pulp, located adjacent to the membrana preformativa (now recognized as the basement membrane beneath the inner enamel organ). It was thought that subsequent waves of new ivory cells added to the incremental growth of dentin.[21]

Most of the advances in dental histology were being made in Europe, where the manufacture and perfection of microscopes was ongoing. Great progress was made in the 50 years after the appearance of Bichat's *Anatomie General* (1801), in which a system of tissue organization was first defined.

The preeminence of German science was exemplified by Albert von Kölliker's *A Manual of Human Microscopic Anatomy*, translated from German and published in London in 1860 with 249 illustrations.[22] It gave the English-speaking medical profession the most outstanding description of microscopic anatomy, including a thorough account of tooth development, with penetrating insights into the formation of enamel and dentin. Kölliker predicted that someday the "molecules which form the cell membrane, the muscular fibrillae, the axial fibres of the nerve, etc." would be discovered and the laws governing the origin, growth, and functional activity of the "elementary parts" (cells and matrices) of which the body was constructed would be elucidated.[22] Kölliker defined his concept of the body as being comprised of elementary parts:

> *These elementary parts, as they are called, are of manifold kinds, some more simple, others compound. The most simple are perfectly homogeneous, without indicating a trace of being composed of heterogeneous particles, and are closely allied to the inorganic forms, the crystalline granules and crystals, which likewise occur in animal organisms. Others present a differentiation, consisting, as they do, of an envelope and special yet homogeneous contents; others, lastly, are still further differentiated even in the contents. The most important of these forms which can be included in the category of simple elementary parts, are the cells, which are not only the starting point of every vegetable and animal organism, but, also, either as cells or after undergoing divers metamorphoses, make up the complete animal body, and, in the most simple vegetable and animal formations (unicellular plants and animals), even possess individuality. Compared with the cells, all the other simple elementary parts possess quite a subordinate importance, as far as their direct participation in the formation of the tissues and organs is concerned: on the other hand, they are undoubtedly of great moment in so far as they are almost all met with in the interior of the cells and participate in their vital processes in a manifold, and, in part, very significant manner.*[22]

Early leaders in the development of cellular and tissue structure, such as Retzius, Nasmyth, Owen, Malassez, and Haverse, pioneered in the development of dental histology. Specific features of enamel, dentin, bone, and soft tissues were named in their honor. Although their work encompassed all areas of human anatomy, they gave attention to the study of enamel and dentin as holding clues to understanding the process of mineralization. Furthermore, the tooth, easily accessible at various stages of its growth, provided a model for conceptualizing fundamental concepts of organogenesis.

Summary

Dental science began in the 16th century with the publication of Vesalius's *De Humani Corporis Fabrica* and Eustachi's *Libellus de Dentibus*. Although dental science was but a small section of an expanding body of medical knowledge, it would grow, albeit at a slow pace, nourished by contributions of Cheselden, Wharton, Malpighi, and Hunter. The invention of the microscope provided a first glance of the structural fabric of the human body, including that of the teeth and gums. Scientists were astonished by the discovery that our environment and even our own bodies were populated by scores of minute living organisms. In the 18th century, the microscopic anatomy of bones, teeth, muscles, nerves, blood vessels, and salivary glands of the mouth was described in a growing number of books. Hunter, in *The Natural History of the Human Teeth*, a landmark text in the history of dental science, applied an experimental approach to prove that teeth were significantly different from bones. He demonstrated that enamel and dentin were avascular yet imbued with a "vital force" enabling successful transplantation. Hérissant's and Blake's studies of tooth development and eruption were fundamental to understanding the transition from primary to secondary dentition. Dental histology, originally concentrated on tooth development, increased in scope with additions from eminent scientists such as Kölliker, Retzius, Nasmyth, and Malassez. Early in the 18th century, Frédéric Cuvier described the diversity of the animal dentition and Richard Owen published his *Odontography; Or, a Treatise on the Comparative Anatomy of the Teeth*. By the middle of the 18th century, it was soon recognized that a substantial body of knowledge relating to teeth and their contiguous tissues formed a scientific foundation for dental practice. It would soon become a required part of the dental curriculum.

References

1. Hoffmann-Axthelm W. History of Dentistry. Chicago: Quintessence, 1981.
2. Cheselden W. The Anatomy of the Human Body. London: William Bowyer, 1740.
3. Baker H. An account of Mr. Leeuwenhoek's microscopes. Philos Trans 1739;41:503–519.
4. Ford BJ. The van Leeuwenhoek specimens. Notes Rec Royal Soc London 1981;36:37–59.
5. Shklar G. Leeuwenhoek and Vermeer, an association of genius. J Hist Dent 1998;46:53–57.
6. Porter JR. Anthony van Leeuwenhoek: Tercentenary of his discovery of bacteria. Bacteriol Rev 1976;40:260–269.
7. Stein JB. On the trail of van Leeuwenhoek. Sci Monthly 1931;32:116–134.
8. Leeuwenhoek A. An abstract of a letter from Mr. Anthony Leeuwenhoek at Delft, dated Sep. 17, 1683. Containing some microscopical observations, about animals in the scurf of the teeth, the substance call'd worms in the nose, the cuticula consisting of scales. Philos Trans 1684;14:568–574.
9. Hoole S. The Selected Works of Anthony van Leeuwenhoek. London: G. Sidney, 1800.
10. Foster M. Lectures on the History of Physiology. Cambridge, UK: Cambridge University, 1901.
11. Libby W. The History of Medicine; In its Salient Features. Boston: Houghton Mifflin, 1922.
12. Paget S. John Hunter, Man of Science and Surgeon, 1728–1793. London: Unwin, 1897.
13. Guerini V. A History of Dentistry from the Most Ancient Times Until the End of the Eighteenth Century. Philadelphia: Lea & Febiger, 1909.
14. Hérissant M. Nouvelles recherches sur la formation de l'email des dents et sur celles des gencives. Histoire de L'Academie Royale des Sciences 1759;1754:59–62,429–434.
15. Blake R. An Essay on the Structure and Formation of the Teeth in Man and Various Animals. Dublin: William Porter, 1801.
16. Cuvier F. Des dents des mammiferes. Strasbourg: F. G. Levrault, 1825.
17. Williams HS. The Story of Nineteeth-Century Science. New York: Harper & Brothers, 1900.
18. Owen R. Odontography; or a Treatise on the Comparative Anatomy of the Teeth. London: Hippolyte Bailliere, 1840–1845.
19. Turp JC. Richard Owen and the comparative anatomy of teeth. J Hist Dent 1997;45:11–16.
20. Zeigler GJ. Periscope of medical and general science in their relations to dentistry. Dent Cosmos 1860;1:433–438.
21. Robin C, Magitot E. Treatise upon the genesis and development of the dental follicles to the epoch of the eruption of the teeth. Dent Cosmos 1861;3:248–257.
22. Kölliker A. A Manual of Human Microscopic Anatomy. London: John W. Parker and Son, 1860.

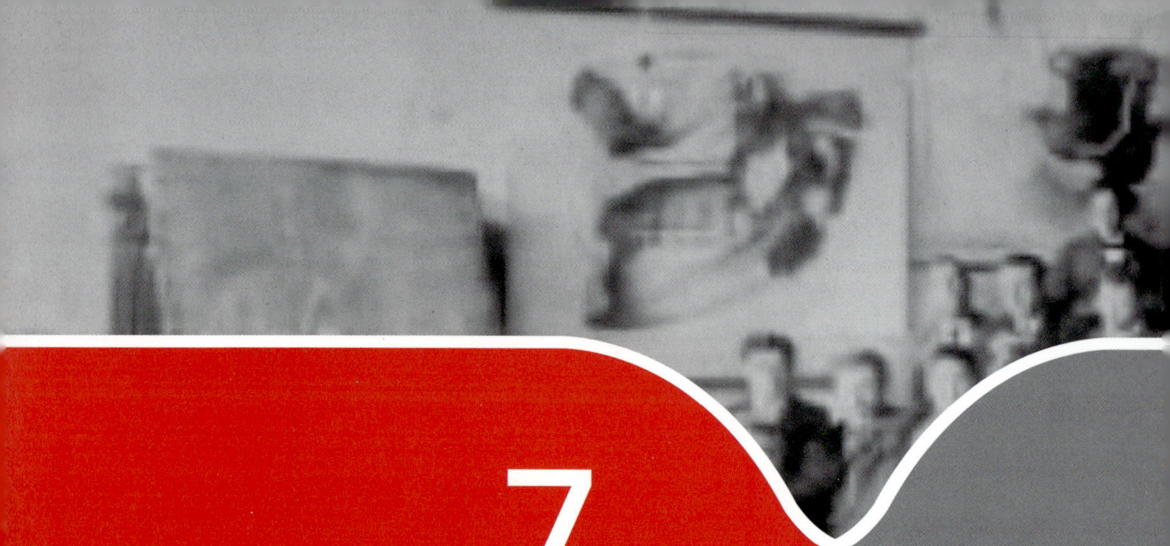

7

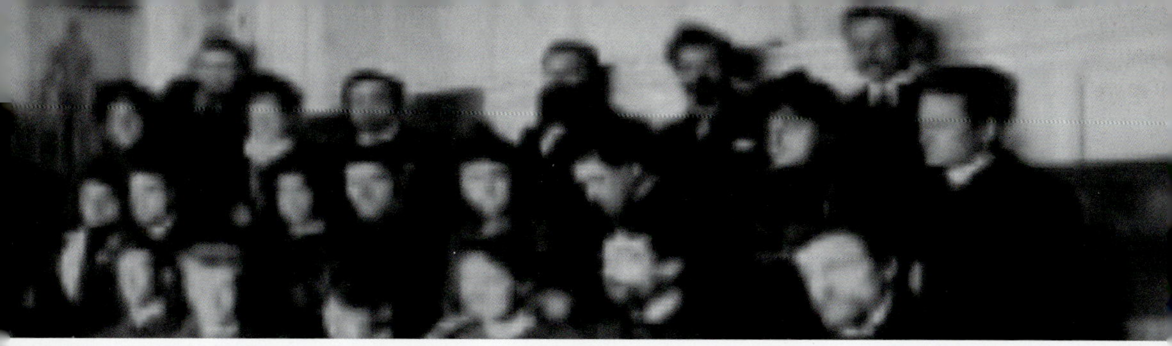

Professionalization of Dentistry in America

Ten years after the opening of the Baltimore College of Dental Surgery, the world's first dental school, Dr E. Townsend, in his address to its alumni in 1850, said the following:

> *Twenty years ago dentistry was practiced as a secret art; its disciples evinced great exclusiveness, and carefully hid from each other the methods by which they attained any individual superiority. The profession was not then a fraternity; it had not the character of a liberal art; it had all the meagerness of a selfish individualism; its spirit was narrow and exclusive, and full of arrogance and pretense, and, while it thus encouraged all that is illiberal in rivalry, it hindered whatever is useful and noble in generous emulation.*[1]

Townsend attributed this fault to infancy and not to meanness of the profession. Dr C. W. Ballard of New York estimated that by the year 1825 the number of dentists in the United States was over 200 and that most of these had started practicing "without any claim upon the public beyond that of having purchased a few secrets from such as possessed them, and were willing to sell, depending upon these secrets, and their own ingenuity and boldness, to help them into practice and out of difficulties."[1]

Before the development of dental schools, the pathway to the practice of dentistry was by apprenticeship to a physician who practiced dentistry or to a dentist who had completed such an apprenticeship. Apprenticeship to a reputed dentist was a privilege and highly costly. Dr L. S. Parmly, a well-respected New York City dentist, charged from $500 to $1,000 in 1820 to share the secrets of his successful practice.[1] Because there were no regulatory laws to ensure uniform acceptance of the apprenticeship system, aggressive individuals could simply call themselves "experts" in dentistry with just a few days of tutoring by some other ill-trained dental practitioner. In learning by trial and error, correcting their mistakes as they went along, these men endangered the public and, as Pierre Fauchard said, gave the field of dentistry a bad name.

Except in the major seaboard cities, dentistry was almost entirely an itinerant practice. According to Dr J. Brockway of Newbury, Vermont, in 1822, dentists were nonexistent "from Canada to Albany, and from the Rocky to the White Mountains."[1]

A rapid rise in the number of dentists in America occurred after the financial troubles of 1835–1836. Men who had lost their employment began practicing dentistry because it required little training and was unregulated. Though the majority of these dentists were empirics who guarded the secrets of their trade from competitors, there were some qualified dentists, such as Horace Hayden and Chapin Harris, who devoted themselves to the betterment of the profession.[1] These leading dentists, mainly from New York and Philadelphia, recognized that in order to establish dentistry as a profession on par with medicine, three things were needed: *(1)* a formal dental education system; *(2)* a dental literature, and *(3)* the formation of dental societies wherein the members could regulate practice and learn through association. Dentistry had evolved as a trade performed by barber-surgeons and associated craftsmen. Not until the latter half of the 19th century would it mature by accrual of a scientific basis and the creation of a dental literature, a combination that gave it status as a newly developing profession. As it sought to establish principles of governance, dentistry was plagued by the conflict between commercialism and the unselfishness inherent to professionalism.

Dental Education

In 1840, under the leadership of Drs Horace Hayden and Chapin Harris, the first dental college opened in Baltimore, Maryland (see chapter 5). Shortly after the establishment of the Baltimore College of Dental Surgery, two more schools were founded in 1845: the Ohio College of Dental Surgery and the Pennsylvania College of Dental Surgery. In 1865, the New York College of Dentistry was founded. The first university-affiliated dental school was founded at Harvard in 1867, followed by the University of Michigan (1875) and the University of Pennsylvania (1878). By 1884, there were 28 dental schools in the United States. Most were privately owned. The leadership of the nascent profession had come to regard a dental school education as a necessary step toward regulating dental practice and protecting the public from incompetent practitioners.

Several factors had to be overcome in developing independent dental schools. Existing medical schools were not in favor of adding dentistry to their educational programs, in part because they lacked the physical space or were not ready to undertake the extra costs of developing a dental clinic. Opposition to the existence of independent dental schools was quick to come from physicians who viewed dental school programs as deficient because of their failing to teach basic medical sciences. Most physicians would not accept a new and separate diploma for dentistry, looking with disdain on dental practitioners who assumed themselves to be doctors without ever having completed a medical curriculum.

In making arguments for a separate dental school system, Dr Chapin Harris stated the following:

> *We should furnish the necessary facilities for those who may design practicing the art, to qualify themselves properly for its duties. Dentistry should be as much a matter of public instruction as medicine or surgery; and to me it has been a matter of much surprise, that the efforts of the better informed of the profession have not been directed to the establishment of an institution for this purpose. An institution of this kind would not only redound to the credit of the whole profession, but it would be instrumental of much general good. Its influence could not be otherwise than salutary, as it would have a tendency to drive from the ranks of the profession ignorant pretenders, and substitute in their places men that would be qualified to practice with credit to themselves, and to the benefit of their patients.*[1]

Dr S. P. Hullihen, in a valedictory address to the graduates of the Baltimore College of Dental Surgery in 1850, blamed the need for independent dental colleges on the neglect of the medical profession:

> *They condemned, without stints a calling they knew not how to practice, and a practice they knew not how to improve. Such of the faculty as were learned in their profession were found always competent and fully prepared to be oculists, aurists, or lithotomists, or to devote*

> *themselves to any other branch of the profession which their interest, inclination, or talents might determine, except that of dental surgery. This branch seemed to require something more than medical knowledge; it required great mechanical skill—education of the hand as well as of the head—a kind of education they had not received, and knew not where to acquire, and yet affected to despise. The necessities of the community cried aloud to them for help—a help which they could not bestow. This drove many sufferers to seek dental aid out of the medical profession, and to obtain that help which mechanical genius alone could supply. At this the profession seemed mortified and chagrined, and loudly mocked at those who dared to supply their delinquencies, and united as one man in deriding the uneducated dental mechanic. They first created the necessity for an empiric, and then croaked forth their withering contempt on the creature their own ignorance had made.*[1]

Despite setbacks and opposition, many physicians who practiced a limited form of dentistry did help to establish separate dental schools. They provided the nucleus of the faculties of the new dental schools. For example, the members of the Harvard medical faculty actively participated in the development of the dental school, served as teaching faculty, and generously provided space for clinical instruction in the outpatient clinics of the Massachusetts General Hospital.[2]

The following anecdote illustrates difficulties encountered in developing a school of dentistry at the University of Pennsylvania. In 1878, as classes were about to start in the newly established dental department, with 53 students on board, Dr Edwin Darby, a founding member of the faculty, recounted his experience:

> *The University approved 20 dental chairs but only 10 were delivered. When the dental faculty arrived at the Medical School (Medical Hall) to inquire the location of the dental facility, the janitor, cross and impolite, ushered them to the basement where they could establish their clinic and mechanical lab, and use the old chemical room as a lecture room in conjunction with the medical students. When the professor of chemistry objected, the dental faculty was offered an old physiology dog kennel for a dental lecture hall.*[3]

Notwithstanding such difficulties, dental schools proliferated in the latter half of the 19th century. Now three pathways to a dental career existed: *(1)* completion of a 5-year apprenticeship with a dentist or physician (who practiced dentistry); *(2)* graduation from a dental college (2-year course); or *(3)* graduation from medical school and completion of the second (clinical) year of dental college. In 1870, 85% of the nation's dentists had been trained under apprenticeships or had simply proclaimed themselves to be dentists. Most practicing dentists favored the apprenticeship system and were opposed to the requirement that a dental school diploma was a prerequisite for practice, because practicing without a diploma implied a lower status and a decline in income. Arguing that the apprenticeships were inadequate amounted to arguing that the majority of existing practitioners were ill-trained. An additional factor in support of the apprenticeship system was that established dentists profited financially by acting as preceptors.

There were numerous abuses of the apprenticeship system, such as poor supervision of the apprentices and apprentices practicing without completion of the required 5-year period. A fundamental problem with the apprenticeship system was its failure to provide education in the sciences—there were no provisions for exposure to anatomy, physiology, and chemistry. In an editorial to *Dental Cosmos* in 1860, Dr John McQuillen touched on the deficiencies in the apprenticeship system and the poor state of education of individuals who were permitted to enter as apprentices:

> *That numbers of dental students have been admitted in the offices of their preceptors who were deficient in the most common branches of an English education, and that a proper inquiry into the fitness of young men to become students is, even now, seldom instituted, are positions which can scarcely be controverted.... In our country, with the facilities now afforded by cheap books and free schools, an individual who attains to manhood without acquiring, in addition to the elementary branches of learning, a fair acquaintance with natural philosophy, chemistry, etc., and is content to remain so possesses neither the aspirations, energy, or industry requisite to make him a thorough practitioner or a successful cultivator of dental science, and it would therefore be a kindness to him, as well as an act of justice to the public and the profession to advise him to devote his energies in some other direction.... Preceptors sometimes fail to perform their duty on another point. Affording their students every facility, encouragement, and direction with regard to mechanic and occasional opportunities to witness and manipulate in operative dentistry, they provide little or no means for acquiring a knowledge of the science of the profession.... The preceptor rarely institutes a regular series of examinations and explanations in the course of studies entered upon, but leaves the inexperienced mind of the student to regulate its own pursuits, and after a probation of a few months, or year at best, the student enters upon the practice of the profession only to find that he has yet to educate himself.*[4]

Minimal progress had been made to elevate the status of dentistry 35 years after the development of the first dental school. Dr James Truman, speaking before the New York Odontological Society in 1875, gave the following description of the deplorable state of the dental profession:

> *We are supposed to number from ten to thirteen thousand operators of all grades; a large army when we consider the comparatively limited period of its development. Of this number some two thousand have received the degree from colleges, and a still fewer number can be regarded as having passed through the studies assigned by those institutions. The result is that from eight to eleven thousand persons are engaged in the practice of the profession who have not the degree, and of whose general intelligence we have no means of knowing. It is very safe to assume that a very large proportion are men whose attainments do not extend beyond the mere practical routine of mechanical operation, and a very large number are by no means experts in these directions.*[5]

Admission requirements were nonexistent until 1865, when several schools required that entering students have a good English education, but it was not until 1889 that 1 year of high school became a prerequisite for admission and not until 1908 that graduation from high school was adopted by the National Association of Dental Faculties as a prerequisite to dental school.[6] Progress was made in the last quarter of the 19th century as the duration and content of the dental school curriculum grew from a 1-year program (with or without an associated period of apprenticeship) to a 3-year self-standing program by the turn of the 20th century[7] (Table 7-1). But without national standards, what constituted a year of instruction ranged from 16 to 28 weeks among various schools.

Conditions in the medical schools of the United States had followed a similar but earlier period of troubled growth. The first medical school was established in 1765 at the University of Pennsylvania by Drs John Morgan and W. Shippen, both of whom had studied with William and John Hunter in London.[8] By 1904, there were 166 medical schools, most proprietary in nature, with a 2-year curriculum (5 months per year) consisting of lectures and clinical demonstrations.[8] With the exception of some of the leading schools, there were no laboratories, except for anatomy. Expenses were kept to a minimum, and professorial pay was generated by selling tickets to lectures. In an editorial of the *Philadelphia Medical Times*, it was reported that medical schools were in competition for students and that the winning schools were those that offered the easiest and quickest path to the diploma.[9] Needless to say, there were many poorly trained physicians let loose on the public.

In 1871, Harvard Medical School abolished the common custom of allowing a 5-year practice to be equivalent to the first year of study.[2] The academic year was extended from September to June and written evaluation examinations were introduced at Harvard in 1875. By the turn of the 20th century, laboratory exercises in physiology, pathology,

TABLE 7-1 A typical dental school curriculum at the end of the 19th century

Year 1		Year 2		Year 3	
Subject	**Hrs/wk**	**Subject**	**Hrs/wk**	**Subject**	**Hrs/wk**
Anatomy and dissection	2	Regional anatomy	1	Therapeutics	1
Physiology	2	Comparative anatomy	1	Pathology	1
Inorganic chemistry	2	Physiology	2	Oral surgery	1
Chemistry lab	4	Organic chemistry	2	General surgery	1
Dental anatomy	2	Chemistry lab	4	Jurisprudence	0.5
Prosthetic technique	10	Metallurgy didactic	1	Orthodontics didactic	1
Histology	4	Metallurgy lab	2	Orthodontics practical	1
Materia medica	*	Materia medica	1	Operative dentistry	2
Comparative anatomy	*	Operative technique	4	Prosthetic dentistry	2
		Bacteriology	4	Electricity	*
		Operative dentistry didactic	2	Ethics	*
		Orthodontic technique	1	History	*
		Pathology	2		
		Clinical		**Clinical**	
		Prosthetic dentistry	5	Operative dentistry	6
		Crown and bridge	3	Prosthetic dentistry	15
				Crown and bridge	4

*—unknown, but less than 1 hour per week. (Adapted from Taft.[7])

and pharmacology were established at better medical schools.[8] With the introduction of more rigid standards by the Council on Medical Education of the American Medical Association in the early 20th century, and in accord with the recommendations of the Carnegie Foundation's Flexner Report, the number of medical schools dropped from 166 to 110. At that time, the leading centers of medical research were found in Europe, especially in France and Germany.

During the last quarter of the 19th century, the movement to reform dental education gathered momentum as representatives of a number of the dental colleges met in New York on August 4, 1884 to form the National Association of Dental Faculties for the purpose of adopting a uniform standard of graduation. It was resolved that students at the dental colleges be required to attend two full regular courses (2 years) of lectures before coming up for graduation and that the clinical studies should be pursued in a dental school infirmary and not in a private dental office. Furthermore, applicants must pass a preliminary examination for entrance to dental college.

Charles W. Eliot, president of Harvard University, in an address to the American Academy of Dental Science in 1878, had called for the extension of dental school to 3 years and to the discontinuance of the recognition of 5 years of practice as an equivalent for any portion of study in dental school. He also wanted an end to the practice of granting dual MD and DDS degrees by certain medical schools, arguing that this practice lowered the standard of both disciplines. In an address to the Harvard Dental School (Fig 7-1), President Eliot expressed his admiration for the progress that had been made in dental education: "I do not think I have seen during my seventy years of observation of the professions and the means of training them, any change so great as that which has taken place in regard to the dental profession and to the means of training."[10]

By the late 1890s, the curriculum of 3 years' duration, with a workweek of 26 to 35 hours of didactic and clinical training, extending over approximately 7 months per year, became the standard (see Table 7-1). In 1903, the National Association of Dental Faculties proposed extending the course of studies to 4 years of 6 months each. After much debate and the potential disintegration of the Association, a compromise was reached to extend the dental curriculum to 3 years of 30 weeks each (including Saturday sessions).[6]

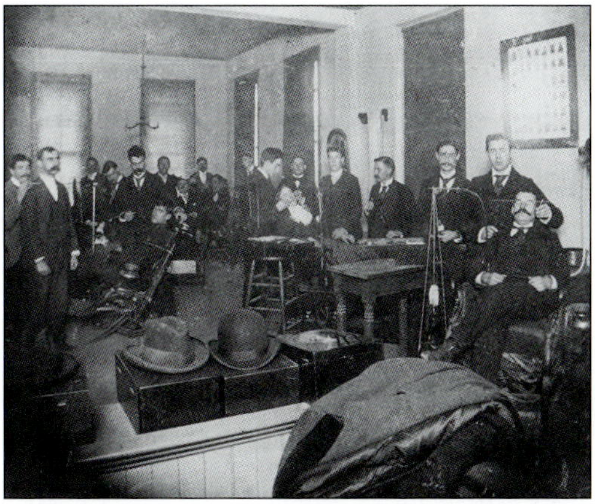

Fig 7-1 A clinic of the Harvard Dental School, 1895. (Courtesy of the Harvard Medical Library in the Francis A. Countway Library of Medicine.)

Commercialization of dental education

During the 1880s and 1890s, dozens of freestanding proprietary (for-profit) schools were founded in the United States. In Illinois alone, 28 dental schools were chartered between 1883 and 1902. A major impetus for the rapid growth in proprietary dental schools was the adoption of state laws regulating dental practice. In some states, dental practice laws granted graduates of dental schools a license to practice without requiring independent qualifying examinations. The failure to examine, coupled with the power of the diploma, increased the number of applicants to proprietary schools. By 1900, there were 57 proprietary dental schools in the United States. The profit motive for founders of proprietary dental schools was also a contributing factor to their growth. Dr Thomas Chandler, professor of mechanical dentistry and dean of the Harvard School of Dental Medicine, speaking on dental education at the New York Odontological Society in 1875, expressed his criticism of the proliferation of dental schools and the lack of standards in these words:

> *A bad omen for good results of our aims is the multiplication of dental schools, or colleges, as they are ambitiously termed, and the consequent*

> *division of the energies of our profession among a multitude of feeble plants, which, applied properly, would serve to nourish a few good and noble trees. A tendency of this division, and the consequent competition for support, is the lowering of the standard of education, flooding the land with half-educated men, and a depreciation of the value of the diploma which attests their acquirements.... There is another evil under the sun in connection with dental schools. Among the requisites for graduation of all but one or two, is a clause which says that three or five years' practice shall be considered as equivalent for one term. Nothing is said or hinted of reputable practice, and the student has only to bring a certificate from his minister or deacon, or the selectman of his village, to the effect that he has practiced to his knowledge so many years, and the thing is done.*[11]

Dr Arthur Black, son of Dr G. V. Black, deplored the commercialization of dental education:

> *But when as has been done with the great majority of our dental colleges, the object of the institution is made a commercial rather than educational one, then I say that honesty and justice are lost sight of to the detriment not only of the profession, but of the public at large. Too many of our colleges have first the commercial aim of earning money for the stockholders, and incidentally the education of students, and in these days the so-called successful colleges are those which boast the greatest number of matriculates.*[12]

In this early period of nonregulation, there were opportunities for dishonesty in dental education. Scandals arose when some dental schools (and some medical schools as well) fell into the business of awarding degrees without examination and in some cases selling diplomas. The most notorious case arose in Philadelphia. In 1845, the newly established Pennsylvania Association of Dental Surgeons attempted to form a dental school, but they were denied a charter by the state legislature. A few years later, Jesse Burden, a member of the Pennsylvania State Legislature and the president of the Philadelphia College of Medicine, obtained a charter to form a dental school. He offered the charter to the Pennsylvania Association of Dental Surgeons on the conditions that he be appointed president of the dental school and that he retain the right to appoint the board of governors.[3] The association would retain the right to appoint the faculty. Agreement was reached in 1852, and the Philadelphia College of Dental Surgery was established with Jesse Burden as president.

The Philadelphia College of Medicine, with Jesse Burden as its president, had been loose in applying its standards for granting degrees, and when Burden tried to introduce the same laxity at the dental college, the faculty balked. Claiming that the faculty alone (not dean Burden) was competent to set the qualifications of the DDS candidates, the faculty resigned, reorganized, and successfully sought a new charter from the state. In 1856, they formed the new Pennsylvania College of Dental Surgery with a new charter containing the following clause: "No degree shall be conferred, whether honorary or upon the qualified students of the college, without the written request of the faculty." This all-important stipulation stands in effect today in that it is the faculty's responsibility to set the curriculum and to approve the granting of academic degrees. Eventually, the proliferation of proprietary schools prompted new state practice acts requiring that graduates of dental schools take licensure examinations and that only graduates of reputable schools be permitted to take such examinations.

At most of the better dental schools, a requirement for graduation included the submission of a written thesis on a selected area of dental science or clinical condition. For example, at the second annual commencement of the Harvard Dental School, the twelve graduates submitted papers on a variety of topics, including the chemistry of the mouth, prevention of caries, and neuralgia, among others. At the Philadelphia College of Dental Surgery's 1870 commencement, 74 graduates submitted papers on a wide range of subjects, including topics such as professional duty. The disappearance of written research papers from the requirements for graduation is unfortunate in that such exercises emphasize the importance of communication in professional life.

Mechanical arts versus sciences

In its early development, dentistry was viewed as a simple mechanical art. Most dental students saw the sciences as an unnecessary interruption in their pursuit of the technical aspects of the trade. From the beginning of dental school instruction, the pull between the mechanical arts (operative dentistry and prosthetics) and the sciences (eg, anatomy and physiology) was apparent.[1] As early as 1851, Dr Chapin Harris wrote that "there is a general tendency evinced by dental students to devote extra time to the practical departments at the expense of the regular lectures, and that it has required the stringent laws of the institution, and effort on the part of the faculty, to counteract this tendency." He also wrote that:

> *The infirmary and mechanical rooms are so attractive, that it requires all the talent of our colleagues, and the stringent regulations of the school, to obtain sufficient consideration for the medical branches. The habit of dentists, such as dentists have been, and for the most part*

yet are, is to undervalue collateral scientific acquirements and make dentistry, as far as possible, a mechanical art.[1]

Because many areas of the country had no dental supply houses, dentists had to make many of their instruments, and thus dental students were required to attend lectures on metallurgy and instruction on forging dental instruments (see Table 7-1). In that time period, a dental student needed a hammer, a small forge, an anvil with bellows, files, and blanks. A student at the University of Pennsylvania Dental Department recalled a lecture demonstration by Dr Darby:

> *On a table in front of the class was an assortment which included a hammer, a small forge and bellows, an anvil, some files and a handful of blanks, i.e. instruments to be. Darby explained that because many areas of the country had no dental supply houses to call upon if one broke an instrument or if one needed a special type it was advantageous to know how to fabricate an instrument. Thereupon he withdrew a red-hot blank from his forge, laid it on the anvil and formed it with a few taps of his hammer, finished shaping it with files and finally tempered it by quenching it in water. Talking steadily, he fashioned a set of excavators and chisels in the span of one hour.*[3]

Prior to the reforms of the early 20th century, dental education suffered from the following deficiencies: lack of illustrative teaching materials, granting diplomas without examination of candidates, insufficient or no entrance requirements, and the bestowal of diplomas by dental societies. Furthermore, department chairpersons were often filled by nonpracticing dentists (MDs), and dental programs were started without appropriate dental equipment.[13]

The annual report of the Pennsylvania College of Dental Surgery for 1860 provides a picture of the type of services provided by the dental school infirmary of that period. All services were divided into Operative Services and Mechanical Services. The Operative Department reported 4,055 operations performed on 308 patients. Extractions (2,858) constituted more than 50% of all services provided by the Operative Department. Gold fillings (612) and tin fillings (310) formed the other operative services. Only 6 amalgam fillings were reported. The Mechanical Department reported that 138 sets of teeth were fabricated. Presumably, the bulk of these services were provided by the graduating class, then comprising 21 individuals.[14]

Based on these outcomes, it was claimed that dentists were being educated as mechanics and tooth fillers but poorly or not at all in the sciences, and on that basis their equality with general medicine should be rightly denied.[1] In 1848, the New York Academy of Medicine refused to admit dental practitioners to membership, stating that dentists were unequal in the more scientific and theoretic parts of the science of healing.[1]

Dr Robert Arthur, in his presidential address to members of the Southern Dental Association at their annual meeting in St Louis, Missouri, in the summer of 1874, asked whether dentists in their pursuit of the practical features of restoring teeth had not neglected higher considerations (ie, the study of general medical sciences) and in the process forfeited their right to hold doctoral degrees.[15] He questioned: "Should mere toothpullers and toothpluggers be called doctors?" Arthur quoted from editorials appearing in the *Medical Times of Philadelphia* of 1874, where it was stated:

> *The higher education, the wider culture of the physician, although it may contribute, is in no case a necessity to such (dentistry's) success, and just so long as this is true will a very large proportion of dentists neglect that culture, which, while it may be an ornament, is not a necessity, for the practice of their profession. Here, it seems, the matter rests. Dentists—we mean the general mass—have at present no claim to be recognized as representatives of a branch of our profession (medicine). Many dentists are doctors; some of them 'oral surgeons' and as such we receive them into the brotherhood; but the great mass must probably remain, as they are at present, dentists, worthy citizens,—we do them no disrespect,—artists of ability many of them, but yet in no sense practitioners of medicine; in no sense entitled to recognition as such.*[16]

Arthur faulted the curriculum of most dental schools as being deficient in teaching general medical principles (eg, general pathology). In comparing the programs of instruction at three dental schools (Harvard School of Dental Medicine, Philadelphia College of Dental Surgery, and the Pennsylvania College of Dental Surgery), Arthur found Harvard's association with its medical school as especially promising, yet he found that its curriculum offered insufficient time to the study of general medicine and pathology. Furthermore, these subjects were taught at the expense of technical instruction in dentistry and thus compromised the essential nature of the dental program. None of the three schools, each being among the best in the country, were in his opinion preparing dental students to take a position of equality with physicians.[17]

In taking this position, Arthur had roused the anger of many of his dental colleagues, who rose to defend their colleges. George T. Barker, professor of dental pathology and therapeutics in the Pennsylvania College of Dental Surgery, accused Arthur of having failed to gather sufficient data and of being unfair and unjust in his criticism.[13]

TABLE 7-2 Number of physicians and dentists compared with population in America from 1850 to 1895

Year	Population	Physicians	Pop./physicians	Dentists	Pop./dentists
1850	23,191,876	40,765	570	2,923	7,934
1860	31,443,322	55,159	570	5,606	5,607
1870	38,558,371	62,446	617	7,839	4,918
1880	50,155,783	85,671	586	12,314	4,154
1890	62,622,250	104,803	597	17,498	3,579
1895	70,500,000	120,000	586	25,000	3,134

(Adapted from Stainton.[18])

Despite his critical judgment of dentists, Dr Arthur went on to make cogent arguments for regarding dentistry as a specialty of medicine. He noted that dentists were often faced with disorders that were not confined to the teeth but affected distant organs, and likewise abnormal conditions in the general system affected normal development of the dentition.[15] He urged dentists to become acquainted with the general principles of medicine, especially in the areas of inflammation and facial neuralgia. In the same speech, Dr Arthur lamented the fact that medical schools gave their students no exposure to dental problems, leaving physicians in practice to rely on mostly outdated textbooks of medicine when it came to dealing with oral diseases. This situation, he argued, was not conducive to prompt and effective treatment of patients who presented with oral or dental complaints at a medical practice.

In concluding his address, Dr Arthur stressed that dentistry needed the higher education and the broader culture of the physician: "When this kind of culture is demanded by public opinion, a different class of men from those who now confine themselves to the manual requirements of dentistry will enter the ranks of the dental profession."[15] It would take many more years of reform, culminating with the implementation of the recommendations of the Gies Report of 1926, before equality was achieved (see chapter 17).

By 1895, the American Dental Association concluded that the number of dentists was adequate to meet demand. The number of dentists had increased from just under 3,000 in 1850 to 25,000 in 1895 (Table 7-2).[18] During this same period, the ratio of population to number of physicians remained stable, while the ratio of popula-

TABLE 7-3 Number of dentists in major American cities in 1895

City	Population	Dentists	Pop./dentists
New York	2,000,000	1,200	1,666
Boston	500,000	325	1,538
Washington, DC	270,000	226	1,194
Denver	120,000	85	1,411
Omaha	140,000	25	5,600

(Adapted from Stainton.[18])

tion to number of dentists was cut by more than half. Western cities were underserved, while the Eastern cities had highly favorable numbers of dentists (Table 7-3).[18] Many dentists claimed that overproduction produced cheap and nasty practitioners. Dr I. P. Wilson stated that "Never before has quackery developed itself in high places so boldly as at the present day. I mean by this that fairly well educated men, dental college graduates, who are devoid of principle, are swindling the public, degrading the profession, and endangering human life as never before." Dr Arthur Black noted that the output of dentists was greater than the demand for services, the result being that more graduates were willing to work for dental companies. He viewed the trend with alarm: "In the growth and financial success of the dental companies…the employer devotes his time to building up the business on strictly business lines and gives no heed to the ideas of honor which influence the professional man."

Output declined as many schools were forced to close as a result of increasing requirements in equipment, supplies, teaching, and research. In Illinois alone, 22 schools lost their charters because of curricular inadequacies. It was increasingly apparent that dental education was failing to keep pace with advances in science and that if it continued to produce mechanics instead of educating men equipped with the scientific knowledge to develop preventive strategies for dental and oral diseases, it would lose its public (and university) support. It was observed that European dental specialists were producing an aggregate of scientific work in dentistry that far exceeded the output of the United States. In 1894, Dr E. S. Talbot urged American dentistry to raise its standards and "make its reputation as a scientific specialty of medicine, and not a manual art."[19]

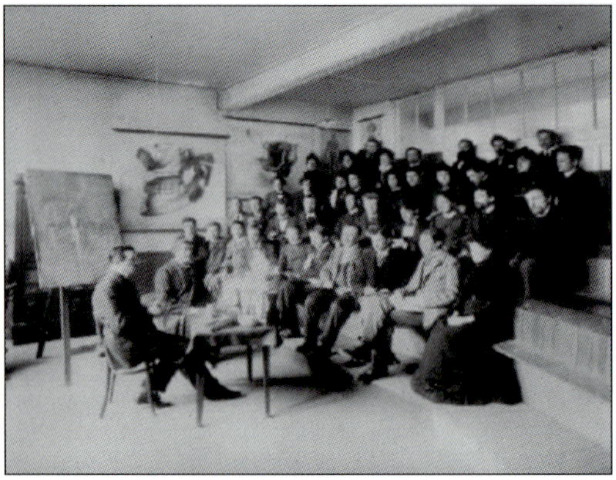

Fig 7-2 A dental school class in Paris, 1911.

At the end of the 19th century, dental education was conducted along two general pathways: the American type, conducted independent of medical faculty control; and the European stomatologic model, wherein dental education followed the completion of the medical degree. In effect, the graduates of American dental schools achieved better mechanical skills, while the European graduates were better educated in medicine but were often lacking in the mechanical aspects of dental restorative care. The first dental school in Germany was founded in Berlin in 1855 as a private clinic for oral diseases. In London, lectures on dentistry were introduced in hospitals (Joseph Fox at Guy's Hospital). In 1858, the Dental Hospital of London was founded. The following year it was renamed the London School of Dentistry. In 1880, a private facility, the Ecole Dentaire, was opened in Geneva. In Paris, the first educational program for training stomatologists opened in 1909 as the Institut de Stomotologie de la Faculte de Medicine (Fig 7-2).

The Development and Importance of Dental Societies

During the formative period from the Civil War to the end of the 19th century, dental societies joined with state governing bodies to ensure that the public was served by competent practitioners. Acting like the guilds of old, dental societies set ethical and technical standards of practice, regulated who should be allowed to practice, and provided a structure for education of their members. The first dental society to be formed in America was the Society of Surgeon Dentists of the City and State of New York. It was founded in 1834 with the purpose of elevating the quality of practice and discouraging the use of amalgam, the chief material in use by unqualified dentists.[20] Shortly thereafter, the American Society of Dental Surgeons was formed in 1840 in New York City. It was the first dental society to be organized on a national level. The same men who had joined together to establish the Baltimore College of Dental Surgery served as the nucleus of this society. Horace Hayden served as its first president. To give its members special status and to distinguish them from the growing number of unscrupulous dental practitioners, the society conferred the degree of Doctor of Dental Surgery (DDS). When the New York State Legislature ruled against the Society's practice of granting degrees, the Society then began to provide diplomas to its members, but this practice soon became the sole right of accredited dental schools.[20] The American Society of Dental Surgeons had specific aims:

> *The objects of this society are to promote union and harmony among all respectable and well-informed Dental Surgeons; to advance the science by free communication and interchange of sentiments, either written or verbal, between members of the Society, both in this and other counties; in fine, to give character and respectability to the profession, by establishing a line of distinction between the truly meritorious and skillful, and such as riot in the ill-gotten fruit of unblushing impudence and empiricism.*[1]

New members had to be 21 years of age and of exceptional moral character and must have practiced for 2 full years with a dentist known to the society or possess a diploma from a dental college. In their drive to curb the malpractice of dentistry, the society became divided over the use of gold versus amalgam as an appropriate filling material. When the society required its members to sign a pledge not to use amalgam in their practice, the membership fell into decline and ultimately folded in 1856.[1]

Other examples of early dental societies were the Virginia Society of Dental Surgeons founded in 1842, the Mississippi Valley Association of Dental Surgeons established in 1844, the Pennsylvania Association of Dental Surgeons founded in 1845, and the New York State Society of Dental Surgeons formed in 1848. Each of these organizations set out to expose quackery and shoddy dentistry and to elevate the profession through education of its members. The Virginia Society of Dental Surgeons adopted a resolution to "distinguish and reward merit and discountenance and expose quackery and charlatanism."[1]

In 1855, leaders of the New York State Society of Dental Surgeons, seeing a need for a nationwide association of dentists, moved to create the American Dental Convention. In the hope of including as many practicing dentists and "auxiliary branches of science" as possible, no constitutional obstacles to membership were adopted. At its fourth annual meeting, held in Niagara Falls in 1859, the leaders of the American Dental Convention, seeing a need for a more formal and better organized structure, formed the American Dental Association based on the model of the American Medical Association.[1] By 1870, delegates from 47 state and regional dental associations and 3 dental colleges were in attendance at the annual convention of the American Dental Association. One of its first official acts was the adoption of a code of ethics for the dental profession.

The rapid growth of the dental association movement led to approximately 85 active state and local organizations by 1875. These groups, meeting on a regular basis, formed the rules and principles by which dentistry was to be practiced and regulated. The proceedings of many of these associations, as recorded in dental journals such as *Dental Cosmos*, provide valuable accounts of the spirit and intensity of the discussions, which centered on issues of education, standards of practice, patient rights, and professional ethics.

The Formation of Faculty Associations

In 1884, faculty representatives from several schools met in New York City to form the National Association of Dental Faculties, with the goals of creating standards for graduation and recommending curricular reforms in line with those implemented at Harvard.[21] When proprietary schools, operating chiefly to generate income, failed to espouse the new ideals, a two-tiered system was soon consolidated. Shortly thereafter, university-based schools (California, Harvard, Iowa, Michigan, Minnesota, and Pennsylvania) formed the Dental Faculties Association of American Universities, whose main purposes were to promote the university-based model and to challenge the controlling influence of the larger number of proprietary schools. In 1923, this group merged with the American Association of Dental Schools.[21] The new association, called the American Dental Education Association, comprised more than 16,000 students, faculty, staff, and administrators from all United States and Canadian dental schools.

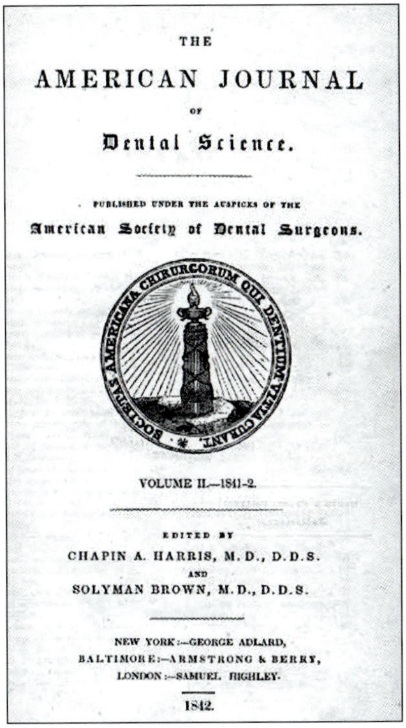
THE
AMERICAN JOURNAL
OF
Dental Science.

PUBLISHED UNDER THE AUSPICES OF THE
American Society of Dental Surgeons.

SOCIETAS AMERICANA CHIRURGORUM QUI DENTIUM VITIA CURANT.

VOLUME II.—1841-2.

EDITED BY
CHAPIN A. HARRIS, M. D., D. D. S.
AND
SOLYMAN BROWN, M. D., D. D. S.

NEW YORK:—GEORGE ADLARD,
BALTIMORE:—ARMSTRONG & BERRY,
LONDON:—SAMUEL HIGHLEY.

1842.

Fig 7-3 *The American Journal of Dental Science*, the first of its kind.

The Growth of Dental Literature

During the mid 19th century, when dental science began its rapid growth, dental practitioners who wished to communicate new techniques or discoveries were obliged to present their work at meetings of local dental societies or to publish in medical journals because there were no periodicals devoted solely to dentistry. The latter approach was not a very effective way of communicating among dentists because most did not subscribe to medical journals. This changed in 1839 with the establishment of the *American Journal of Dental Science* (Fig 7-3), led by Drs Chapin A. Harris of Baltimore, Eleazar Parmly, Elisha Baker, and Solyman Brown of New York City. This monthly journal was devoted exclusively to dental science and clinical literature. In 1841, the journal passed into the hands of the American Society of Dental Surgeons, and the title changed to the *American Journal and Library of Dental Science*. Under the editorial leadership of Solyman Brown and Chapin Harris, it continued until 1850, when it became the sole enterprise of Chapin Harris. Upon his death in 1860, the journal ceased to exist.[21]

Other early entries into the dental literature were the *Dental News Letter*, a quarterly journal published by Jones, White, and McCurdy of Philadelphia, and the *Dental Register of the West*, published by the Mississippi Valley Association of Dental Surgeons.[21] In 1859, the *Dental Register* changed its name to *Dental Cosmos*, a monthly journal published by the S. S. White Company. A new policy was introduced at *Dental Cosmos*, wherein three editors instead of one assumed responsibility for its content. Drs J. H. McQuillen, G. J. Zeigler, and J. D. White shared the editorial work. *Dental Cosmos* helped create a new generation of better-educated dentists by its support of the university-based model of dental education.[21]

These journals provided a place for dentists not only to publish original observations of a scientific and clinical nature but also to report the proceedings of the many state dental associations and local odontologic societies that were forming throughout the nation. Dentists who were unable to attend meetings in person were able to read the news of new discoveries and follow the debates pertaining to current controversies, whether on issues of licensing, standards for granting diplomas, or content of the dental curriculum. Furthermore, the journals printed excerpts from some of the major textbooks available to subscribers. *Dental Cosmos* continued to be published until 1936, providing a record of the growth of American dentistry as a profession. Other dental periodicals, such as *Items of Interest* (1879), *Dental Digest* (1895), and *Dental Brief* (1897), served mainly as sources of information on operative and mechanical dentistry and owed their survival to the financial sponsorship of dental supply houses.[22] Dental literature was also essential for improving practice through the free interchange of ideas and ultimately for decreasing the selling of secrets.

The value of the early dental literature was compromised because the number of contributing authors who had good writing skills was limited to a small number of academics and learned clinicians. The quality of the submissions was said to be deplorable and less than gentlemanly in tone of communication. McQuillen, as editor of *Dental Cosmos*, observed in 1859:

> *In making a retrospective view of dental journals during the past few years, however mortifying the acknowledgment may be, one must admit that whilst there has been much to admire and commend, a certain portion have evinced an unpardonable laxity in those particulars, and the recollection of the sad trash by which they have frequently been*

> *disfigured, cannot but be a subject of regret to properly constituted minds. Papers, faulty in language, defective in structure, and utterly devoid of useful information, which a due regard for the reputation of the writers alone, should have induced the editors to return to them, have been published without comment, correction, or the apology that matter was scarce, and the magazines must be filled.*[23]

Furthermore, the need to fill each issue with new content placed a restraint on applying standards by editors who knew better.

In 1906, members of the New York Institute of Stomatology, the American Academy of Dental Science, the Harvard Odontological Society, and the Metropolitan District of the Massachusetts State Dental Society launched the *Journal of the Allied Societies*. Its aim was to communicate new scientific discoveries to members of the dental profession. In 1919, this journal was revived as the *Journal of Dental Research* by Dr William Gies of Columbia University.[20] Its editorial board of 67 dental scientists and educators assured the high quality of its content.[22] The stature of the *Journal of Dental Research* was further ensured by its freedom from commercial influence, as it was produced without the support of advertising dollars.[22]

The *Journal of the National Dental Association* began publishing in 1913. As the official organ of the National Dental Association, it had a large number of subscribers and was thus a financially independent publication. It evolved into the *Journal of the American Dental Association* in 1922.[20] In 1937, *Dental Cosmos* was merged with the *Journal of the American Dental Association*.[20]

State Boards of Examiners

The first law to regulate dental practice in the United States was passed in Alabama when its legislature ruled in 1841 that to obtain licensure to practice dentistry in Alabama, one had to pass an examination administered by the state medical board, whose membership included one dentist.[20] Although the intent of the law was to decrease the number of ill-trained dentists, Dexter suggested that if this law suppressed some irregular practitioners, it had little effect in elevating the overall standards of the dental profession.[1] Progress in elevating standards would come through the establishment of journalism and dental colleges, a process begun by Chapin Harris in 1840 with the founding of the Baltimore College of Dental Surgery and the appearance of the first dental periodicals.

Chapin Harris objected to placing dental licensure in the hands of the medical profession:

> *The insuperable objection to committing the interests of dental surgery into the keeping of the general surgeon and the physician is, that gentlemen who are only medically educated, as far as it regards dental surgery are oftentimes as ignorant as the most unlearned. The medical colleges have never taught this branch of surgery in its most important and difficult operations, and hundreds of (medical) students are graduated yearly who do not really know how to extract a tooth scientifically.*[1]

Harris's preferred remedy for regulating dental practice was through the union of educated dentists in state dental societies backed by law. Despite the growth of dental schools and the increased numbers of dental graduates from 1840 to 1860, there was a demand to legitimize dentists who were not graduates of dental colleges through examination by appointed State Boards of Examiners. In 1859, in support of this change, Dr A. Westcott argued before the New York State Dental Association:

> *My position was, and is, that a certain number of years' practice as a dental surgeon should render one eligible, not necessarily to a degree, but simply to an examination. The more I have reflected upon the subject of the best method of elevating the standard of the profession, the more I am impressed with the belief that it can never be done without some agency by which we can assert the practitioners already in the field.... If a State Institute can be established with a competent board of directors, who shall, from year to year, appoint an able and impartial Board of examiners, before whom the qualifications of all, say of five years' standing, may be fully tested, will it not tend to draw a line of demarcation between those who are worthy, and those who are not. It would furnish a scale by which each could get his true weight or measure, and a legal certificate, if he came up to a proper stand.*[24]

Change came in 1868 with the passage of legislation to incorporate the Dental Society of the State of New York with powers to appoint a board of censors for the purpose of examining candidates for licensure. Successful candidates were granted a diploma and the degree of Master of Dental Surgery. Graduates of dental colleges were licensed without examination. By 1876, Ohio, Georgia, New Jersey, and Pennsylvania had passed laws regulating the practice of dentistry through examination and/or graduation from a reputable dental college.[1]

The power of the state boards to rule on the status of a dental college and to invalidate its diplomas was tested in 1883 before the Supreme Court of Illinois in the case of Isaac Sheppard, a graduate of the Indiana Dental College who was denied a license to practice in Illinois on the basis that the Indiana Dental College was not a "reputable" college.[25]

Sheppard vs the State of Illinois

The dental practice act of the State of Illinois made it unlawful for any person to practice dentistry unless he had received a diploma from a reputable dental college or had been granted a license from the State Board of Dental Examiners upon satisfactory completion of its examination. The examination could be waived, for a fee, for a graduate of a reputable college. Isaac Sheppard, a graduate of the Indiana Dental College, was refused a license to practice by the Illinois State Board of Dental Examiners on the grounds that the Indiana Dental College was not a reputable school. Sheppard petitioned the Illinois Supreme Court for a license without examination on the basis that the Board of Examiners had no authority to decide the issue of whether a school was reputable or not.

In a landmark decision, the Supreme Court of Illinois upheld the State Board of Dental Examiners' discretionary power to determine the status of a dental college and the value of its diploma. At the trial, Judge Scholfield explained that the term "reputable" was meant to express the fact that there were some factors beyond matters of curriculum that characterized a school's merit. The sale of diplomas without recognition of scholarship was a factor that could cause a school to drop from the ranks of the reputable. The court explained that whether a college is reputable is a question of fact to be decided by the Board, that the responsibility of investigation, judgment, and discretion—of ascertaining and determining the facts—rested with it and that no other tribunal was authorized to review, set aside, or confirm the exercise of that discretion by the Board.

The Board having decided that in its judgment the curriculum of study and requirements for graduation of the Indiana Dental College were not such as to entitle it to be classed as a "reputable" dental college, the petition for a mandamus was therefore denied. The grounds for the refusal by the Board was that the Indiana Dental College, although it prescribed regular courses of study, did not require actual attendance at its lectures before graduation but granted diplomas on evidence of the fitness of the candidate to practice as determined by examination, without reference to when or where the fitness was acquired. The Board contended that such power is dangerously liable to abuse.

The editors of *Dental Cosmos* wrote that the judicial power of state boards "to determine questions of fact is, we think, essential to the carrying out of the legislative intention in the enactment of laws to ensure the better education of practitioners of dental surgery and to regulate the practice of dentistry, and the profession is to be congratulated upon the legal confirmation of their powers in this respect."

Backed by law, the State Boards of Dental Examiners were able to check the growth of low-quality schools by rejecting their graduates from entrance to the licensure examinations. They also eliminated the granting of diplomas by dental societies. The examiners also influenced the dental curriculum through the content of written examinations.

In 1883, members of several state boards met to establish the National Association of Dental Examiners.[26] This body was instrumental in creating standards for the examination of candidates and assisted new states in creating regulatory legislation. The National Association of Dental Examiners created uniform standards for the written examinations and abolished the practice of granting degrees and diplomas by local state boards.

Throughout the 19th century, the growth of dental associations at the local and state levels provided a framework for setting rules of professional conduct and standards of clinical performance. Through the interchanges of ideas at state and national meetings, a construct was forged for American dentistry. In 1895, the National Association of Dental Examiners adopted a plan to improve the quality of dental education by insisting on a minimal composition of the faculty for schools joining the Association after 1895. Every school was required to have at least three professors to teach operative dentistry, dental prosthetics, and dental pathology and therapeutics. Five professors were required to teach the basic medical sciences: anatomy, physiology, chemistry, general pathology, and materia medica.[27] Schools were required to have laboratories to teach chemistry, bacteriology, and anatomy. Prosthetic laboratories and clinical infirmaries came under closer scrutiny. On-site examinations by state board representatives led to improvements in physical facilities as well as in the organization and administration of the academic programs.

Summary

By the 1920s, in one short generation, dentistry had undergone a metamorphosis from a practice dominated by an ideal that was mechanical and artistic to a biologic orientation as the element of primary importance in dentistry.[10] But it was not until the completion of the Carnegie survey of dental schools conducted in the 1920s that major changes were put in place to elevate dental education to the same plane as medical education. The Gies Report on dental education (see chapter 17), modeled after the Flexner Report on medical education, stimulated a reformation within dental schools that led to the establishment of research-oriented dental schools staffed by scientists and full-time clinicians.

References

1. Dexter JE. A History of Dental and Oral Science in America. Philadelphia: S. S. White, 1876.
2. Hapgood RL. History of the Harvard Dental School. Boston: Harvard University, 1930.
3. Asbell MB. A Century of Dentistry: A History of the University of Pennsylvania School of Dental Medicine. Philadelphia: University of Pennsylvania, 1977.
4. McQuillen JH. Dental education. Dent Cosmos 1860;1:650–652.
5. Truman J. Dental education. Dent Cosmos 1875;17:358–362.
6. Brophy TW. Dental education. Dent Rev 1916;30:581–597.
7. Taft J. Report from the committee on curriculum. Proceedings of the National Association of Dental Faculties. Dent Cosmos 1899;41:907–908.
8. Lusk G. Medical education in the United States. Science 1913;38:491–499.
9. Garretson JE. Periscope (medical education). Dent Cosmos 1875;17:28.
10. Kirk E. The vital question. Dent Cosmos 1926;68:17–22.
11. Chandler TH. Dental education. Dent Cosmos 1875;17:362–364.
12. Black GV. A Work on Operative Dentistry, ed 3. Chicago: Medico-Dental, 1917.
13. Barker GT. Dental education. Dent Cosmos 1873;15:25–28.
14. Barker GT. Dental commencement. Dent Cosmos 1860;1:477–479.
15. Arthur R. Opening address, sixth annual meeting of the Southern Dental Association. Dent Cosmos 1875;17:57–72.
16. Arthur R. Opening address, partly delivered at the Sixth Annual Meeting of the Southern Dental Association held at St Louis, July 28, 1874. Dent Cosmos 1875;17:57–72.
17. Arthur R. Dental education. Dent Cosmos 1876;18:62–69.
18. Stainton CW. Ought the formation of dental schools be limited? Dent Cosmos 1895;37:778–782.
19. Talbot ES. Science in dentistry. Dent Cosmos 1894;36:737–739.
20. Lufkin AW. A History of Dentistry. Philadelphia: Lea & Febiger, 1948.
21. Ward ML. Landmarks in dental education. Dent Cosmos 1934;76:3–23.
22. Taylor JA. History of Dentistry. Philadelphia: Lea and Febiger, 1922.
23. McQuillen JH. Dental journals. Dent Cosmos 1859;1:135–137.
24. Westcott A. New York State Dental Association (proceedings). Dent Cosmos 1859;1:133–135.
25. The power of state boards of dental examiners. Dent Cosmos 1884;26:438–440.
26. National Association of Dental Examiners. Dent Cosmos 1883;25:455–457.
27. National Association of Dental Examiners. Dent Cosmos 1895;37:866–868.

8

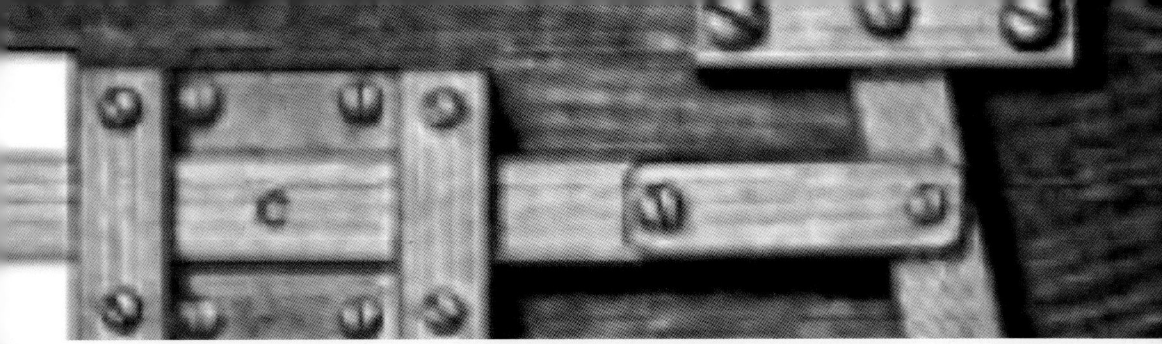

Exemplars of the New Profession

Every profession has its pioneers, men and women who demonstrated vision, determination, intelligence, and unusual energy in leading their contemporaries toward a more perfect construct of their chosen field of activity, whether it be in medicine, law, architecture, or any other branch of human endeavor. Dentistry has its heroes, men who shaped the profession, often in the face of opposition and criticism. The following men made their mark during the last half of the 19th century, the crucial formative years of the dental profession, as dental schools, examining boards, and professional societies were taking shape. They represent but a few of the men who dedicated enormous energy to bring dentistry out of an unregulated, unscientific, and chaotic past to its modern state of professionalism.

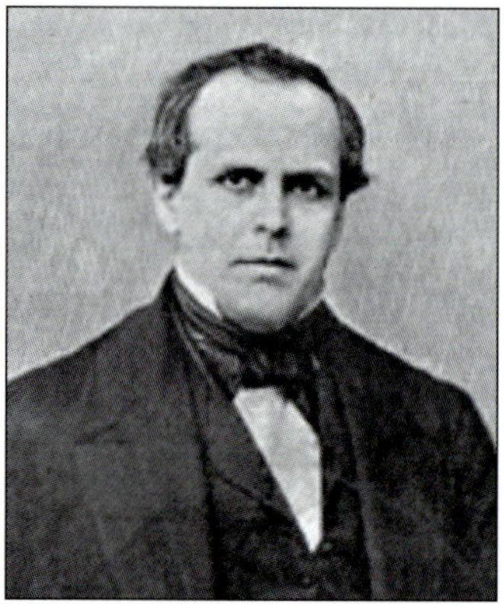

Fig 8-1 Chapin Harris, 1806–1860.

Chapin A. Harris: Reformer, Educator, and Visionary

Chapin A. Harris (Fig 8-1) was born in Pompey, New York in 1806. He learned medicine and dentistry as an apprentice to his older brother, Dr John Harris, a practitioner of medicine in Madison, Ohio.[1] John Harris must have placed importance on the dental health of his patients and must have been convinced that dental practice constituted a viable profession, because he served as preceptor to Chapin Harris, James Taylor, and John Allen and thus deserves credit for assisting the early development of dental education.[2]

After passing the State of Ohio's Board of Medical Censor's examination in 1824, Chapin Harris opened a medical practice in Greenfield, Ohio. He developed a strong interest in the dental component of medical practice, and after several years of practicing medicine in Ohio, his practice had become almost exclusively limited to dentistry. In 1833, he took further steps to strengthen his expertise in dentistry by studying with Dr Horace H. Hayden in Baltimore, Maryland. Hayden had been practicing dentistry in Baltimore for nearly 30 years. He held a license from the Medical and Surgical Faculty of Maryland, where he lectured on dentistry to students of the medical school.[3] Eugene Cordell of the University of Maryland, writing in his history of that institution, stated that Horace Hayden "was accustomed to hold classes in dentistry in his offices at night with no light but the fallow dip.... That dentists should be educated like other

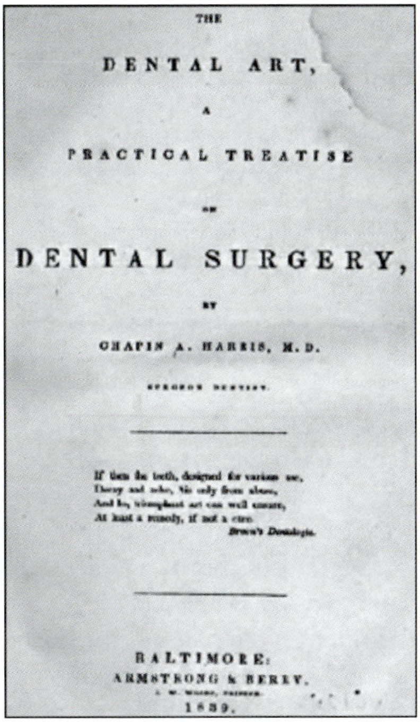
THE

DENTAL ART,

A

PRACTICAL TREATISE

ON

DENTAL SURGERY,

BY

CHAPIN A. HARRIS, M.D.

[illegible]

BALTIMORE:

ARMSTRONG & BERRY.

1839.

Fig 8-2 Harris's textbook on dental practice, the first of its kind in America.

professional men in schools and colleges was a thought often brought out by Hayden in his conversation, and he always regarded dentistry to be a mere branch of medicine."[4]

Chapin Harris settled in Baltimore in 1835 and obtained a license from the Medical and Surgical Faculty of Maryland to practice medicine and dentistry. One of Harris's early interests was in writing articles for the medical literature. His broad knowledge and his belief that it should be shared soon led to the publication of his first book, *The Dental Art, A Practical Treatise on Dental Surgery* (Fig 8-2), in 1839.[1] In the preface to his book, Harris noted that "for a long time [I have] thought that there was still wanting a treatise, that should possess a more practical character, especially as regards mechanical dentistry, than any that have hitherto been published in America."

Harris deplored the current state of mechanical dentistry being practiced by many of his colleagues:

> *The construction and insertion of artificial teeth is an operation which, though acknowledged to be of great importance, and performed by everyone having any pretension to a knowledge of dentistry, is, unfortunately, but little understood by the majority of practitioners. Notwithstanding the triumphs of Mechanical Dentistry, and the high state of excellence to which it has arrived, at no previous time was there ever so much injury inflicted, and suffering occasioned by artificial teeth, as at present—resulting solely from their bad construction and incorrect application. That such should be the case, when there are so many scientific and skillful dentists in every city, and in many of the villages of the country, may seem strange, but the fact is nevertheless undeniable.*[1]

Harris explained that the deplorable condition of dentistry was due, in part, to an insufficient development of intelligent and skilled dental practitioners, a problem that in his view could be corrected by the establishment of dental schools and dental journals. In recognition of the need for special schools of dental education, Drs Harris and Hayden, joined by several medical colleagues, moved to create a dental school in Baltimore, Maryland. Initially, they petitioned the Medical Department of the University of Maryland to establish a subdivision for dental education within the medical program. The failure of this attempt was in part due to the Medical Department's financial difficulties related to a long-standing lawsuit, and in the medical faculty's opinion, dentistry was an "insignificant subject," inconsequential to medicine.[4] For most physicians, dentistry was a trade, too young and unscientific to earn the respect of the medical establishment:

> *The professional dentist occupied a curious position…a harmless quack who was endeavoring to perform a certain work which in part they had previously performed, but as it was disagreeable work and not especially remunerative moreover, they were quite willing that the dentist should have it, and smiled complacently when he answered to the title of doctor.*[5]

Harris and Hayden were not deterred, and with the signatures of numerous citizens and prominent dental practitioners, they petitioned the Maryland State Legislature for a statute for the incorporation of an independent College of Dental Surgery in Baltimore[1,4] (Fig 8-3). A legislative charter was approved in 1839, and the world's first dental school was opened in 1840 with Hayden as dean (1839–1840), who was followed in that post by Harris from 1840 to 1842. The act of incorporation named Horace Hayden as professor of dental pathology and physiology, Chapin Harris as professor of practi-

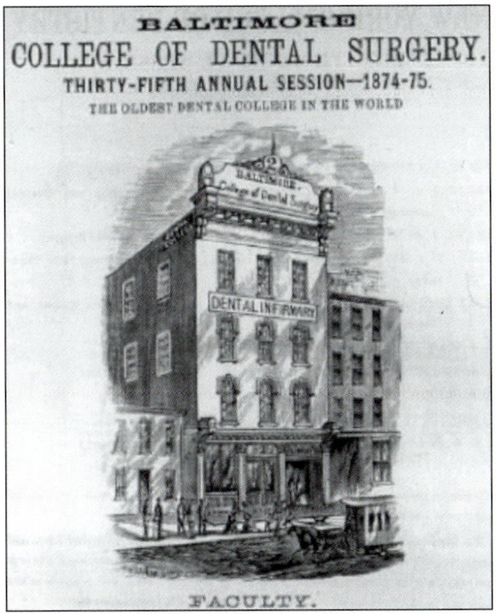

Fig 8-3 The second home of the Baltimore College of Dental Surgery.

cal dentistry, Thomas Bond as professor of special dental pathology and therapeutics, and H. Willis Baxley as professor of special dental anatomy and physiology.[6] Solyman Brown and Eleazar Parmly were also among the promoters of the new school.

In recognizing the importance of Chapin Harris in the early development of the dental profession, one must give equal credit to Horace Hayden, because Harris modeled himself after the older and more experienced clinician.[7] It was said of Hayden that he was "the strong man and the power behind the throne in organizing dentistry from a trade into a truly scientific profession. It was Hayden who furnished the gray matter."[8,9] Taylor stated that it was the "ripe thought and experience of Dr. Hayden combined with the unlimited activity and power for work of the youthful Dr. Harris" that elevated American dentistry to a position of prominence.[1]

The same nucleus of men who founded the world's first dental school also started the first national dental organization, the American Society of Dental Surgeons, in 1840. Chapin Harris served as its first corresponding secretary and in 1844 as its president. The mission of the society was to improve the profession of dentistry through better education and regulation of practice. It strived to eliminate charlatanism and to diminish faulty dental services, often attributed to the use of amalgam as a restorative material. Most members of the society were staunch supporters of the use of gold as the best dental restorative material and outspoken hard-liners against the use of plastic (amalgam) filling materials. The value of gold versus silver-amalgam as a filling material was hotly debated in the mid 19th century, as was the use of the newly developed vulcanite as a cheap replacement for costly precious-metal denture bases. Harris and his colleagues agreed with old-guard conservatives that there was no better material than gold foil for permanent filling of teeth. He viewed amalgam as abominable: "It is the most pernicious material that has ever been employed for filling teeth." His low opinion of amalgam continued to be expressed throughout his life, as noted in the eighth edition of his textbook, wherein he stated: "In the first edition of this work, the author expressed his disapprobation of the employment of this article; since which time he has had abundant opportunity of observing its effects, and is fully confirmed in the unfavorable opinion which he then expressed with regard to it." Harris stressed that mercury was "the mischievous ingredient" capable of injuring tissues and discoloring the teeth.

Although Harris and his colleagues discouraged the widespread use of amalgam in dental practice, and thus an affordable treatment for less affluent patients, they did promote high standards of care by education and vigilance and in the process elevated the dental profession.

The second edition of Harris's textbook, entitled *Principles and Practice of Dental Surgery,* went through 11 editions, serving as the most used textbook in American dental education during the last half of the 19th century. Each edition of this textbook contained new material adapted from the work of many of the most important contemporary scientists and clinicians. In his coverage of what was then known of the basic science of dental tissues, Harris revealed his acquaintance with the latest discoveries and controversies, citing the histologic studies of Tomes, Nasmyth, Purkinje, Raschkow, Kölliker, Hunter, and Retzius. The enlarged and revised eighth edition (1863), published 3 years after his death, was a monumental work of 890 pages encompassing all aspects of the basic science and clinical disciplines of dental practice.[10] It was divided into seven parts: anatomy and physiology, physical characteristics, diseases of the teeth and their treatment, diseases of the gums and alveolar processes, mechanical dentistry (including operative, surgical, and prosthetics), and diseases and defects of the palate. It contained everything that a dental student needed to learn during his brief time in dental school.

The year 1840 was another turning point in the history of dentistry in that Dr Harris founded the world's first dental periodical, *The American Journal of Dental Science*. He served as its editor until his death in 1860. In 1849, Harris published a 779-page *Dictionary of Dental Surgery, Biography, Bibliography and Medical Terminology*, believed to have been the first of its kind. In the preface to the second edition of this dictionary, Harris admitted that he had erred in the first edition by not including purely medical and collateral science terms:

> *A more extended view of the subject was necessary, since the scope of professional education for the dentist has become so widened that general Medicine and Collateral Science are now, to a considerable extent, embraced in the curriculum of dental study. He has therefore, introduced into the present edition, not only the words and phrases purposely omitted in the first, but also those that have been added to the literature of the above-mentioned department of science, thus making it a complete Dictionary of Medicine as well as of Dental Surgery.*[1]

The DDS degree was conferred on Dr Harris by virtue of his membership in the American Society of Dental Surgeons. Prior to state statutes legalizing the conferring of dental degrees solely by accredited dental colleges, dental societies granted DDS degrees to members who had met specified apprenticeships and/or medical school training. In 1838, while serving as a professor at Washington Medical College in Baltimore, Harris was the recipient of an honorary MD degree from that institution.

Dr Harris is said to have been a generous soul, who, despite his large dental practice, died a poor man in Baltimore in 1860. Dr Charles McManus wrote that Dr Harris "not only labored harder, but spent more time and money for the advancement of his profession, than any other man."[11]

Dr Chapin Harris was instrumental in creating the first dental college, the first dental journal, and the first formal dental society—the tripod on which a profession is established. For these advances, he is regarded as a leader in the development of the dental profession.

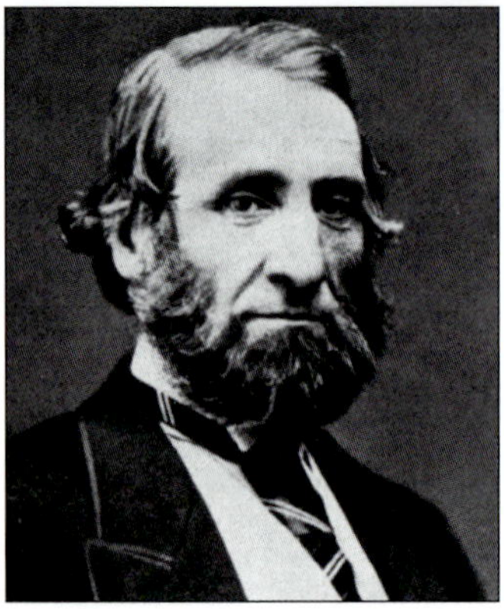

Fig 8-4 Sir John Tomes.

Sir John Tomes: Leading British Dental Scientist and Clinician

Sir John Tomes (Fig 8-4) deserves to be included among the pioneers whose dedicated service elevated dentistry to its scientific and professional status. Tomes, a complete professional, encompassed research, clinical practice, and professional leadership, sharing the same stature as G. V. Black, his American counterpart.

John Tomes attended schools in Stratford upon Avon and Evesham, England, where at the age of 21 years he was apprenticed to Thomas F. Smith, a physician.[12] After 5 years of apprenticeship, he began medical school courses in 1836 at London's King's College and at the Middlesex Hospital, where he served as house surgeon from 1839 to 1840. From 1840 to 1843, he was a dental surgeon at King's College Hospital, and for the next 30 years he practiced dental surgery at Middlesex Hospital.[12]

From the time he began his medical studies, Tomes was intrigued by the microscopic anatomy of dental tissues. In 1838, while still a student, he presented his first paper to the Royal Society. According to his son, Charles S. Tomes, many of John Tomes's evenings were spent in studies and discussions of microscopic anatomy with a group of enthusiasts.[13] He soon became a member of the newly established Microscopical Society. Through careful management of his income, he managed to purchase a Powell microscope, considered to be among the best made at the time. As house surgeon at King's College Hospital and later at Middlesex Hospital, he had a steady supply of extracted teeth for study.[13]

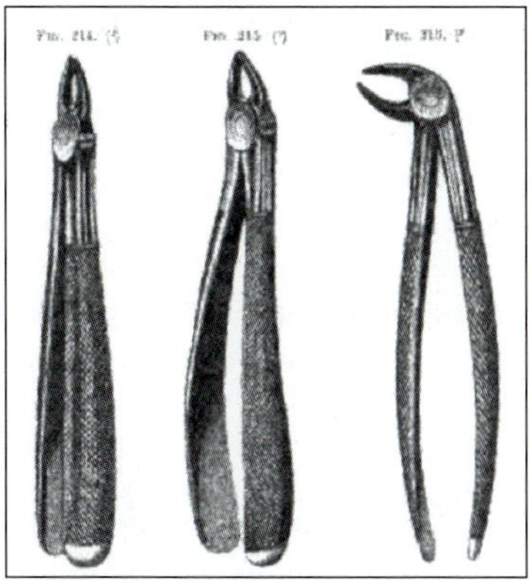

Fig 8-5 Special extraction forceps designed by John Tomes.

His expertise in dental surgery led to a request in 1845 from the officers of the Middlesex Hospital School of Medicine that he give a series of lectures on dental physiology and surgery to the medical students. These lectures were assembled and published in 1848,[14] later forming the basis for his 1859 *A System of Dental Surgery*.[15] This book covered all aspects of dental histopathology as well as the newly developing basic science of dentistry. It describes mid 19th century diagnosis and treatment for irregularities in the development and eruption of the teeth, caries, periosteal and alveolar inflammation, dental abscesses, cysts, neuralgias, and other pathologic conditions of the jaws.[15] Mechanical dentistry and the fabrication of dentures were described in a separate publication by Tomes.[16] In addition to revealing wide clinical experience, Tomes also demonstrated his inventiveness, describing newly designed forceps specially adapted to each tooth type[15] (Fig 8-5). These forceps became widely popular and have been in use since their invention. Tomes also described a new machine called the "dentifactor," which he designed for the shaping of denture bases. It used the same principle as the lathe for shaping wood or other material.

Tomes noted that there was no practical use for the transplantation of teeth. He observed that most transplanted teeth were lost within a few years as a result of root resorption. Furthermore, in his opinion, the risk of transmission of syphilis precluded any consideration of this operation.

In 1849, he reported to the Royal Society his observations on the teeth of marsupials, wherein he took exception to the prior work of Sir Richard Owen.[1] Tomes noted that the dentinal tubules of marsupials coursed from dentine into the enamel:

> *The enamel presents a very strongly-marked peculiarity, common (so far as I have examined), with one exception only, to all marsupial teeth, and present only in a very limited number of other mammalian teeth. The main peculiarity to which I allude, is that the greater number, if not all, of the dentinal tubes are continued into, and constitute a considerable portion of the enamel.*

In 1850, Tomes presented his work on the microscopic anatomy of the dental tissues of the order Rodentia.[17] He reported on upwards of 60 members of this order, noting a structural peculiarity, the lamellated arrangement of the fibrils (prisms) in the inner zone of the enamel.

His most famous discovery was the presence of dentinal fibrils within the dentinal tubules[18] (Fig 8-6). In his 1856 report to the Royal Society, he stated the following:

> *On reviewing the various circumstances under which dentine evinces sensibility, and those under which that sensibility is lost, it is difficult to avoid the conclusion, that the dentinal tubes are in some way the medium through which sensation is distributed through the substance of the tissue. But if the sole office of the tubes be the conveyance of nutrient fluid derived from the pulp, the difficulty of accounting for the sensitiveness of the dentine remains, inasmuch as we have no instance of sensation being manifested in a fluid. We might seem to get out of the difficulty by assuming that the dentinal tubes are constantly filled by fluid, and that pressure made upon the exposed ends of the tubes is felt by the pulp at their inner extremities. This assumption does not, however, account for all the circumstances of the case, failing altogether to explain the greater sensibility of the dentine at one part of the tooth than at another. The want of accordance between the views usually entertained upon the structure of dentine and the physiological conditions manifested by that tissue when in connexion with the body, has wholly arisen from assuming that the dentinal tubes are solely for the conveyance of fluid, and that they are otherwise empty. With the hope of gaining some further knowledge upon this point, I commenced a series of observations, the results of which it is the main purpose of this paper to communicate. When these investigations were commenced, I had but little expectation of finding that one of the most important parts in dental structure had been overlooked, namely, that each dentinal tube is permanently tenanted by a soft fibril, which after passing from the pulp into the tubes, follows their ramifications.*[18]

[1] Owen R. Odontography; Or, A Treatise on the Comparative Anatomy of Teeth. London: H. Bailliere, 1840–1845.

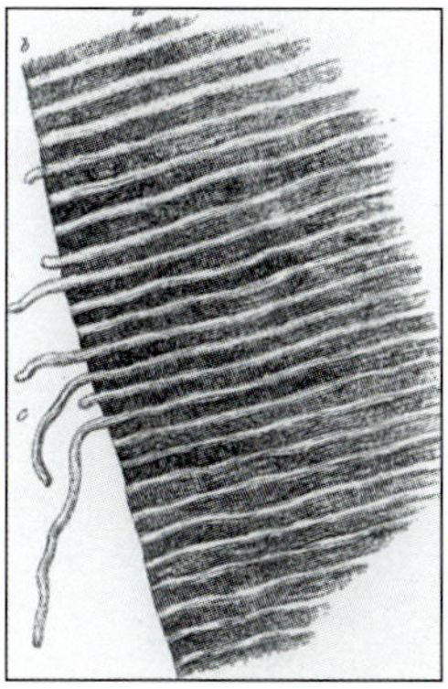

Fig 8-6 Dentinal fibrils, as drawn by Tomes.

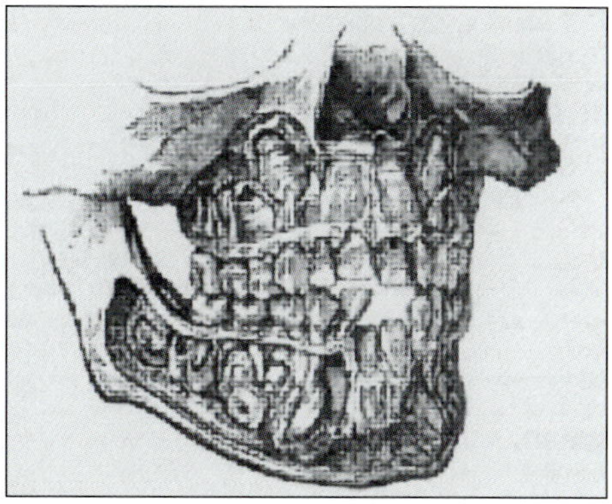

Fig 8-7 Mixed dentition illustrated by Tomes.

The "dentinal soft fibril" is a cytoplasmic process or extension of the odontoblast. In addition to the presence of the odontoblast process within the dentinal tubule, nerve fibrils also occupy parts of the dentinal tubules. Although Tomes was unable to clarify the exact nature of the dentinal fibril, he was perceptive in linking pain sensation to the dentinal tubules and the soft fibrils. Tomes concluded: "That dentine owes its sensation to the presence of the dentinal fibrils cannot, I think, be readily doubted, seeing that if their connexion with the pulp be cut off by the destruction of the latter, all sensation is at once lost."[18]

The first section of *A System of Dental Surgery* devotes 117 pages to a comprehensive discussion of "teething," or the development and eruption of the primary and permanent teeth. The discussion is beautifully illustrated by numerous engravings depicting the relationship between the teeth in each jaw during growth from infancy to young adulthood (Fig 8-7). Tomes notes:

> *It would perhaps be difficult to find a more interesting subject for investigation, than the progressive changes in form and of relative proportion between the various parts of the jaws during infancy which occur as necessary consequences of their mode of growth, and are connected with the development and arrangement of the teeth.*[15]

In his studies of the shedding of primary teeth, Tomes noted that the nature of the resorption of the hard tissues was of "great physiological interest." In cementum, dentin, and enamel, where the teeth are undergoing resorption, Tomes saw "the same characteristic surface as that shown by bone when undergoing a similar action—namely a surface full of deep indentations, as though they had been

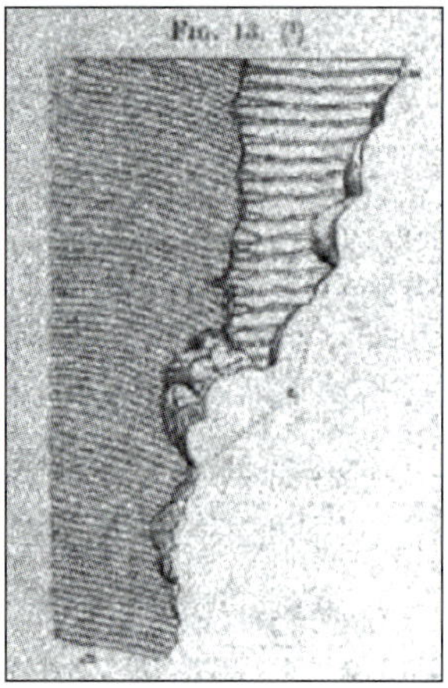

Fig 8-8 Gouged-out surface of dentin of an exfoliating primary tooth, as drawn by Tomes (1873).

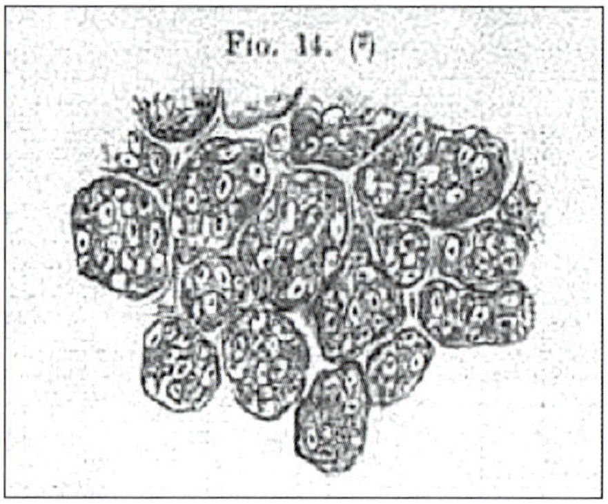

Fig 8-9 En-face view of cell clusters (giant cells) on the surface of resorbing dentin, as drawn by Tomes (1873).

made by a sharp piercing instrument, having a semicircular extremity" (Fig 8-8). Within these indentations, he observed the presence of "peculiar multiform cells, each one being composed of several smaller cells, the number varying from two or three to as many as fourteen or fifteen"[19] (Fig 8-9). These have since been established to be multinucleated osteoclasts. He observed the same cells in contact with resorbing bone, cementum, and enamel. Tomes was "irresistibly led... to the conclusion that the superficial compound cells are the immediate agents by which the tissues are removed." Although he admitted that "The precise nature of the action by which the cells eat away the hard tooth structures still remains a matter of great uncertainty," he had made some remarkable observations, and his interpretations were at the forefront of physiologic and histologic studies of his day.

From his microscopic studies of normal dentinal tissues, he turned his attention to investigate the nature of dentinal caries.[2] He noted the growth of microorganisms within the dentinal tubules at the advancing front of the caries lesion. Tomes recognized the correctness of Miller's research demonstrating the bacterial production of acid as the key factor in the demineralization of enamel and dentin, concluding that "a decalcification of enamel and subjacent dentine having been effected, these or other bacteria enter the tubes of the dentine, and, acting from thence, effect the solution of the decalcified matrix by a kind of peptonising action."[20]

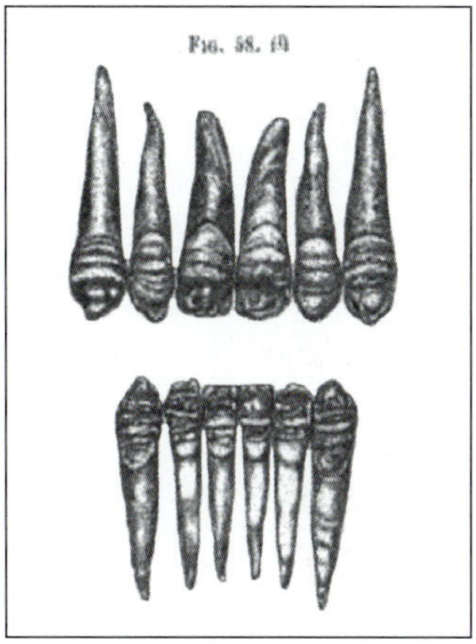

Fig 8-10 Incisors and canines marked by horizontal grooves and ridges caused by systemic disease, as drawn by Tomes.

In *A System of Dental Surgery*, Tomes reported extensively on developmental defects. Here he correctly recognized the pernicious action of systemic diseases or metabolic stress upon the development of enamel and dentin. He described cases of teeth marked

> *by grooves and ridges, very regularly disposed [Fig 8-10]. The grooves are the result of imperfect, and the ridges of perfect development of the enamel and subjacent dentine.... Although in many, it is not in all cases easy to trace this ridged, or pitted, or honeycombed condition of the teeth to the presence of serious indisposition of the patient during the period when the defective portions of the teeth were being developed; it can, however, be scarcely doubted that an imperfect organization of the teeth, if not the result of some special disease, such as measles, influencing the system generally, is yet consequent upon a constitutional condition. The fact that if one tooth is affected, those parts of other teeth which correspond in respect to the period of formation will present a similar condition, precludes the supposition that the effect has been produced*

[2] Charles S. Tomes (1846–1928), the son of John Tomes (1815–1895), completed medical school before entering into a long collaboration with his father in clinical dentistry, research, and dental education. Charles was co-author of the second (1873) and subsequent editions of *A System of Dental Surgery*. In the publication of the revised second edition, the contributions of John and Charles are conflated to such a degree that any effort to assign primacy of discovery or thought to either man is almost impossible. Both men shared a keen interest in dental histology, dental pathology, operative and mechanical dentistry, and dental education, all of which is expounded upon in the 1873 and later editions of the *System*. It must be assumed that with each edition, Charles's contributions grew both in number and importance, and thus the son must get a good deal of credit for the enlightened observations contained in their classic textbook. The observations on microbes and dental caries contained in the 1897 edition are likely to have been those of Charles Tomes.

by a merely local cause. The evidence points to a general cause, but it will not uncommonly be very difficult to discover the precise nature of that cause.[19]

Both John's and his son Charles's curiosity was not confined to histology; they were just as enthusiastically involved with matters of clinical practice. At a time when there was considerable discussion over the appropriate use of amalgam as a restorative material, they expressed the opinion that each filling material had its advantages:

It may, I think, be assumed as a settled point, that for dental purposes a pure metal, such as gold, or even tin, is in all respects preferable to any mixtures of metals at present known. But there are cases in which the one can be used while the other cannot. The American writers on dental surgery have urged every possible argument against the use of amalgams, and have gone, so far as to pass rules for the expulsion from dental societies of members who would not pledge themselves to discontinue the use of mercurial fillings (mercury-containing amalgams). Yet there are teeth the condition of which is such that gold fillings cannot be inserted with any chance of success, but which, if plugged with a good amalgam, will last for years, and be perfectly effective for a long period.[15]

Up until the mid 19th century in England, there were no specific qualifications for dental practice. Dental care was conducted by barbers, wigmakers, silversmiths, apothecaries, and a smaller number of practitioners who held diplomas from the Royal College of Surgeons.[21] John Tomes was ever concerned with the large number of unqualified individuals who practiced dentistry on Londoners. Tomes summarized the situation as follows:

At this time there were a limited number of practitioners of education and well-earned eminence, others of humbler educational rank, and a strong contingent of advertising dentists. Then there was no prescribed dental education, each person who would be a dentist had to learn the science and art with the assistance of a teacher or master, or by the exercise of his own powers of observation in the conduct of such practice as came within his reach.[12]

From 1843 onward, John Tomes, leading a small group of prominent dentists, worked to correct this situation by petitioning the Royal College of Surgeons to create a specific examination for licensure in dental surgery. He was instrumental in forming the Odontological Society of London in 1856 and the London School of Dental Surgery in 1859.[12] Through the efforts of John Tomes and a few of his colleagues, the LDS degree (License in Dental Surgery) was instituted as a prerequisite for admission to the department of dental surgery

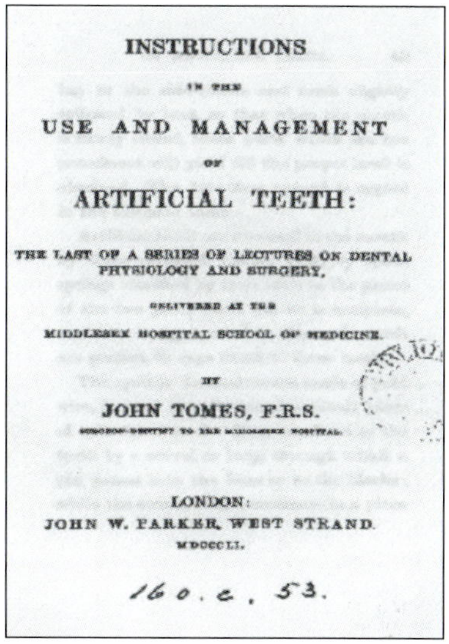
INSTRUCTIONS

IN THE

USE AND MANAGEMENT

OF

ARTIFICIAL TEETH:

THE LAST OF A SERIES OF LECTURES ON DENTAL PHYSIOLOGY AND SURGERY,

DELIVERED AT THE

MIDDLESEX HOSPITAL SCHOOL OF MEDICINE.

BY

JOHN TOMES, F.R.S.

SURGEON-DENTIST TO THE MIDDLESEX HOSPITAL.

LONDON:
JOHN W. PARKER, WEST STRAND.
MDCCCLI.

160.c.53.

Fig 8-11 Tomes's textbook describing his clinical techniques for the construction of artificial teeth.

of the Royal College of Surgeons. Under this agreement, a board of examiners consisting of three licensed dentists (Tomes among them) and three surgeons of the Royal College of Surgeons conducted the first LDS examinations in 1860.[21] In that year, 43 members of the dental profession successfully passed this examination. Tomes had played a key role in achieving formal recognition for dentistry and had established a professional rapprochement between dental surgeons and the medical establishment represented by the Royal College of Surgeons.[12]

However, it was not until 1878 that the government entered the picture, again after the petitioning by John Tomes and his colleagues, by instituting the Dentists Act of 1878, which called for a dentist registry under the control of the government's General Medical Council.[21] The Dentists Register of 1879 listed slightly more than 5,000 practitioners of which only 483 held the LDS degree. Unregistered dentists continued to practice in England until 1921, when a new Practice Act was passed to limit dental practice to only those registered and qualified practitioners.[21] John Tomes was also among the leaders who formed the British Dental Association in 1880.

Based on his contributions to the science and practice of dentistry (Fig 8-11), his advancement of the literature through his many publications, and most importantly his successful efforts to regulate the practice of dentistry, John Tomes led the advancement of the profession and set standards to be emulated by others in the coming 20th century.

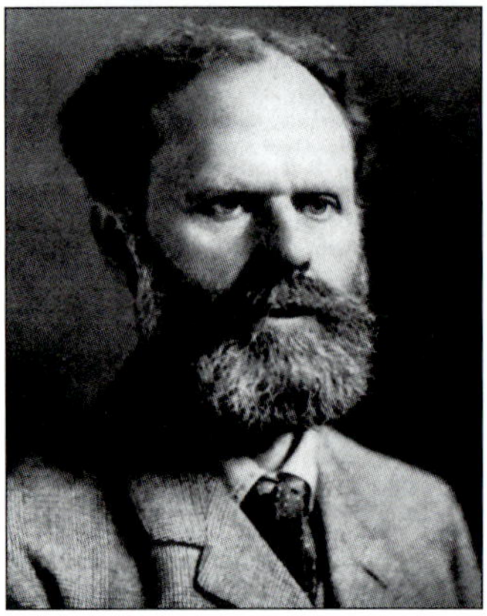

Fig 8-12 W. D. Miller.

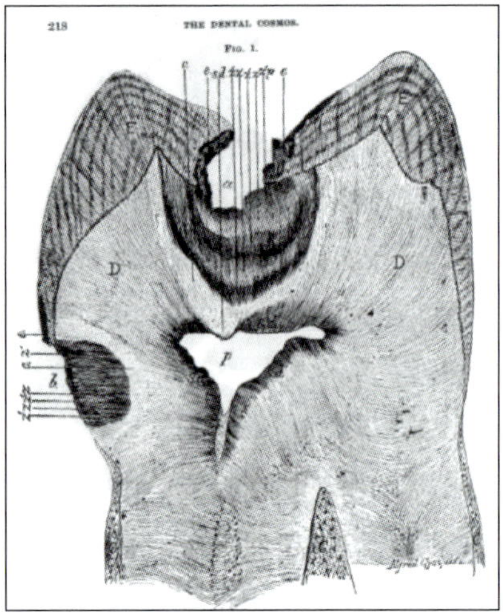

Fig 8-13 Section of human tooth depicting dental decay. (Adapted from Gysi.[22])

Willoughby D. Miller: Father of Scientific Dentistry

W. D. Miller (Fig 8-12) is considered to be the "father of scientific dentistry." As the first well-educated research scientist within the dental profession, he achieved fame by unlocking the true nature of dental decay (Fig 8-13). Miller was born in 1853 in Licking County, Ohio, not far from the city of Alexandria, where he was raised on the family farm. After the Miller family moved to Newark, Ohio, he graduated from high school in 1871 and went off to continue his education at the University of Michigan. At Michigan he majored in organic chemistry, graduating with honors in 1875. In that same year, Miller took a major step by moving to Edinburgh, Scotland. He enrolled in the University of Edinburgh to further his studies in chemistry, mathematics, and natural philosophy under Professor Sir William Thomson. What prompted him to make that move and how he was able to afford living abroad is unclear. Miller, at the young age of 22 years, knew that his future success would require advanced studies at the best universities in Europe. It has been suggested that at that time he was planning a career as a mining engineer.

After completing courses at Edinburgh, Miller traveled to Berlin, Germany, to continue his studies of the physical sciences. Berlin was a vibrant center of cultural activity with an excellent reputation in the industrial arts and physical sciences. Its population of over 1 million was enjoying an economic revival following Germany's victory in the Franco-German War of 1870–1871. Shortly after his arrival in Berlin, Miller suffered a nervous breakdown, which forced him to take leave from his studies for several months.[9,23]

At that time, there were many Americans living in Berlin, attracted by its culture and the ample opportunities for advancement in its growing industrial empire. Among the Americans living there was Dr F. P. Abbot, an American-trained dentist who was conducting a flourishing dental practice among the upper classes. Abbot had married the daughter of the American Minister to Germany and was well known among the Americans living in Berlin. Visitors from America were received at his home, and it was natural that Miller would eventually meet Dr Abbot. Miller, a young, attractive, and well-educated young man, would soon be introduced to Dr Abbot's only daughter, Caroline, an event that would set off chemical reactions new to the young chemist. With time, the two fell in love, vowing to live together in marriage. But Dr Abbot was not easily given to accepting the marriage proposal, because he feared that Caroline would return to America with her new husband.[23]

As Miller spent more and more of his time with the Abbot family, he became interested in dentistry, and, as a young scientist, he began to ponder some of the scientific questions that dentists hoped to answer. In 1877, less than 2 years after his arrival in Berlin, Miller returned to the United States to study dentistry at the Pennsylvania College of Dental Surgery (1877–1878), graduating in 1879 from the newly organized Dental Department of the University of Pennsylvania.[24] A model student, Miller was awarded a prize for best essay for his "Conservative Treatment of the Dental Pulp." With his DDS degree in hand, he promptly returned to Berlin as an associate in Dr Abbot's dental practice and soon-to-be son-in-law of the family.[23] But Miller's natural curiosity and scientific thinking did not end with his new career as a practicing dentist.

While in dental school, Miller had been exposed to the prevailing concepts of the causes of dental caries and periodontal disease. He must have learned of the new cellular concept of pathology and the exciting discoveries in the new science of bacteriology. Once back in Berlin, Miller began to study medicine, starting with a course in bacteriology with the now famous Dr Robert Koch.[9] Koch, while conducting a busy medical practice, performed research in his own small research laboratory that would lead to the proof that anthrax was caused by a microorganism (*Bacillus anthracis*) and its spores. In 1880, Koch moved to Berlin to accept a government post in the Imperial Health Bureau. This new appointment included a research laboratory, later known as the Institute of Hygiene, where he took on students and research assistants and continued to advance the technical aspects of bacteriology. In this institute, Koch conducted investigations on the germs that caused cholera and tuberculosis. It was in this institute that Miller learned the microbiologic techniques and the postulates (Koch's postulates) that led him to describe for the first time the mechanisms whereby dental decay was produced by microbial infection.

Nearby to the Institute of Hygiene was the more famous Virchow Institute of Pathology. It was here that the cellular theory of disease was confirmed. Medical students attending the lectures of Rudolf Virchow were taught that diseases consisted of the destruction, proliferation, or alteration of the cells, which constituted diseased tissues. It was a revolutionary concept equaling new discoveries in the bacteriology of infectious diseases. Miller must have sat in on Virchow's lectures while studying medicine, his MD degree conferred in 1885.[25]

The germ theory of diseases was capturing the attention of the entire civilized world as new findings were being announced from the Pasteur Institute in Paris and the laboratories of Virchow and Koch in Berlin. Led by the scientific findings of Louis Pasteur in France and Rudolf Virchow in Germany, the science of bacteriology was in the forefront of medical science, leading to new explanations of the causation of diseases. Miller's curiosity and formal training in bacteriology led him to investigate the role of bacteria as etiologic agents of dental caries. At that time, there were several theories of the cause of dental caries. Many advanced the notion that caries was caused by a form of inflammation, proposing that enamel, being situated at a distance from its nutrient supply (the pulpal blood vessels), was especially prone to break down during pulpal inflammation. It was similarly believed that internal caries of dentin could develop from the same causes. This explanation was first offered in the 18th century as the "vital" theory. Others advanced the theory that caries developed from the action of acids in the mouth (the chemical theory). Robertson in 1835 claimed that acids were derived from abnormal secretions and the fermentation of trapped food particles.[26] It was also proposed that caries was the outcome of the combined action of acids and internal inflammation (the chemico-vital theory). Another school advanced the chemico-parasitic theory, wherein acid

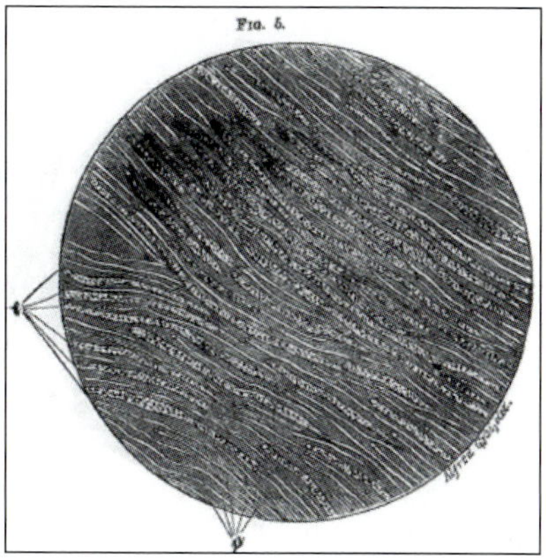

Fig 8-14 Dentinal tubules infected by micrococci. (Adapted from Gysi.[22])

decalcification of the tooth opened the way for bacterial invasion and subsequent destruction of the organic matter by bacterial secretions.

Evidence suggestive of a role for bacteria as a cause of dental caries came from microscopic study of ground sections of carious teeth.[22] When caries lesions were viewed at high magnification, bacteria were observed within the dentinal tubules. In 1868, Drs Leber and Rottenstein advanced the theory that caries was caused by "fungi," known then as *Leptothrix buccalis*.[27] Furthermore, at the International Medical Congress, held in London in 1881, Drs Miles and Underwood reported that the development of dental caries was dependent on the presence and proliferation of "organisms." They proposed the so-called septic theory, claiming that dental caries was caused by direct action of microorganisms that penetrate the dentinal tubules and destroy the organic component of the dentin, leaving the inorganic parts to be broken down and washed away in fluids of the mouth. Others, such as Dr Frank Abbott, a professor at the New York College of Dentistry, considered the presence of bacteria in carious dentin to be a secondary phenomenon, common to all decomposing organic material.[28]

Miller had also studied caries lesions by microscopy and had described the penetration of dentinal tubules by bacteria[29,30] (Fig 8-14). In examining approximately 1,000 sections of dentin, he reported that bacteria were found in every section. Miller reported a widening and distention of the tubules by growing bacterial colonies. He suggested that acid demineralization of enamel and dentin exposed the organic matrix of the tooth to a liquefaction and decomposition resulting from the necessary action of the microbes. Reporting in the journal *Dental Cosmos* in 1883, Miller stated: "I am not an advocate

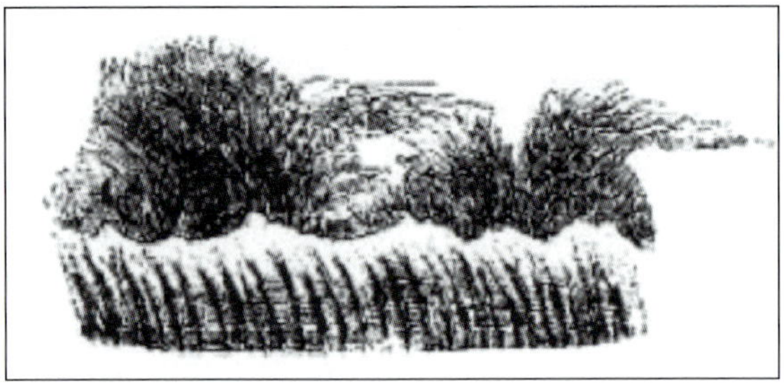

Fig 8-15 Leptothrix threads on the border of decayed dentin. (Reprinted from Miller.[31])

of the pure acid theory of caries nor of the pure germ theory; I believe rather that both acids and fungi are concerned in producing caries, that the tendency of late has been to under-estimate the former and over-estimate the latter."[27]

From a series of experiments, Miller concluded the following:

> *The general results which I have arrived at may be summed up in the following paragraphs, partly in accordance with and partly contrary to the commonly-accepted views: 1. The first stage of caries of the teeth, i. e., the extraction of the lime-salts, is for the most part caused by those acids which are generated in the mouth by fermentation. 2. Decalcification of the enamel signifies total destruction of that tissue; of dentine there remains after decalcification a tough spongy mass, which becomes subject to the invasion of enormous numbers of fungi (leptothrix-threads, bacilli, micrococci, etc.) [see Figs 8-15 to 8-17]. 3. The leptothrix-threads are found, with rare exceptions, only upon the surface, or in the superficial layers of the softened dentine, and appear to take but small part in the invasion. The bacilli, on the other hand, penetrate far into the dentine, even into the finest branches of the canaliculi. Micrococci penetrate furthest. 4. In the separate tubules is frequently to be seen a gradual change from leptothrix-threads to long bacilli, from long to short bacilli, and from the latter to micrococci. 5. The fungi produce anatomical and pathological changes in the deeper layers, stop up the canaliculi, and necessarily lead sooner or later to the death of the dentinal fibrils. The outer layers of dentine, thereby deprived of nourishment, die and fall a prey to putrefactive agents. 6. The invasion of the fungi is always preceded by the extraction of the lime-salts. 7. The fungi have not the power either to penetrate or to decalcify sound dentine, so that the infection of a perfectly sound tooth by a carious one seems to be excluded. 8. We may accordingly look upon*

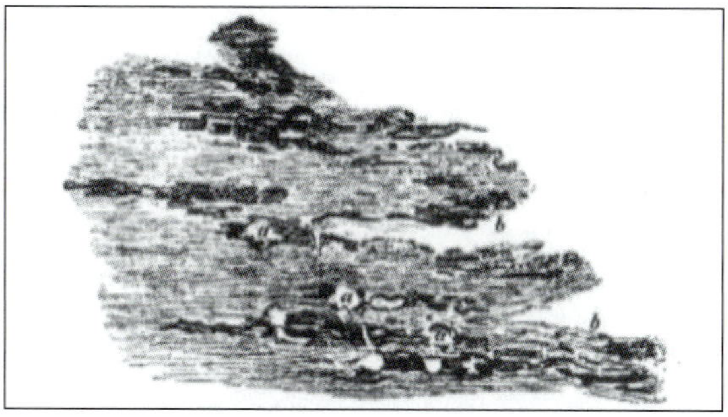

Fig 8-16 Decayed dentin showing distended tubules and invading organisms. (Reprinted from Miller.[30])

caries of the teeth as consisting of three stages: (1) decalcification; (2) infection and devitalization of the decalcified dentine; (3) putrefaction of the devitalized dentine; though it would not be easy to say just where one stage ceases and the other begins.[29]

Miller's studies of dental decay in human teeth led him to examine whether or not the teeth of different animals were susceptible to similar diseases. He confirmed that the teeth of domestic animals and more exotic animals kept in zoos did indeed undergo decay. In 1892, he reported that teeth of monkeys in captivity were highly susceptible to development of dental decay. Microscopic examinations of the decayed tissues revealed the familiar process of destruction, characterized by distended dentin tubules filled with bacteria[32] (Fig 8-16). An unusual case presented itself when he was permitted to study two manatee skulls in the Berlin Dental Institute:

I laid one of the carious teeth in water for twenty four hours in order to soften the carious dentine, which had become exceedingly dry and hard. After this time I scraped out a small piece with a spoon excavator, and prepared sections of it on the freezing microtome, which were then colored after the Gram-Gunther method. They showed under the microscope the same appearance with which we are familiar from the study of caries of human teeth.[33]

When Miller learned that an elephant in the Berlin Zoo had undergone an amputation of a tusk, he obtained a segment of the tusk for histologic study. Although elephant tusks never decayed, Miller became interested in the numerous pathologic calcifications (nodules) that were a common occurrence in the pulps of tusks. In de-

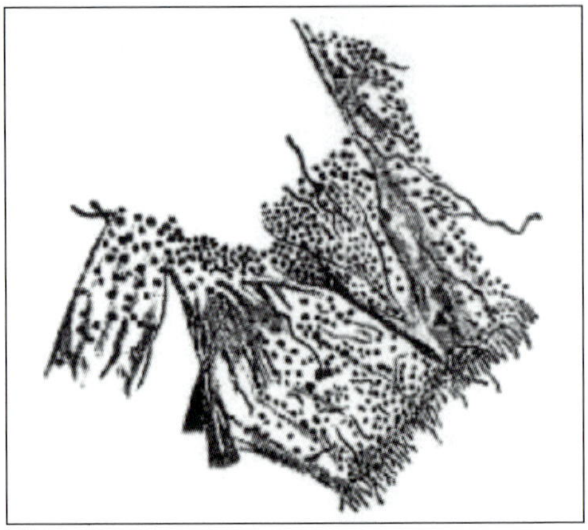

Fig 8-17 Enamel cuticle permeated by bacteria. (Reprinted from Miller.[31])

scribing his observations, Miller contributed to the discussion of the origin of the nodules and the potential for cells of the pulp to form mineralized tissues.[34]

Miller investigated the enamel cuticle, an organic deposit on the surface of teeth, as a possible substrate for the growth of bacteria. Miller observed that "the enamel cuticle in the early stages of caries forms a matrix for immense numbers of bacteria, and that the thickening of this tissue is chiefly due to growth of bacteria in or upon it"[31] (Fig 8-17). The potential significance of the cuticle and its associated bacterial growth was given impetus by the report of Williams and Black, suggesting that the "softening" of enamel in caries was caused by acids excreted by bacteria in situ. Miller had observed that areas of caries activity were almost always associated with an overlying adherent bacterial layer (a bacterial plaque). Other pioneering dental scientists, including G. V. Black, had developed the theory that the cuticle, and possibly a "gelatinous matrix" contributed by the associated microorganisms, shielded bacterial acids from the neutralizing action of saliva. Miller suspected that the importance of the gelatinous matrix had been overrated. From investigation of hundreds of teeth, Miller concluded that bacteria could establish themselves on enamel surfaces devoid of cuticle. Miller was unsure of the composition of the cuticle, and of the associated bacterial matrix, and he questioned whether the matrix could protect acids from the action of saliva.[31]

After experimenting with methods for disinfection of the mouth with various antiseptics, Miller concluded that a mouthwash consisting of a mixture of saccharine and benzoic acid, sometimes in combination with hydrogen peroxide, provided a significant reduction in oral bacteria without harming the mucosal tissues.[27] He noted that the constant presence of microorganisms in the mouth necessitated strict adherence of antiseptic procedures during oral operations and that all instruments and accessory equipment needed to be free of infectious agents.

Hans Block of Dresden, Germany, writing in *Dental Cosmos* in 1893, attacked the general concept that the cause of dental caries was the activity of microorganisms. He argued that "The real principles of etiology have to be founded upon general hygiene, and not upon microscopy...not out of observations made on little glass slabs." Hans Block did not mention the work of W. D. Miller by name, but he pitched his attack directly at the microbiologists: "The value of an antiseptic treatment of the mouth, with disregard of the much more important dietetic and hygienic regimen, is here unmasked as an irrelevant, if not a burlesque accessory."[35] One wonders if Block was not among the Germans who were jealous of the important place that the American dentist, W. D. Miller, had come to occupy in Berlin's university and medical circle. Miller's research on dental caries surpassed that of his contemporaries by his systematic and exhaustive efforts to isolate and culture the various organisms found in dental lesions. Using the classic techniques of the Koch laboratory, Miller identified 22 different species of microorganisms within the mouth, noting that 16 were capable of producing lactic acid from fermentable substances.

At the 24th annual session of the American Dental Association, Dr W. C. Barrett, chairman of the section on physiology and etiology, read a report on the etiology of dental caries in which he described Miller's work as "a course of experiments and observations such as were new to the history of dentistry." Barrett noted how Miller had made pure cultures of the bacteria isolated from caries lesions; how he studied the morphologic, physiologic, and chemical nature of these microorganisms; and how he produced artificial caries through the action of these microorganisms.[36]

Miller distinguished himself from others who had studied dental caries by his scientific approach; he relied on experimentation, not on observation alone. The accuracy of his work was supported by Koch and later confirmed by G. V. Black.[37] In 1888, the American Dental Association awarded W. D. Miller a $200 prize for the best essay on the etiology of dental caries. Dr James Truman, in a review of Miller's monograph published in *Dental Cosmos* in 1890, stated the following:

> *In closing the examination of this work of Prof. Miller, it is impossible to avoid the conclusion that it has no counterpart in dental literature. That to the author belongs the credit of finally solving the great problem of dental caries, there can be no question; but this honor must be shared with a long list of able men who laid the foundation for the final solution. Caries has been too long the opprobrium of dentistry, and it seemed, at one time, as though a solution would never be reached by one of our profession. This danger, happily, is now passed.*[38]

Dr W. C. Barrett wrote:

> *Dr Miller's views were determinedly fought, for they were in direct opposition to everything then believed. But his experience was unanswerable, and soon the best men who were examining the question, found that his arguments, and more especially his demonstrations, were irrefutable. The Germans were forced to accept his views; England followed; France was a little slower; and America finally awakened to the fact she had furnished to the world the man who had solved the problem which had been the professional question of the ages.*[23]

Miller's discoveries were widely acclaimed and soon became a favorite topic of discussion at professional meetings. At a meeting of the New York Odontological Society, held in January of 1889, Dr Robert Ormiston read a paper describing the experimental basis of Miller's germ theory of dental caries. After enumerating the many failed theories of the late 18th and early 19th centuries, Ormiston described how Miller had fulfilled Koch's postulates to prove beyond doubt that dental caries was of bacterial origin.[39]

In 1884, Miller received an appointment as Royal Professor of Operative Dentistry in the newly established German Dental Institute of the University of Berlin. Upon completion of his medical studies in 1887, Miller passed the "Rigorosum" examinations with magna cum laude honors. This success led to an additional appointment as Professor Extraordinarius in the Medical School of the University of Berlin and helped to quiet the opposition from German dentists who were jealous of Americans. They had been unsuccessful in petitioning the Minister of Education to replace him with a German dentist.[23] When it became necessary that he give up his American citizenship and become a naturalized German citizen to retain his professorship, he returned to the United States in 1907, accepting the deanship of the Dental College at the University of Michigan.

Throughout his stay in Germany, Miller practiced dentistry in association with Abbot. Well respected as a clinician, Miller treated several members of the German royal family, including the crown princess.[9] Overcoming initial opposition from German dentists, he rose in popularity and fame among his dental colleagues. As an enthusiastic member of the local professional societies, he was elected president of the Association of Dental Faculties of Germany and in 1904 president of the Federation Dentaire Internationale (FDI). He received numerous awards for his research and contributions to dentistry from dental societies throughout Europe and America, including gold medals from the FDI and the Dental Society of the State of New York. He received an honorary PhD degree from the University of Michigan and a Doctor of Science from the University of Pennsylvania. In 1906, the German Emperor recognized his accomplishment by conferring him with an appointment of Privy Counselor to the Emperor.

Miller published his classic 364-page monograph, *The Microorganisms of the Human Mouth* in 1890. Papers describing his work in dental bacteriology, pathology, and histology appeared in such journals as *Dental Cosmos*, *Independent Practitioner*, and several German-language publications. Also remarkable is the fact that despite his arduous schedule, Miller found time to play golf, becoming good enough to win the championship of Germany and Austria![40]

In 1907, soon after returning to the United States to assume the deanship of the University of Michigan, Miller suffered an attack of appendicitis. He died on July 27, several days after unsuccessful surgery.[25] On August 6, the president of the W. D. Miller Dental Club of Berlin read the following resolutions:

> *Whereas, Geheim Medizinalrat Professor Dr. Willoughby D. Miller, the great scientist and beloved friend for whom our club was named, has been removed by death; therefore, RESOLVED, That in common with all the members of our profession we deeply mourn our irreparable loss; and RESOLVED, That as we were united to him not only by the admiration and respect which his scientific work spontaneously evolved, but also by the ties of warm personal friendship, we hereby pledge ourselves to cherish forever the memory of his example, which shall inspire us to higher devotion to our profession, to broader charity, to nobler living, and to deeper compassion toward suffering humanity, whom he served so well and so unselfishly.*[41]

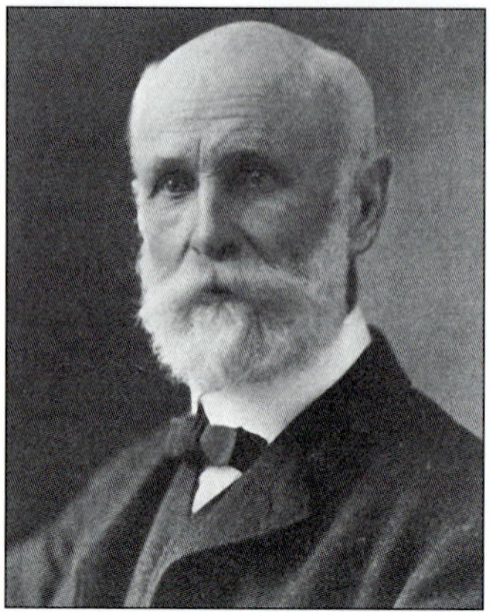

Fig 8-18 Greene Vardiman Black.

Greene Vardiman Black: Educator, Scientist, Inventor, and Clinician

Greene Vardiman Black (Fig 8-18) was a key figure in leading the dental profession out of a period of tumultuous and unregulated growth, marked by entrepreneurship and outright hucksterism, into a time of relative stability, where reliance on research, invention, scholarship, and ethical practice gave dentistry respectability. G. V. Black possessed the ideal characteristics of self-learning, scientific inquiry, and organizational skill, attributes that led to his becoming a most reputed educator, inventor, and clinician.

G. V. Black was born on a farm in Scott County, Illinois, in 1836. With nothing more than rural schoolhouse learning, he left home at age 17 years to study medicine in his older brother's medical practice in Clayton, Illinois. As was common in most rural medical practices at that time, Thomas Black's practice would have included some dentistry, and it has been suggested that the mechanical aspects associated with dentistry must have appealed to the younger G. V. Black, a naturally gifted craftsman. After 4 years of study with his brother, G. V. Black moved to Mt Sterling, Illinois, where he joined the dental practice of J. C. Speer. Shortly thereafter, he set out on his own to establish a dental practice in Winchester, Illinois.

Black's practice was interrupted in 1862 when he joined the Union Army. He served as a scout for the 129th infantry regiment throughout Kentucky and later in garrison at Mitchellville, Kentucky. While serving with the North, G. V. Black suffered a double tragedy, the loss

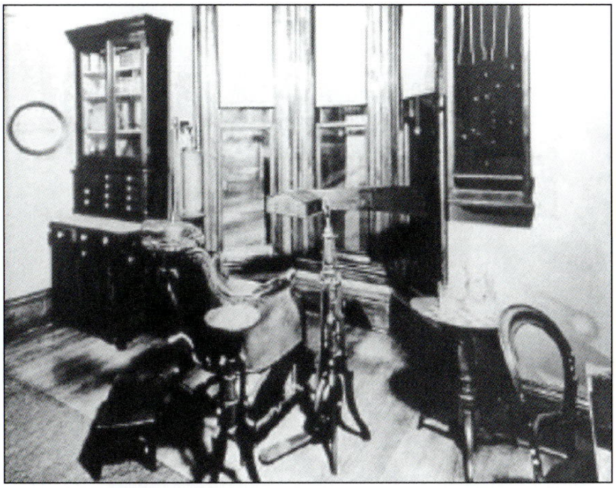

Fig 8-19 G. V. Black's dental office.

of his wife and infant son from pulmonary consumption (tuberculosis). Following a disabling injury to his knee, he was discharged from the Union Army in 1863 to settle in Jacksonville, Illinois, where he practiced dentistry from 1864 to 1897[42] (Fig 8-19). Although G. V. Black limited his practice to dentistry, he was eligible to register as a physician in Illinois due to his having completed an apprenticeship in his brother's medical practice. In 1878, after the passage of the Illinois Medical Practice Act that required all physicians to be licensed and registered, Black passed the medical licensure examination and was legally permitted to practice medicine in Illinois. Three years later, G. V. Black played an instrumental role in preparing legislation that led to the passage of the Illinois Dental Practice Act of 1881. In recognition of his leadership in passage of this act, he was appointed president of the Illinois State Board of Dental Examiners from 1881 to 1887.

Active in both the local dental and medical societies, Black's circle of professional colleagues grew. His scientific curiosity was stimulated by association with other educated men, and his process of self-education accelerated and took on more significance in shaping his career. He was reported to be a voracious reader of medical, dental, and biologic books, mostly borrowed from professional colleagues. He helped establish clubs for the study of chemistry and microscopy.

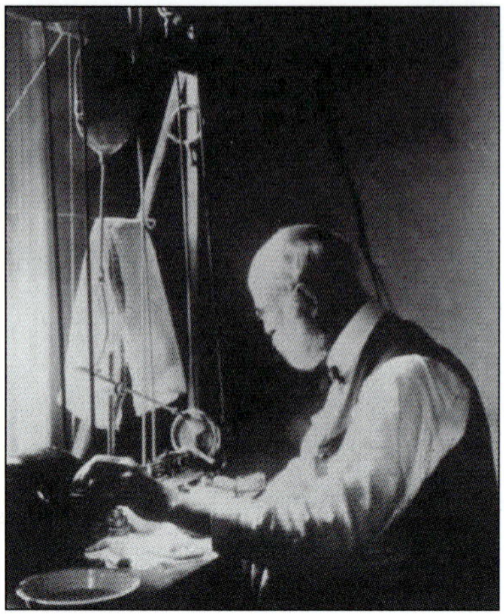

Fig 8-20 G.V. Black at work in his dental laboratory.

Black set up a laboratory for chemical and metallurgic experiments above his dental office in Jacksonville (Fig 8-20). A visitor described the laboratory as follows:

> *There I saw all sorts of things, a big foot-turning lathe, fine tools of all kinds, an anvil and things that go with it, mechanical drawings on the walls, some moving clockwork causing a fluid to flow slowly over some teeth suspended in a jar, which I afterwards learned was an effort to produce chemical erosion of the teeth. I also saw test tubes and other chemical apparatus, and a blackboard with chemical symbols on it. He was teaching chemistry to a class in this room those days. There were gas bags and other things too numerous to mention. I gazed at all these things in wonder.*[42]

One of his first research projects was an investigation of the properties of gold foil and other metals as restorative filling materials. His first scientific report, read before the Illinois State Dental Society in 1869, was an account of his investigations on the cohesive properties of gold foil. Black reported that certain atmospheric gases reacted with pure gold, rendering it less cohesive.[42] He found that by heating the gold before its use, its adhesiveness was returned and its placement and use as a filling material was improved.

For decades, a great controversy existed within the profession over the use of amalgam. For conservative members, the use of gold was equated with excellence of practice, while the use of amalgam represented poor dentistry. The debate was intense and came to be known as the Amalgam War. In 1859, Jonathan Taft, in his popular textbook of operative dentistry, enumerated many deficiencies of amalgam and concluded that "so great and so numerous are the objections to this material (amalgam), that it is but little used by reliable operators." The implication was clear: Any dentist willing to use amalgam was practicing shoddy dentistry. According to Taft, gold possessed more of the requisite properties than any other filling material. The disadvantage to the public was its high cost and the potential harm to the tooth pulp during condensation of the gold filling. The Amalgam War lasted for about 50 years, until Black (and others) finally formulated better amalgams and defined new models of cavity preparation.

Even before the advances introduced by G. V. Black, there were many dentists who came to recognize that by restricting themselves to the use of gold fillings, they were of necessity sacrificing many teeth to extraction that otherwise could have been saved by use of amalgam. Teeth with large areas of decay were unsuitable for gold foil restoration. Furthermore, the trauma to the pulp generated by malleting gold into large cavities often led to inflammation and death of the pulp. Several men questioned whether gold fillings were best for the patient and for the population at large. Dr J. Foster Flagg asked if the goal of the profession was to save as many teeth as possible or to demonstrate high technical skill in manipulation of precious metal. At a dental convention held in Niagara Falls in 1878, Dr Flagg made a powerful argument for increased use of amalgam in place of gold in operative dentistry:

> *I recognize as well as you do the high appreciation which the whole world extends to American dentistry. I recognize as well as you do the wonderful manipulative skill of our "best operators." I recognize as well as you do the vast amount of good which has been done to the community and the world by all this hearty effort, but I also recognize that in despite of it our people are semi-edentulous, and that the whole civilized world is flooded with artificial dentures. Dentures on celluloid, dentures on rubber, dentures on silver, and dentures on gold, dentures on porcelain, and dentures on platinum, dentures on everything except the roots which God designed for their support. Is it too much for me to claim that this result is due largely to the teaching that gold is the best material with which to save teeth?*

Flagg went on to recount that he had abandoned the use of gold in his practice and in its place used gutta-percha, cements, and amalgam to restore decayed teeth. He claimed to have saved more teeth and consequently made fewer dentures, and for this there had been "outcroppings of gratitude and satisfaction" from his patients.

By the turn of the 20th century, the philosophy expressed by Flagg and his fellow "new departurists" was widely accepted. This was in large measure due to the research and teachings of G. V. Black. Black's research led to long-lasting amalgam restorations that were provided at a reasonable cost, thereby significantly improving the dental health of the general public. His studies on the composition of amalgam, its handling properties, and its degree of contraction led to the development of the best available formulation for use of amalgam as a filling material. Black published his results for the benefit of all practitioners without any desire to profit from his discoveries through the patent process.

G. V. Black's academic career began in 1870, when he was invited to teach at the Missouri Dental College in St Louis. For the next 10 years, he spent several days per week at the college, where he lectured on histology, pathology, and operative dentistry. It was a trek from Jacksonville of some 100 miles, the first 25 on horseback and the rest by riverboat on the Illinois and Mississippi Rivers.[42] From 1883 to 1889, he served as professor of pathology at the Chicago College of Dental Surgery. Throughout this period, he continued to educate himself by reading the works of European biologists. Cognizant of the growing importance of Germany's progress in biologic and medical sciences, Black taught himself to read German. He became so deeply influenced by Virchow's discoveries in cellular pathology that he purchased a microscope and set out to investigate dental tissues. As his observations extended beyond dental tissues, his reputation grew, and, before long, physicians called on him for his general knowledge of tissue histopathology.

Black became especially impressed with the new research supporting the growing importance of microorganisms as pathologic agents. This led to his first book, *The Formation of Poisons by Micro-organisms*, published in 1884.[43] It was a compilation of his lectures given at the Chicago College of Dental Surgery describing the development of the new science of microbiology. Black demonstrated his knowledge of the research of Koch, Jenner, Needham, Lister, and Pasteur on the propagation of microorganisms, the antiseptic technique, infection, and pathogenic secretions (poisons). In the last section of the book, Black included his own ideas of the potential importance of microbes and their products in the pathogenesis of disease. In reviewing the relationship between the germ theory of diseases and dental caries,

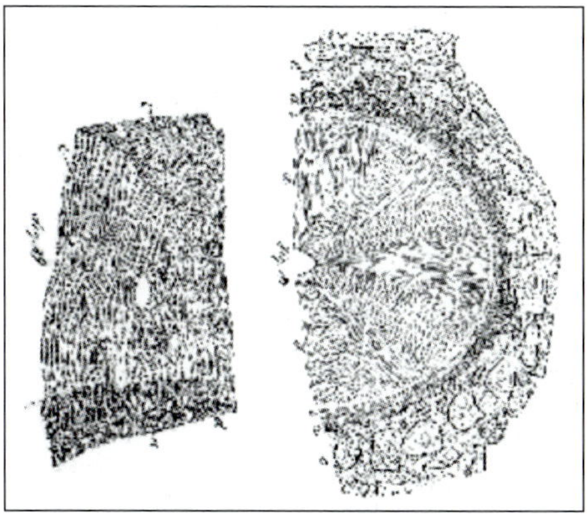

Fig 8-21 Histologic sections of periodontal tissues. (Adapted from Black.[44])

Black concluded that Miller's research was exceptionally significant in resolving the mechanism whereby teeth decayed.

Microscopy was very much in vogue in the mid 19th century, and Black had taken it up with much zeal and had become proficient in preserving, sectioning, and staining tissues for microscopic study.[42] To accomplish these studies, he built a machine for making ground sections of hard mineralized tissues. In 1887, Black published a classical treatise in oral histology, *A Study of the Histological Characters of the Periosteum and Peridental Membrane*.[44] This book was the first detailed description of the microscopic structure of the periodontal membrane, a work noteworthy for its sophistication and significance to the science of connective tissues. Black assembled the results of his histological observations in a clearly written monograph, illustrated by 67 hand-drawn figures (Fig 8-21). Black explained the many reasons why knowledge of the structure and development of the periodontal membrane was needed:

> *Upon the peridental membrane there had not been much written, and there did not seem to be much interest in the subject among the dental specialists. Since then, however, attention has been strongly called to the structure of this membrane from several directions almost simultaneously, and an intense interest awakened. These are, first, the efforts that have been expended in the study of its destructive diseases, which was stimulated primarily by the late Dr. Riggs of Hartford; secondly, by the greater and more general interest recently felt in*

> *the correction of irregularities of the teeth, in which changes in this membrane and the relations of the parts which it unites are brought about; third, by the greater interest that has been manifested by the masses of the dental profession in the retention of pulpless teeth, and roots which have lost their crowns, and which are dependent upon the continued health of the peridental membrane under modified conditions; fourth, by the revival under varied forms of the ancient methods of replanting and transplanting teeth, the success of which is supposed to be dependent, in whole or in part, upon the reconstruction of the peridental membrane, or its re-attachment to the teeth; and, fifth, by the singular fact that has of late been noted more accurately; that a large proportion of the teeth thus replanted with seeming success, are finally lost by absorption of their roots; a matter which seems to depend upon some mal-condition of the tissues of the peridental membrane. All of these considerations call earnestly for an intimate knowledge of the histology and physiology of this membrane as the basis for the formation of correct views of its pathology and recuperative powers when subjected to disease or serious injury.*[44]

In G. V. Black's time, the composition of connective tissues was thought to be limited to white (inelastic) and yellow (elastic) fibers, ground substance, and connective tissue cells. Black described the development of connective tissue, noting that in the process a gelatinous ground substance was transformed into white and yellow fibers. In some tissues, such as the dental pulp, the transformation of its gelatinous substance appeared to be incomplete. Dental pulp and similar tissues contained fine reticular fibers associated with star-shaped reticular cells. In contrast, in dense connective tissue, such as in the submucosa of skin or the periosteum of bone, larger well-defined white fibers were prominent. Black's observation that cells in the peridental membrane were elongated and parallel to the newly developing fibers led him to the conclusion that "fibers arise under the immediate supervision of cells." As evidence of the role of cells in forming fibers, he stated: "I shall, therefore, call such cells fibroblasts." Anticipating the discovery of extracellular proteoglycans, he observed that "fibers are cemented together by an intervening substance."

Black was of the opinion that one could understand the structure and function of the periodontal ligament only after first understanding the nature of the periosteum of bone. He claimed that although the bone-forming activity of the periosteum had been studied in relative detail, the attachment areas of the periosteum to bone had not been adequately examined.[45] Black observed that the periosteum consisted of nonattached and attached segments to the underlying bone substance. The bone surface beneath nonattached periosteum was covered by a layer of osteoblasts, and no fibers were observed to enter the bone. Attached periosteum was present near the junction of long bones and articular surfaces, near the insertion of tendons and ligaments, and where other tissues attached to bone. He showed that in the attached areas, fibers "spring directly out of the bone" and that after passing out of the bone the fibers "break up into a tuft of very fine fibers."

A major part of Black's monograph was devoted to describing the microscopic structure of Haversian bone and its method of development and replacement.[45] It is in this discussion about the nature and function of Sharpey's fibers that Black's keen sense of observation is seen at its best, as well as his readiness to challenge current scientific dogma. According to Black, Sharpey's fibers, or "penetrating fibers," are "not a part of the bone per se, but are the accident of the formation (of bone)." These fibers were implanted in bone by building the bone around them during its formation. He noted that after decalcification of a bone, its penetrating fibers were only loosely connected to the bone matrix and on some surfaces could be pulled out intact from the bone. Black concluded that these fibers were rendered firm and attached to the bone by the mineralization process. He stressed the attachment role of these fibers, while noting that Sharpey viewed them as having a formative or osteogenetic function in directing the growth of new bone. Black was supported in his idea by the fact that there were no penetrating fibers in Haversian bone. These penetrating fibers were also most highly developed along the attached parts of the periosteum and in the periodontal membrane. He made his position clear:

> *The function of these fibers, it seems to me, is physical and entirely passive; that of giving firm attachment to the periosteum and the tissues it supports. I should, therefore, regard the term osteogenic fibers consisting of osteogenetic substance, applied to them by Sharpey and adopted by many histologists, as an error.*[45]

His analysis of the function of the penetrating fibers was important to his concept of the attachment function of the periodontal ligament and cementum.

Few have recognized the exceptional merit of G. V. Black's study of the development of the periodontal membrane.[46] Based on the high quality of Black's histologic work and the clarity of his thinking, he might have achieved fame in that discipline had he not assumed administrative duties and clinical teaching responsibilities. He is much more remembered for his studies of amalgam and his contributions to operative dentistry.

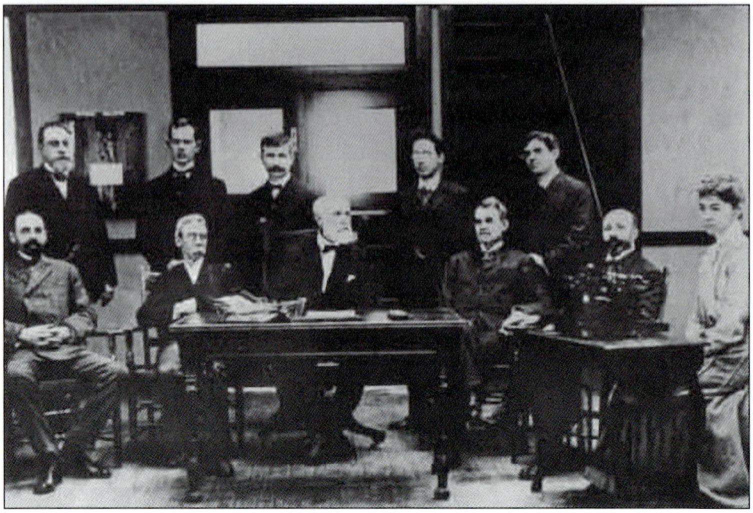

Fig 8-22 G. V. Black seated *(center)* with members of the faculty at Northwestern University Dental College.

In 1890, Black accepted a new post as professor of dental pathology and bacteriology at Northwestern University Dental School (Fig 8-22). Here he perfected his academic contributions to dental anatomy and operative dentistry. His recognition of the need for standardization of nomenclature in dental anatomy and for precision in dental operative procedures led to the publication of his most popular textbooks: *Descriptive Anatomy of the Human Teeth* and a two-volume *Operative Dentistry*[47,48] (Fig 8-23). In the former, he created a systematized nomenclature of the several parts of the teeth: "Such a description will call attention successively to every part of each tooth, as Gray, in his Anatomy, has called attention to every part of each bone, however apparently unimportant." Black made his own illustrations, noting that they were not works of art but accurate representations that took into account the existing variations in human tooth form (Fig 8-24).

His experiments on metal alloys led to improved filling materials and ended the long-standing debate over the appropriate use of amalgam. In the late 1890s, he introduced his concepts for the management of enamel margins and his "extension for prevention" protocol for operative preparation of carious teeth.[49] Black advocated removal of enamel sufficient to ensure the prevention of recurrent decay (ie, the placement of the prepared cavity margin at a point on the

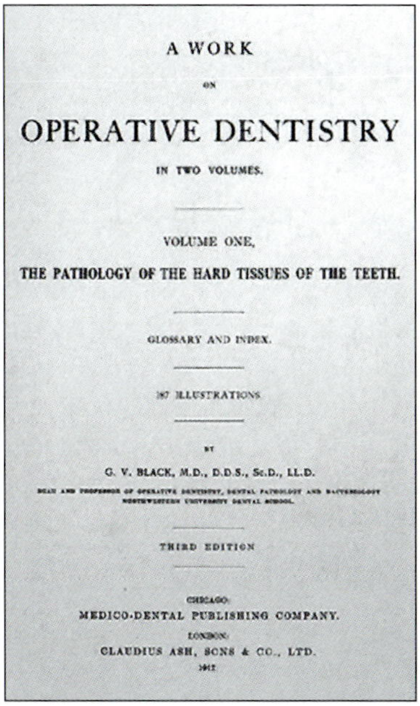

A WORK

ON

OPERATIVE DENTISTRY

IN TWO VOLUMES.

VOLUME ONE,

THE PATHOLOGY OF THE HARD TISSUES OF THE TEETH.

GLOSSARY AND INDEX.

[illegible] ILLUSTRATIONS

BY

G. V. BLACK, M.D., D.D.S., Sc.D., LL.D.

DEAN AND PROFESSOR OF OPERATIVE DENTISTRY, DENTAL PATHOLOGY AND BACTERIOLOGY NORTHWESTERN UNIVERSITY DENTAL SCHOOL.

THIRD EDITION

CHICAGO:

MEDICO-DENTAL PUBLISHING COMPANY.

LONDON:

CLAUDIUS ASH, SONS & CO., LTD.

[illegible]

Fig 8-23 Cover page of Black's textbook on operative dentistry.

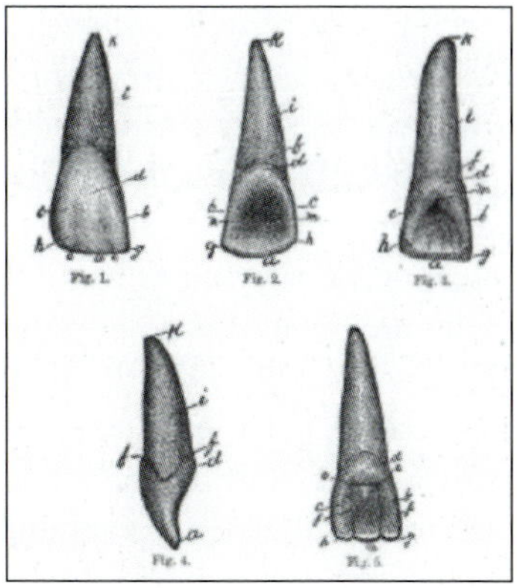

Fig 8-24 Anatomy of human incisors as drawn by G. V. Black.

tooth where there existed less chance for redevelopment of the caries process).[42] Black's cavity preparations involved cutting away sound enamel and dentin:

> *When a cavity has occurred in the occluding surface of a molar, the dentist prepares a filling with the idea that the tissues in this part of the enamel have favored the occurrence of that cavity. For this reason the fissures and grooves adjoining the cavity, even though not decayed, are cut away to such a point as seem to give opportunity for a smooth, even finish of the margins of the filling. This is done as a prevention of future recurrence of decay, because such points have been observed to be more liable to caries than the smooth parts of the enamel. I think that this has become a fixed principle with the large majority of operators; and a failure to do this is regarded as careless operating. The sacrifice is more than justifiable,—it is required for the safety of the operation and the tooth.*

"Extension for prevention" became an axiom in operative dentistry that controlled the technique of cavity preparation for the next two to three generations of dentists. Black's axioms of cavity preparation were elaborated especially in conjunction with the perfection of amalgam and its increasing use for filling teeth.[42] It was not until the development of new composite plastics in the mid 20th century that Black's extension for prevention methods were replaced by new, more conservative approaches to cavity preparation.

In 1895, G. V. Black published a lengthy report in *Dental Cosmos* describing his investigations of the physical properties of teeth.[50] This research was the first of its kind, an endeavor requiring special equipment and great attention to details to avoid introduction of artifacts. Black set out "to find the truth if possible, as to the differences in the density, percentage of lime-salts, strength, etc., occurring in the human teeth, and to find what relation, if any, such differences may bear to dental caries and other diseases of the teeth." Black knew that his research would have clinical implications and hoped that dentists would apply the findings of his work in their practices.

It was commonly believed by the profession and the laity that a lack of lime salts in the dental tissues made the teeth susceptible to caries. In Black's words:

> *It may now be said that the hypothesis that the condition of the tooth-structure, in a large degree, renders the tooth susceptible or unsusceptible to caries exists in full force in the minds of a large proportion of some members of the dental profession. We see constantly in dental literature allusions to "frail teeth," "chalky teeth," "hard teeth," "soft teeth," "dense teeth," that this patient's teeth have become soft and are melting down rapidly; or that that patient's teeth are hard and firm in structure, etc.*[50]

Although it had been known that "earthy matter" (lime salts) made up approximately 72% and that "animal matter" (organic matrix) made up 28% of dentin, there had been no attempt to measure potential differences in the physical composition of teeth in relation to the incidence of dental caries.[51] Black proposed to study a large sample of patients to record the physical characteristics of teeth in relation to dental caries, age, and sex. Because there had been no previous work of this magnitude and precision, he needed to use his ingenuity to devise new protocols and equipment. He observed in preliminary studies that differences in the physical characteristics of teeth were extremely small:

> *So much so that the most delicate instruments would be required for the successful prosecution of the work. Special balances with arrangements for weighing in moist and dry conditions, to weighing differences as low as the tenth of a milligram would be needed [Fig 8-25]. Because of the hygroscopic properties of dentin to absorb water from the atmosphere in humid weather and to give it up in dry weather it was necessary to control humidity and temperature to ensure that measurements were made under like conditions.*

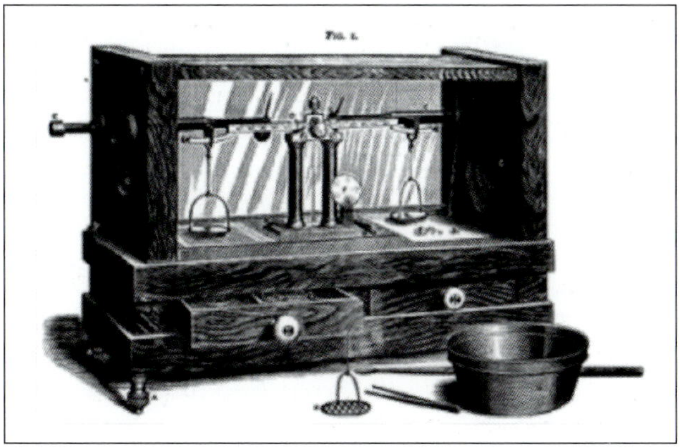

Fig 8-25 Analytical balance of the type used by G. V. Black in measuring the weight of tissue samples.

With a large supply of teeth (268) extracted from 112 individuals from his practice and from that of several "gentlemen who extract many teeth," he cut sections of dentin of about ¹⁄₁₆-inch across the teeth at the gingival line. Each section was analyzed as to the proportion of water, lime salts, and organic matter in dentin, which represented the character of the tooth as a whole: "Each piece of dentin is weighed four times, first, under water, *the submarine weight*; second, in the air wet, *the wet weight*; third, after drying, *the weight dry*; fourth, after calcining, *the weight of the lime-salts*."[50]

Black showed that lime salts accounted for 63.54%, the organic matter for 25.36%, and the water for 11.06% of the average total weight of all teeth. He found that the range in the percentage of lime salts in human dentin was small (61.08% to 65.57%), of little consequence as to hardness or softness, and unrelated to the incidence of dental decay. The notion that some teeth were soft and more prevalent to caries was not supported by the data:

> *Any basis for accounting for caries in this or that case on account of "frail teeth" or "teeth below the medium in structure," "poorly calcified teeth" etc., must disappear, whether it be in connection with the electric theory of caries, the chemical theory of caries, or the microbic theory of caries.... The teeth of persons who suffer much from caries are just as hard, just as dense, just as heavy, and contain just as much lime-salts as the teeth of persons who do not suffer from caries.*[50]

The data also failed to confirm the hypothesis entertained by many that the teeth of women became soft on account of a loss of lime salts during pregnancy and lactation. Furthermore, the hardness of teeth had no relation to the development of periodontal disease.

Despite the detailed evidence provided by G. V. Black, there were those men, such as Hans Block, who would never be convinced:

> *The individual that may be well-nourished in all respects, but any disproportion between the demand and supply of lime-salts may reduce the density of the tooth structures, for instance, during pregnancy or diabetes mellitus, etc. In these cases the demand for all lime-salts is increased beyond normal, and the system establishes a retrogressive metamorphosis. This can also happen under mental overwork, debauchery, sleeplessness, and intemperance, conditions where the expenses are always greater than the income. Many mothers lose a tooth with every child.*[35]

Having established the uniform density of teeth, Black turned his attention to testing the strength of dentin. Using the same set of extracted teeth, Black cut small blocks of dentin and subjected them to pressure in a device he called a dynamometer. In these experiments, he discovered that dentin had elastic properties. Dentin exposed to 100 pounds of stress was compressed by 2.09% of its thickness and upon removal of the stress recovered its original size. The validity of Black's results was demonstrated in 1952 using advanced equipment. Black concluded that variations in the strength of the human dentin were not directly dependent on the density or the percentage of lime salts. The strength of dentin seemed rather to be dependent on the condition of the organic matrix. Dentin of older teeth generally broke with lighter pressure. In comparing crushing stresses of the teeth with their tendency to caries, the result seemed to be that no relation whatever exists.

In pondering the question of why some patients were so susceptible to caries while other individuals appeared totally protected, he offered this view:

> *It seems to be admitted by all who have examined the subject from the standpoint of the bacteriologist, that the caries producing organisms are present in every mouth whether caries occurs or not. I have myself made cultures from the saliva of many people, those in whose teeth caries was making sad havoc, and though in whose teeth no caries whatever appeared, and must say that I have found no mouth that was free from the caries producing organisms. Then, if these microorganisms are present in every human mouth, why is it that they induce caries in the teeth of the one and not in the teeth of another? Why is it that the teeth of the one are quickly destroyed while there are only a few slowly progressive decays in case in the teeth of the other? The popular answer to these questions, both by the profession and the laity, has been,—*

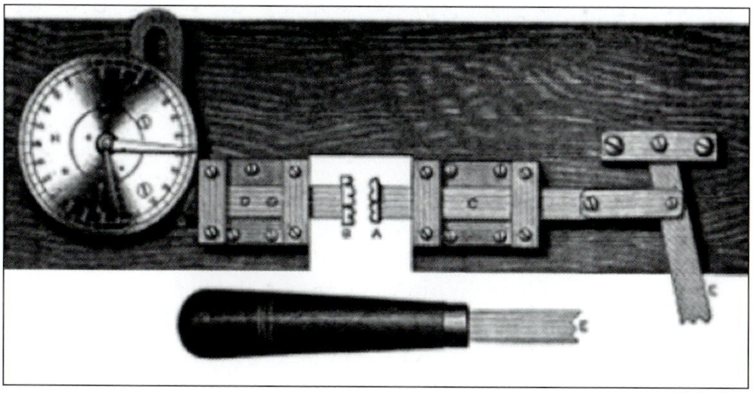

Fig 8-26 Black's phagodynamometer for measuring the forces needed to crush (masticate) various foods.

> *differences in the physical qualities of the teeth. Teeth that contain but a small percentage of lime-salts, soft teeth, have been regarded as most susceptible to caries, while teeth that contain a large percentage of lime-salts, hearty teeth, had been regarded as least susceptible to caries.*[50]

But Black had proven these ideas to be incorrect, and he now sought an answer to why some mouths were protected from dental caries in the new theory of immunity:

> *We must conclude that there is some deterrent action or force operating within the human mouth that acts to hinder the destructive effects of the products of the microorganisms, either by restraining the growth of the organisms, by hindering the production of their typical acid excretions, or by limiting the effects of the acid excreted by the organisms.*[50]

Having disproven the notion that caries was a disease of soft teeth, Black turned his attention to measuring the forces that teeth could withstand during the mastication of food. He measured the forces exerted by the jaws during biting using a device called a *gnathodynamometer*. He found that the amount of pressure that could be exerted on a tooth varied from about 100 pounds for young ladies to upwards of 200 pounds for strong men. Maximum forces were exerted by molar teeth.

An amusing episode in Black's research occurred when he conducted experiments to determine the forces needed to crush various foods. For these studies he used a phagodynamometer, a machine of his own design that incorporated human teeth in a presslike contraption to crush particles of food (Fig 8-26). Black described inviting a small group of fellow dentists to a Chicago restaurant, where the phagodynamometer was put to use crushing samples of beefsteak, broiled ham, mutton chops, and a number of other foods during a 3-hour dinner.[50] Black noted that a light crackling sound could be heard the moment when the fibers of the meat were being forcibly broken up during mastication in the phagodynamometer. One wonders what befuddled looks they received from waiters and fellow diners during this odd performance, as they bent close to the machine's jaws to hear the death throes of ham, mutton, and beefsteak fibers.

In 1897, he was appointed dean of Northwestern University Dental School, a post he held until his death in 1915 (Fig 8-27). While at Northwestern, Black completed his extensive studies of the physical properties of amalgam, considered by many to have had a most pervading influence on operative dentistry. Much of this work was contained in his textbook on operative dentistry[42] (see Fig 8-23). Under his tenure as dean, the Northwestern University Dental School grew to become one of the finest dental schools in the world.

Black did find time for relaxation during his summer vacations, when he sailed his boat, the *Microbe*, in the waters of northern Michigan.[52] In between hunting and fishing, he found time to sketch illustrations for his publications. His travels were recorded in several unpublished papers, such as "From Quebec up the Saguenay and Chicoutimi," "Not Tides but Barometric Waves," and "Studies on Saprophitic Moulds." Music was another of his loves; he led a church choir and played the violin, flute, cello, and piccolo.[52] In reviewing the life of G. V. Black, B. Henderson concluded that Black, more than any of his predecessors, "established dentistry upon a scientific basis and raised it to truly professional status." Henderson listed the following as Black's major accomplishments:

> *He systematized the operative treatment of dental caries, according to certain principles of cavity preparation. Of these, the most important were, (a) the preventative extension of cavity margins, (b) a seven-stage operative sequence, (c) principles of design for mechanical stability and permanence of function, and (d) the application of these principles to the peculiarities of structures associated with different teeth.*[42]

Henderson, in enumerating G. V. Black's many contributions to the development of clinical dentistry, included the discovery of

> *a method of maintaining the cohesive properties of gold foil, and described the physico-chemical principles of its contamination.... He established that the chemical constitution and physical characteristics of teeth are not the determining factor in their susceptibility or immunity to caries. He disproved the notion that the teeth of women are*

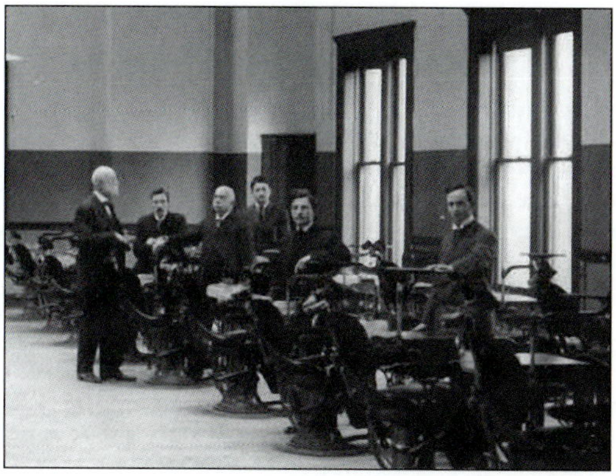

Fig 8-27 G. V. Black *(left)* addressing faculty and/or students at Northwestern University Dental College.

weakened, or made more liable to caries in themselves, by the supposed withdrawal of lime-salts during the child-bearing period, especially during pregnancy.[42]

Summary

The dental profession was lifted from obscurity and low esteem by the vision and determination of a relatively small number of men. These men were more often than not graduates of medical schools, unlike the larger body of practitioners who trained by apprenticeship. They possessed knowledge of biologic science and could visualize the place of dental and oral disease within the larger context of medical science. Furthermore, it is clear that they hoped to practice according to high standards in harmony with the established medical community. Through research, extensive clinical practice, and communication through textbooks and journals, they educated new members of the profession. The individuals highlighted here were positioned at a crucial period, a time when dental schools, national organizations, and regulatory bodies were being created. They had a profound and enabling influence in setting the path that led to the recognition of dentistry as a legitimate medical discipline.

References

1. Taylor JA. History of Dentistry. Philadelphia: Lea & Febiger, 1922.
2. Mills EC. Bainbridge, Ross County, Ohio, the cradle of dental education. J Am Dent Assoc 1932;19:361.
3. Ward ML. Landmarks in dental education. Dent Cosmos 1934;76:3–23.
4. Cordell EF. University of Maryland 1807–1907: Its History, Influence, Equipment and Characteristics. New York: Lewis, 1907.
5. Brophy TW. Address on oral and dental surgery. J Am Med Assoc 1884;1:533–535.
6. Scharf TJ. History of Baltimore City and County. Philadelphia: Louis H. Everts, 1881.
7. Robinson JB. Dr. Horace H. Hayden and his influence on dental education. Dent Cosmos 1932;74:783–787.
8. Thorpe BL. A biographical review of the careers of Hayden and Harris. Trans Fourth Int Dent Congress 1904;3:413–424.
9. Thorpe BL. Biographies of Pioneer American Dentists and their Successors. Chicago: National Art, 1909.
10. Harris CA. The Principles and Practice of Dental Surgery, ed 8. Philadelphia: Lindsay & Blakiston, 1863.
11. McManus C. The makers of dentistry. Dent Cosmos 1902;44:1105–1128.
12. Cope Z. Sir John Tomes: A Pioneer of British Dentistry. London: Dawsons of Pall Mall, 1961.
13. Tomes CS. Sir John Tomes, obituary notice. Proc Royal Soc London 1895; 59:xiii–xiv.
14. Tomes J. A Course of Lectures on Dental Physiology and Surgery. London: John W. Parker, 1848.
15. Tomes J. A System of Dental Surgery. London: J. Churchill, 1859.
16. Tomes J. Instructions in the Use and Management of Artificial Teeth. London: Savill and Edwards, 1851.
17. Tomes J. On the structure of the dental tissues of Rodentia. Abstr Pap Communicated Royal Soc London 1843;5:951–952.
18. Tomes J. On the presence of fibrils of soft tissue in the dentinal tubes. Philos Trans Royal Soc London 1856;146:515–522.
19. Tomes J, Tomes CS. A System of Dental Surgery, ed 2. London: J. & A. Churchill, 1873.
20. Tomes J, Tomes CS. A System of Dental Surgery, ed 4. Philadelphia: Blakiston, Sons, and Co, 1897.
21. Gelbier S. 125 years of developments in dentistry, 1800–2005. Part 2: Law and the dental profession. Br Dent J 2005;199:470–473.
22. Gysi A. Dental caries under the microscope. Dent Cosmos 1887;29:218–232.
23. Barrett WC. W. D. Miller, A.B., Ph.D., M.D., D.D.S. Dominion Dent J 1891;3: 41–49.
24. Thorpe BL. A brief review of the prominent pioneer manipulators of gold foil. Dent Cosmos 1906;48:389–399.
25. Webster JO, Barrows ED. Obituary: W. D. Miller. Dent Cosmos 1907;49:1009–1014.
26. Robertson W. A Practical Treatise on the Diseases of the Teeth, in which the Origin and Nature of Decay are Explained; and the Means of Prevention Pointed Out. London: Longman, Rees, Orme, Brown, Green & Longman, 1835.
27. Miller WD. The agency of acids in the production of caries of the human teeth, with comparative analysis of carious dentine and dentine softened by acids. Dent Cosmos 1883;25:337–344.
28. Abbott F. Caries of human teeth. Dent Cosmos 1879;21:184–192.
29. Miller WD. Agency of micro-organisms in decay of human teeth. Dent Cosmos 1883;25:1–12.
30. Miller WD. Decay of a replanted tooth. Dent Cosmos 1891;33:253–256.

31. Miller WD. The presence of bacterial plaques on the surface of the teeth and their significance. Dent Cosmos 1902;44:425–446.
32. Miller WD. Microscopic examination of a case of caries of a monkey's tooth. Dent Cosmos 1892;34:892–893.
33. Miller WD. Caries of the teeth in an African manatee *(Manatus senegalensis)*. Dent Cosmos 1893;35:519–521.
34. Miller WD. Studies on the anatomy and pathology of the tusks of the elephant. Dent Cosmos 1891;33:169–175,421–440.
35. Block H. The causes of dental caries. Dent Cosmos 1893;35:597–612.
36. Barrett WC. Proceedings of the American Dental Association. Dent Cosmos 1884;26:595–610.
37. Ismail AI, Hasson H, Sohn W. Dental Caries in the Second Millennium. In: NIH Consensus Development Conference on Dental Caries Diagnosis and Management. Bethesda, MD: National Institute of Dental and Craniofacial Research, 2001.
38. Truman J. Review of "Die Mikroorganismen der Mundhole." Dent Cosmos 1890;32:70–78.
39. Ormiston R. The new epoch in medicine. (A paper read before the New York Odontological Society). Dent Cosmos 1889;31:256–263.
40. Thorpe BL, Melendy AR, McManus J. In memoriam of Willoughby Dayton Miller, A.B., D.D.S., M.D., Ph.D., Sc.D. Dent Cosmos 1908;50:395–396.
41. Webster JO, Barrows ED. W. D. Miller Dental Club of Berlin, Germany, resolutions. J Allied Dent Soc 1907;2:215.
42. Henderson D. Greene Vardiman Black (1836–1915), the grand old man of dentistry. Med Hist 1961;5:132–143.
43. Black GV. The Formation of Poisons by Micro-organisms. A Biological Study of the Germ Theory of Disease. Philadelphia: P. Blakiston, Son, & Co, 1884.
44. Black GV. A Study of the Histological Characters of the Periosteum and Peridental Membrane. Chicago: W. T. Keener, 1887.
45. Garant PR. G. V. Black's contribution to the structural biology of the periodontium. Periodontal Clin Investig 1995;17:16–20.
46. Held AJ. Periodontology from Its Origins up to 1980: A Survey. Basel: Birkhauser, 1989.
47. Black GV. Descriptive Anatomy of the Human Teeth. Philadelphia: S. S. White, 1897.
48. Black GV. A Work on Operative Dentistry, ed 3. Chicago: Medico-Dental, 1917.
49. Black GV. A Work on Operative Dentistry. Chicago: Medico-Dental, 1908.
50. Black GV. An investigation of the physical characters of the human teeth in relation to their diseases, and to practical dental operations, together with the physical characters of filling-materials. Dent Cosmos 1895;37:353–421,469–484,553–571,637–661,737–758.
51. St John FE. Physiological observations on the teeth. Dent Rep 1858;1:59–65.
52. Dunning WB. Greene Vardiman Black. J Allied Dent Soc 1915;10:409–417.

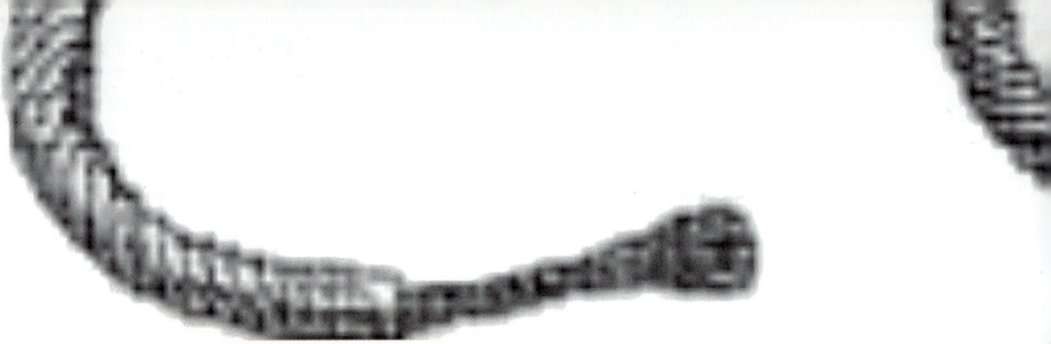

9

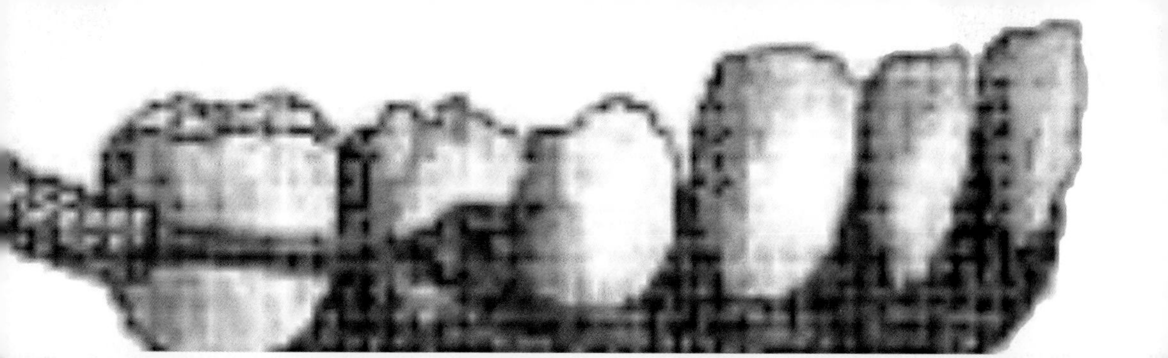

Mechanical Dentistry

Mechanical dentistry encompasses the techniques for replacing lost teeth with prosthetic devices, consisting in its simplest form of a single tooth or in its more complex form of multiple teeth (partial denture) or an entire arch (complete denture). Prior to the invention of porcelain teeth, prosthetic replacements were made from human teeth or carved from blocks of bone and ivory, normally obtained from animal tusks or hippopotamus teeth.

Examination of a late 18th to early 19th century dental laboratory workshop reveals the work that dentists performed and how they adapted the tools of other craftsmen, such as jewelers, silversmiths, and clockmakers, to their work. Fauchard was the first to provide illustrations of some of the tools he used to fabricate artificial teeth and dentures, but it is C. F. Delabarre's many illustrations that allow for a more complete picture of the delicate work required to provide advanced dental prosthetic services.[1] When one examines the techniques employed in early restorative dentistry, it is easy to see how men who were primarily engaged in making jewelry, clocks, fine woodwork, and other delicate items were inclined to try their hand at dental work.

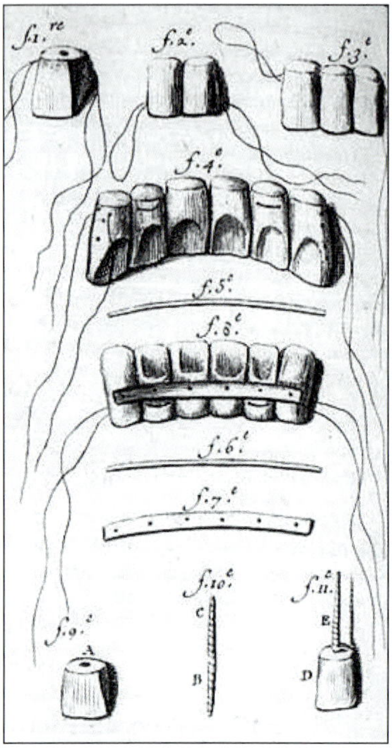

Fig 9-1 *(center)* Partial denture (f8) consisting of six crowns attached by pins to a gold or silver lingual bar to be secured to natural abutment teeth by silk or gold threads. *(bottom)* Pivot crown (f9), pivot (f10), and unit assembled (f11). (From Fauchard.[2])

Tooth Replacement

Replacement of a single tooth was a fairly simple procedure. A suitable crown was selected from a pool of teeth previously extracted from other patients (or perhaps obtained from cadavers). The crown of the replacement tooth was often simply fastened with silk or gold wire ligatures to adjacent natural abutment teeth (top left in Fig 9-1). A more stable and more permanent procedure was to secure the replacement crown to a retained root with a pin. In this method, the donor crown was attached to the patient's exposed root via a pivot or dowel made of wire or wood (bottom right in Fig 9-1). Good front teeth were not always available; Le Mayeur, a Philadelphia dentist, in a newspaper announcement offered two guineas for sound front teeth.

Partial and complete dentures were carved from single blocks of bone or ivory, shaped to adapt to the contours of the jaw. Fauchard described how a partial denture could be fabricated with multiple human replacement teeth secured to a metal lingual bar via metal pins

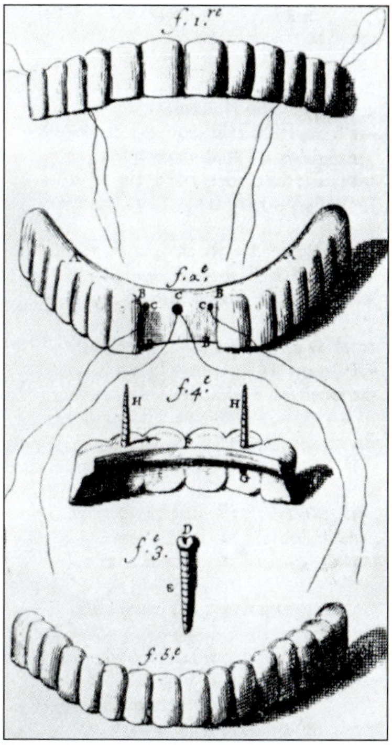

Fig 9-2 Block dentures to be secured to abutment teeth by threads or by pins to retained roots. (From Fauchard.[2])

(center in Fig 9-1). He noted that when dentures were secured to pivot teeth, they could last for 20 years or more. Often the anatomical details of the teeth were imitated by simply making vertical cuts in a block of ivory or bone, ignoring the normal anatomical cuspal inclines. In some cases, these block dentures were secured by pivoting into retained roots or fastened to natural teeth with silk or gold ligatures and later by wire clasps (Fig 9-2).

M. Mouton, in 1746, wrote the first book exclusively devoted to the art of fabricating dentures, in which he hoped to dispel the contemporary prejudice against the use of artificial dentures. He noted that when made by a competent dentist, dentures and pivot teeth were indeed useful in the mastication of food and were not likely to become loose or to be accidentally expelled from the mouth. The notion that dentures had to be removed from the mouth during sleep for fear of swallowing them was also said to be false. Guerini points out that Mouton introduced two advances: the gold cap or crown and the use of clasps for securing artificial teeth and partial dentures.[3]

Pivot Teeth

Fauchard described a rather simple method for securing replacement teeth using pivots.[2] After the root canal was cleaned of all pulp tissue and decayed dentin, the canal was enlarged with an instrument used by clockmakers to enlarge holes in metal (Fig 9-3). These pointed instruments had four sharp edges that could cut away dentin when rotated in the canal. Fauchard then filled the enlarged root canal with lead and, using a stiletto, formed a long, straight hole in the lead to receive the pivot. The pivots were made of gold or silver, with a roughened surface to better adhere to the mastic used to secure them within the canal.

Joseph Fox, in his 1806 treatise, succinctly described the use of pivot teeth as replacements for crowns irreparably damaged by dental caries:

> *The incisors and cuspidati of the upper jaw are very frequently affected with caries, and the crowns of the teeth decay, so as to leave little more than the fangs in the sockets. When the teeth are in this situation, if there be no disease in the socket, new teeth may be fixed to the fangs of the decayed ones, without any attachment to other teeth being required. This operation is to be performed as follows. All the ragged or carious remains of the crown of the tooth are to be filed away close to the gum; the hole in the fang, which forms the natural cavity, is then to be prepared for receiving the pivot, by which the new tooth is to be fastened; this is done by passing a small instrument, called a broach, into the cavity, and drilling it into a smooth, round hole. The fang being thus prepared, the crown of a human tooth, corresponding with the one that has been filed off, is to be fitted to the fang, a hole is then to be drilled, and a piece of gold wire screwed firmly into it; the wire being left of a length equal to the hole in the fang, and filed to the exact size, is to be introduced, and, being made tight, it may continue for many years without occasioning any trouble, or requiring any repair. In this mode, several teeth belonging to the same person may be replaced, which cannot be discerned upon the most minute inspection.*[4]

One of the first steps in the insertion of a pivot tooth was the preparation of the retained root. Of primary concern was the elimination of the pulpal nerve. This was accomplished by inserting a red-hot probe into the root canal to cauterize the tissues. Delabarre described an alternate procedure to extirpate the nerve with barbed gold or steel needles spun between the fingers to cause the needles to sink deeper and to entangle the nerve tissues:

> *A gold needle or untempered steel tip makes the work easy: The surgeon spins the tool between his fingers to make it penetrate the root canal as*

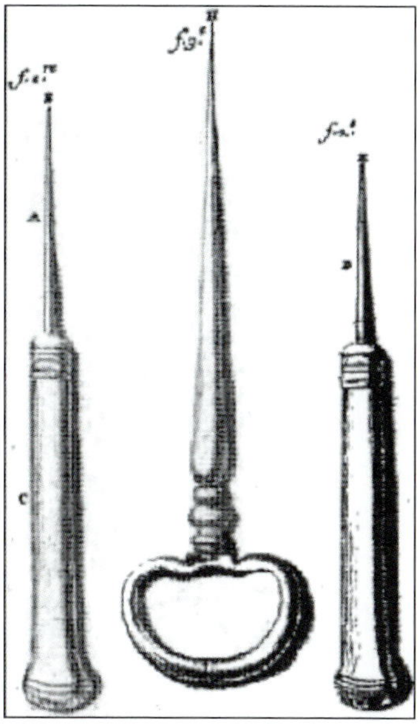

Fig 9-3 Instruments used to enlarge a root canal and to pierce a lead-filled canal. (From Fauchard.[2])

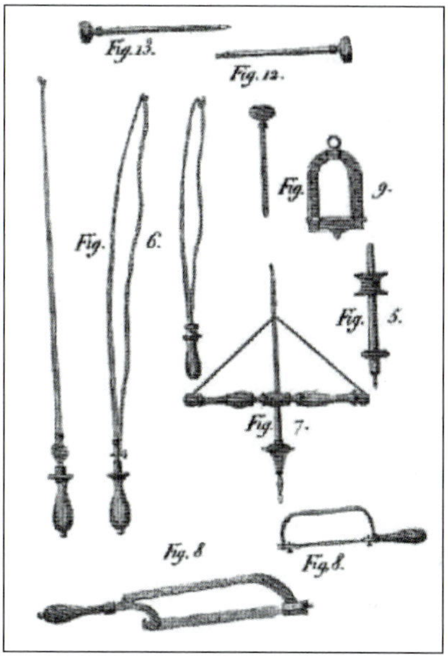

Fig 9-4 Jeweler's drills, drill bows, and handsaws used in dental work. (From Delabarre.[1])

> *far as it will go. It is good to bend the end of the instrument to form a hook so that during rotation the nerve is twisted and can be extirpated without much trouble.*

Such procedures were performed rapidly to minimize the pain. In some cases, if the pain was too great or the nerve was too dispersed or inaccessible, it was best to destroy the nerve with one or more applications of silver nitrate.[1]

Delabarre used a small drill to enlarge the canal to accommodate a cylindric post or pivot (Fig 9-4). He cautioned that care must be taken not to break the drill bit in the canal, because they were difficult to remove. In addition, the operator must avoid drilling beyond the root apex, because this could cause inflammation and development of a fistula. Delabarre noted that it was sometimes necessary to open or enlarge the apex to create an exit for a purulent inflammatory exudate. In cases where the root canal was too wide at the cervical end, it was necessary to build a new support by obturating the opening with condensed gold foil or with fusible metal and later to create a

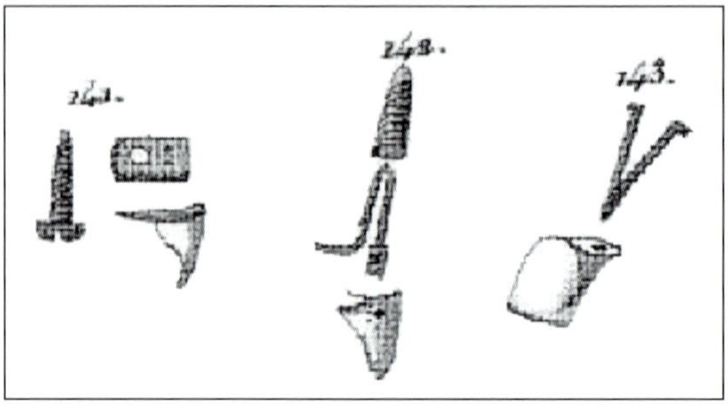

Fig 9-5 Screw-type pivot *(left)* and Maggiolo clip or spring pivot *(right)*. (From Delabarre.[1])

new opening for insertion of the pivot. Although Delabarre indicated a preference for molten metal, he also described the use of wooden inserts prepared in the following complex manner: A wax impression of the canal was used to create a steel screw with which to shape the interior walls of the canal. Care must be taken not to crack the root. The steel screw was advanced and retreated repeatedly within the canal until the proper depth was reached. Using a lathelike instrument, the steel screw was then used to form an identical wooden screw, which was then screwed carefully into the canal to the end point and then backed off one-half turn to account for subsequent swelling of the wood. Excess wood at the cervical end was removed with a small saw, and a central canal was made in the wood (with instruments similar to those depicted in Fig 9-3) to receive the pivoted crown. Delabarre stated that he had achieved a 10-year success rate using this technique in several cases.[1]

A variety of pivot designs were employed, such as the ingenious design attributed to Maggiolo of a cliplike pivot that attached to the inside of a metal tube inserted into the canal (Fig 9-5). This device permitted the removal of the artificial tooth for cleaning. Delabarre did not recommend this method because he was of the opinion that if one had a tight-fitting pivot it was best not to disturb it. Delabarre described special pivot designs used in situations where the crown did not match the position or angulation of the retained root (Fig 9-6). He also noted that his favorite pivot was the screw type. Delabarre considered that the diversity of methods used by dentists to secure artificial teeth to roots was a clear indication of the difficulty encountered in obtaining a stable attachment that did not cause damage to the root. Pivot teeth were used without much change in technique well into the 19th century.

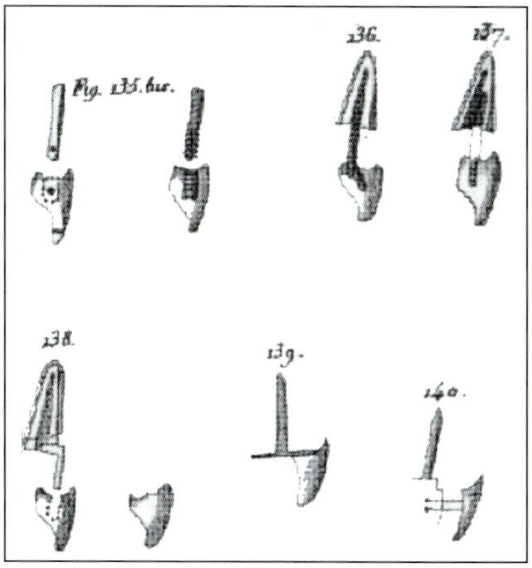

Fig 9-6 Screw-type pin (135r), angular pins (136–138), and pivots to be used with horizontal pins. (From Delabarre.[1])

Chapin Harris, in the first American textbook of dentistry, recommended the insertion of a gold tube into the canal to function as a receptacle for the pivot. He described his method as follows:

> *First, the crown of the natural tooth is removed, the nerve, if alive, destroyed, and the canal in the root enlarged as before directed. Secondly, a screw-tap is then introduced for the purpose of cutting a screw on its inner walls. Thirdly, a corresponding screw-thread is then cut on a piece of hollow gold wire, during which process the gold tube is filled with steel wire to prevent compression. This done, it may be screwed into the root about a quarter of an inch; the wire on the inside of it is then withdrawn, and the lower or protruding extremity dressed off even with the root with a very fine file. Fourthly, an artificial tooth is selected, of the right size, shape and color, and fitted to the root; after which a gold pivot fixed in it in the manner before described, corresponding in size and length to the gold tube in the root. Having proceeded thus far, the operation is completed by applying the tooth to the root, but little pressure being required to force up the pivot.*[5]

Delicate work of this type was undertaken by only the most capable operators and was provided to those few patients who were willing to submit to long and painful operations. Surely, less complex and less durable procedures were probably used by many dentists, resulting in poorly fitted pivots and subsequent infection and suppuration within the canal.

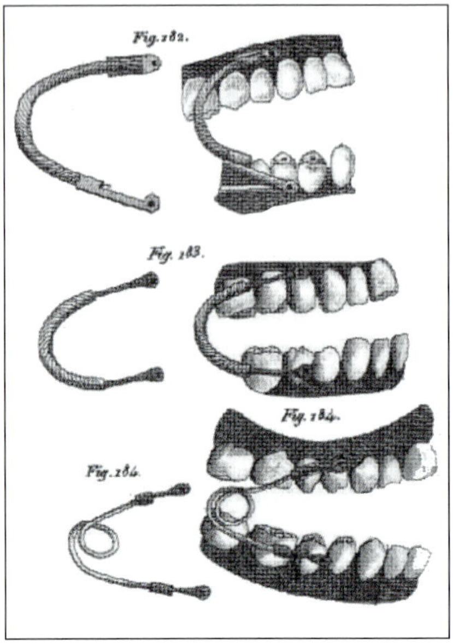

Fig 9-7 Spring-supported dentures. (From Delabarre.[1])

Dentures

In the fabrication of dentures, a dentition was carved from blocks of bone or ivory or was assembled from human and mineral teeth anchored by pins or soldered to a baseplate designed to fit on the gums. To construct the baseplate, a model of the surface anatomy of the patient's edentulous jaw was made by taking an impression with soft plaster of Paris. When the plaster impression had hardened (set), a reverse imprint was cast in stone. Using this stone model, the dentist formed the baseplate from a block of bone or ivory by carving and grinding the underside of the block to fit the contours of the stone model of the jaw. By applying various dyes to the model, the dentist could mark the high points of contact on the underside of the baseplate and then sculpt away. Repeating this process allowed for a wider and more uniform contact between the baseplate and the jaw (model). The next step was a trial in the patient's mouth. The opposite surface of the base was then carved to resemble teeth or prepared so that it could hold artificial teeth.

Retention of full maxillary dentures, always a special challenge, was improved by the use of springs; as early as 1728, Fauchard reported success with this method.[2] Delabarre demonstrated several designs for fabricating retention springs[1] (Fig 9-7). On the whole,

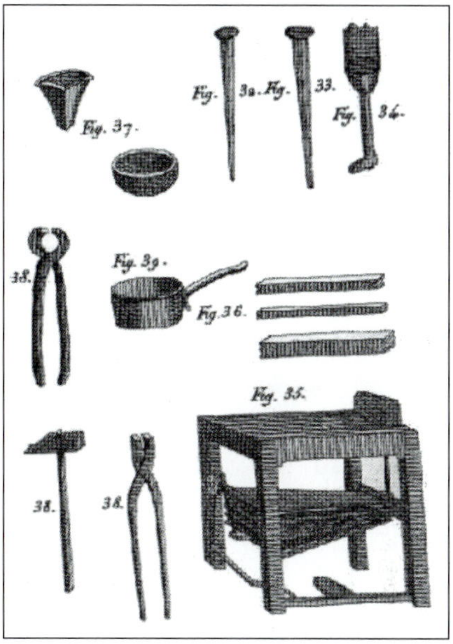

Fig 9-8 Tools used in metal work: forge (35), metal slabs (36), crucibles (37), hammer and pliers (38), and metal pot (39). (From Delabarre.[1])

these arrangements were uncomfortable and difficult to keep clean, with salivary deposits and food constantly becoming trapped in the springs. James Gardette, around 1800, made a serendipitous observation that atmospheric pressure could act to secure a maxillary denture. The "suction plates" worked only when there was accurate and close adaptation between the plate and the palatal tissue. Chapin Harris improved on this idea by creating a depression in the surface of the plate to form an "air chamber."[5]

Artificial dentures made to replace anterior teeth may have aided in pronunciation and beautified the smile, but they were almost totally useless to withstand the forces of mastication in eating food. Another serious limitation of artificial dentures was their susceptibility to decay caused by the porous nature of bone and ivory. The action of saliva and the decomposition of microscopic food particles retained within and/or adherent to the pores of the open interstitial spaces of the bone or the dentinal tubules of the ivory led to deterioration of the dentures as well as to bad odor and taste. Because of the susceptibility of bone and ivory to deterioration in the mouth, a more durable substitute for fabricating baseplates was sought. Many dentists experimented with gold, silver, aluminum, tin, and platinum, either as thin plates hammered to shape or poured as molten metal.

For such operations, dentists needed skills in working with metals, and the dental laboratory reflected this activity (Figs 9-8 and 9-9).

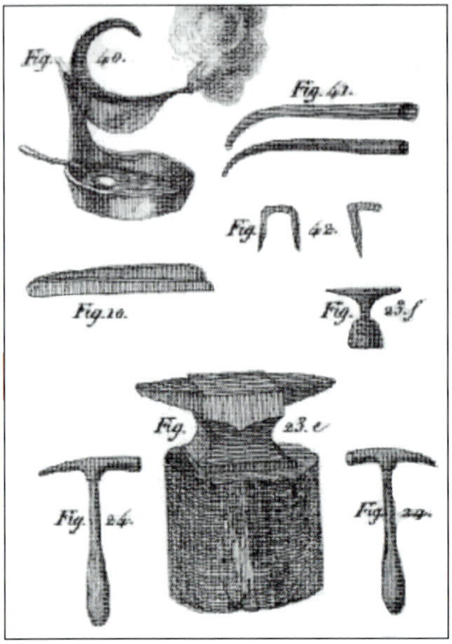

Fig 9-9 Anvils (23), hammers (24), a soldering lamp (40), blow pipes (41), pins (42), and pincers (10) for metalwork. (From Delabarre.[1])

According to Chapin Harris, every mechanical laboratory "should have the necessary fixtures for melting and working this metal into the various forms required for dental purposes. The principal of these are, a small furnace, with crucibles and tongs, ingot molds, an anvil and hammers, and a rolling mill; a plate gauge, draw-plate, and bench-vice; fluxing and refining chemicals."[5] Before gold plate was commercially available, dentists needed to know how to purify gold from coins. Chapin Harris stated that

> *most dentists did not have a sufficient knowledge of chemistry to undertake the chemical purification of gold and were forced to use the less preferred method of refining by fire.... By this method of refining gold, known as the dry process, or "refining by fire," sufficiently accurate results will be obtained for many of the practical purposes of mechanical dentistry; since the variation of an eighth or a quarter of a carat in the fineness of gold-plate is not often a matter of much consequence. Comparing the two classes of refining processes—the humid, by acids; and the dry, by fire—the first is the more accurate, and the only way to remove platina or silver; but it is the most troublesome, and requires a familiarity with chemical details, which, unfortunately, many dentists are totally ignorant of. The second may remove the lead, tin, zinc, antimony and bismuth, if in small quantity; and if continued for a sufficient length of time, with a free use of nitre, may remove a large proportion of copper. It can scarcely be depended upon if the object is to*

> *make an ingot of pure gold, but will answer admirably if the purpose is merely to lessen the alloy or remove certain impurities.*[5]

Harris noted that the dentist will often have occasion to use the dry process and gave the following description of the method pursued by Dr Elliot of Montreal:

> *The following implements are necessary for this purpose a small draught furnace, a quantity of fine hard-wood coal, a clean crucible with a sheet-iron cover (a lump of charcoal is better), a light pair of crucible-tongs, an ingot-mold made of soapstone, a little nitrate of potash, carbonate of potash, borax and oil. The fire-place of the furnace should be about ten inches in diameter, and eight or ten deep; this should be connected by means of a pipe with the chimney, so that a powerful draught may be made to pass through the coal. A blast-furnace is objectionable, for the reason that the bellows burns out the coal immediately under the crucible, and it is, therefore, constantly dropping down, which is not the case with the draught-furnace; besides, the draught-furnace produces a more even fire, a quality equally indispensable. In preparing for a heat, the furnace should be filled about half full of coal, and after it is well ignited, it should be consolidated as much as practicable without choking the draught. The crucible containing the metal and a little borax may then be set on, and more coal placed around and over it, the door of the furnace closed, and the damper opened. It should remain in this way until the gold is perfectly fused. The coal may then be removed from over the crucible, and a bit of nitrate of potash dropped in, quantity equal to the size of a pea to every ounce of gold, and the crucible immediately covered with a plate of iron. More coal may then be placed over and around the crucible, and the gold kept in a fused state at a high temperature, until the scoria ceases to pass off', which it will do in the course of five or six minutes. The ingot-mold having been previously warmed, should be placed in a convenient position for pouring, and filled about half full of lamp-oil. The cover should now be thrown off quickly, the crucible seized with the tongs, and at the same instant another small bit of nitrate of potash should be thrown into it, and the gold rapidly, but carefully, poured into the mold.*[5]

It is quite easy to see why physicians, with a long history of aversion to manual (surgical) operations, would shy away from dentistry, being perfectly comfortable in leaving it to others.

Dentists who worked with gold needed to understand the process of alloying gold with copper and silver to produce gold of different degrees of hardness and malleability. Harris recommended that 20-carat gold be used for maxillary plates, 21-carat gold for mandibular plates, and 18-carat gold for clasps and spiral springs. Many steps were required to fabricate a gold baseplate for a partial or full denture (Fig 9-10). From the poured model of the patient's jaw, a die and counterdie were made from fusible metal such as lead or zinc. A thin,

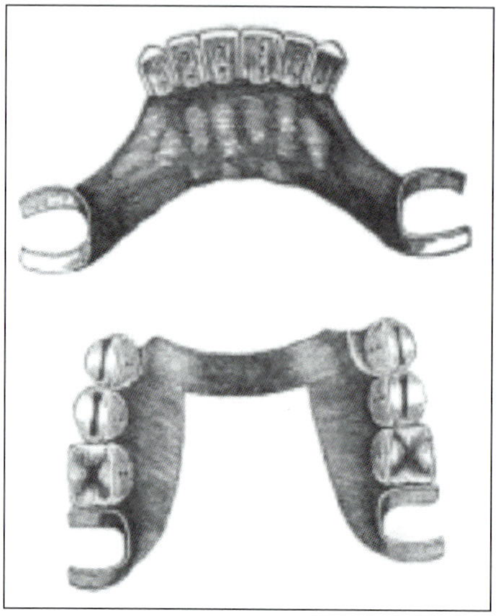

Fig 9-10 Partial metal plates secured by metal clasps. (From Harris.[5])

malleable sheet of gold, trimmed and roughly adapted to fit the edentulous area of the model, was swaged to an exact shape as follows:

> *The plate having been thus almost fitted by hammers and partial counters, it should be trimmed to its exact shape, and then placed between a fresh die and the full counter-die, and carried "home" by several firm blows of the hammer, given directly upon the center of the die. The hammer should not weigh more than three pounds, with a handle about a foot long. It is a great mistake to use a very heavy or a very long handled hammer. The "striking block" may be an anvil or a large wooden block set in sand, and the base of the counter-die must rest steadily upon it. Throughout the entire process of swaging the plate must be frequently annealed. It may be suddenly cooled after all except the final annealing; when the cooling must be very gradual so as to avoid warping or springing. After fitting the plate to the metallic die, it is applied to the mouth, for the purpose of ascertaining if the impression from which the model was procured is correct. It sometimes happens that this is imperfect; in which case, a new one will have to be taken, and the whole process of procuring plaster and metallic models and counter-models again gone through with; hence the propriety of the precaution of trying it in the mouth before the clasps and teeth are attached.*[5]

With the baseplate completed, it was ready for attachment of artificial teeth.

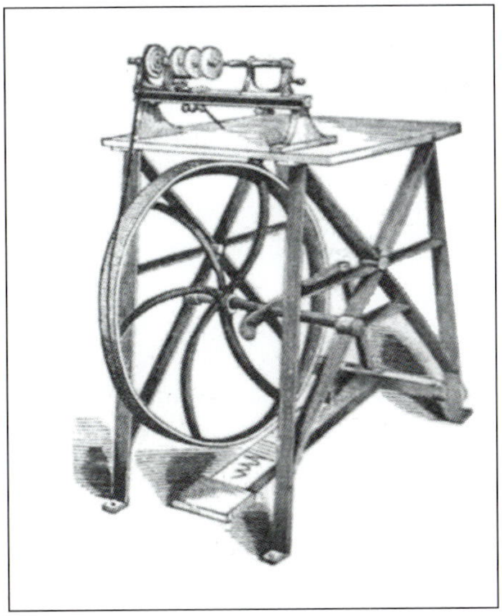

Fig 9-11 Foot lathe equipped with carborundum wheels for grinding natural and artificial teeth. (From Harris.[5])

By the mid 19th century, three kinds of plate teeth (plain, gum, and sections) were available from manufacturers. Harris claimed that in strength, durability, and facility of repair, plain teeth were superior to the others and more readily adapted to the plate. They were arranged on the plate, retained in place by a piece of wax, and, in a delicate process requiring precision, riveted and soldered to the plate. If the teeth did not fit closely to the plate or gums, they "must be ground on emery or corundum wheels until accurately fitted, and so arranged as to meet the teeth with which they are intended to antagonize, at the same instant around the entire arch in full cases; in partial cases the natural teeth should touch their antagonists more decidedly than the artificial ones."[5] Lastly, the plate must undergo a finishing process to remove excess solder and to polish all external surfaces with burnishers or revolving brushes and jewelers rouge. Foot-operated lathes (Fig 9-11) were used to trim teeth, shape pivots, and polish metal surfaces.

Dentures made with precious metals were obviously a costly item for the few patients that could afford them. The famed violinist, A. Paganini, dramatically underscored this point. He had been edentulous for years and had often complained of his inability to eat his favorite foods. After much encouragement from his friends and without bothering to ask about cost, he agreed to have himself fitted for a denture. Pleased with his superb dentures, he ordered a second set.

Shortly thereafter, the dentist's clerk arrived at Paganini's home to present the bill. Just finishing his bath and still wrapped in a towel, Paganini glanced at the bill and let out an outrageous cry, and with wild gesticulations he dropped his towel in the excitement, crumpled the bill, and threw it to the floor, all the while hurling invectives at the poor messenger. The dentures were charged at 1,000 francs apiece. No doubt the work of a virtuoso![6]

Porcelain teeth

Porcelain, or mineral, teeth were introduced into the American colonies from Paris by Dr A. A. Plantou. Early mineral teeth had a "split bean" shape with a rounded labial surface and a flat lingual or palatal surface, on which a semicircular groove was made to hold two small platinum pins before firing of the paste. In use, the mineral teeth were either soldered to a gold wire (via the platinum pins) and subsequently fastened to adjacent natural teeth with the gold wire or attached to a baseplate carved from ivory or bone, again using gold wire. These early mineral teeth were opaque and brittle. Following Plantou's early work, the fabrication of porcelain teeth was taken up by several individuals, not all of whom were dentists. Charles W. Peale, foremost portrait painter of Philadelphia, perhaps best known for his portrait of George Washington, made mineral teeth around 1822. Within a few decades, several dentists, including S. Spooner (New York), J. F. Flagg (Boston), and E. Wildman (Philadelphia), established a reputation for this type of work.

Samuel W. Stockton began an enterprise to supply mineral teeth on a commercial basis in 1835. Despite batches of varying quality, his production reached 500,000 teeth per year by 1845. Wildman, in Philadelphia, experimenting with different mineral compositions and firing temperatures, ultimately produced outstanding porcelain teeth with lifelike gingival surfaces. He is regarded to have given the process its scientific basis. But in this rapidly moving business, it was Samuel S. White who achieved the pinnacle of success. White, a nephew of Samuel Stockton and trainee in Stockton's business, began producing artificial teeth on his own. He introduced new pin designs, better heat resistance to soldering, and minimization of bulk and weight. Improvements in texture, color, and transparency made his product more physiologically and anatomically correct. To improve the appearance of dentures, the "continuous gum" denture was developed, in which the artificial teeth were attached to a previously baked porcelain baseplate by a second paste that fused at a lower temperature. Single and block teeth with colored gums (gum teeth) were introduced by numerous dentists, most of whom filed for patent rights to their inventions.

Vulcanization

Around the middle of the 19th century, baseplates of gutta-percha were introduced. These had the advantage of lower cost and could be colored to match the natural gingiva. In 1851, Nelson Goodyear published a method for hardening rubber compound. This process, called *vulcanization*, was carried out by exposing the rubber to high heat and sulfur. The hardened product was stable and resistant to heat, cold, and acids. Thomas Evans, a notable American dentist practicing in Paris, had recognized the potential use of vulcanized rubber in dentistry and had mentioned it in 1852 to Nelson Goodyear, the discoverer of vulcanization.[7] This method proved to have great benefits for the fabrication of dentures, because the soft rubber compound could be easily adapted to the model and the artificial teeth could be positioned in the soft rubber prior to hardening by vulcanization. Furthermore, the product was light, durable, and could be colored to mimic the pink tones of the oral tissues.

In the fabrication of vulcanite dentures, a temporary baseplate was made by molding softened gutta-percha or wax onto a plaster of Paris model of the patient's edentulous jaw.[8] Next, the artificial teeth (crowns fitted with platinum pins) were placed in the temporary plate, using wax to hold them in place (see Fig 9-12b). After confirmation of the correct articulation to the opposing dentition with models mounted in an articulator and by trial in the patient's mouth, the temporary plate was ready to be packed in a three-part vulcanizing flask (Fig 9-12a). After the exposed surfaces of the plate (but not the teeth) were coated with oil, the plate was mounted on its model and placed in chamber A of the flask (Fig 9-12b). Plaster of Paris was added just to the edge of the plate and rim and allowed to set. Now chambers B and D were assembled over chamber A and were filled with plaster of Paris. All three chambers were clamped tightly with bolts using a clamping device.

Once the plaster was fully hardened, the flask was taken apart. Now chamber B of the flask contained the gutta-percha plate with the teeth in their correct alignment and with pins exposed to the surface (Fig 9-12c). The gutta-percha and wax were removed with instruments to expose the underlying surface of the model and the base of the artificial teeth with exposed pins, and radiating and marginal outlet grooves were carved in the surface of the plaster to permit the flow of excess rubber during the vulcanization step (see Fig 9-12c). Small

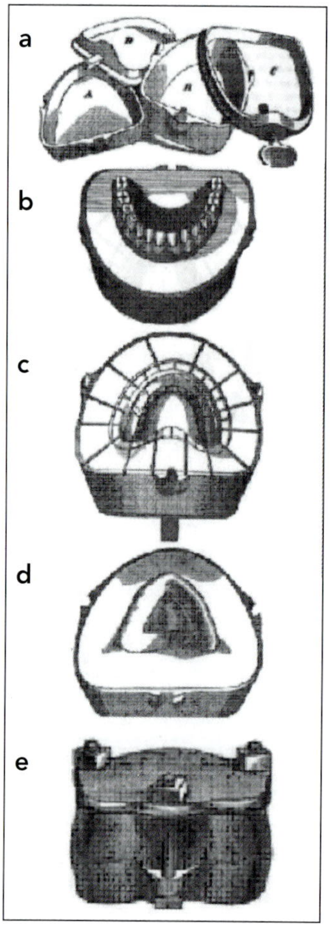

Fig 9-12 Steps for fabricating a vulcanite denture using the tripartite flask, as described by Richardson.[8]

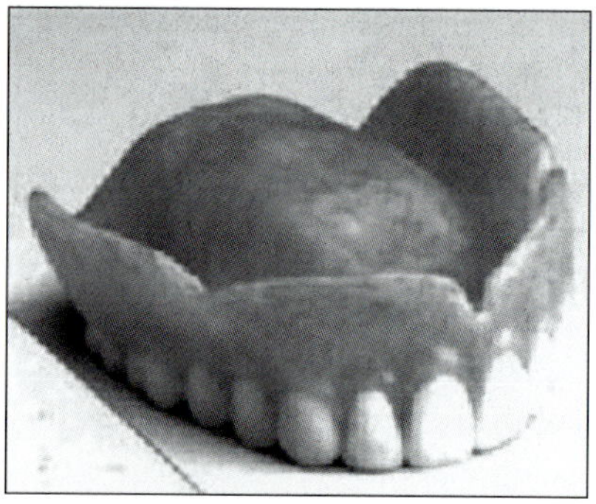

Fig 9-13 Completed vulcanite denture.

pieces of soft, vulcanizable rubber matrix were now applied to the exposed pins and undersurface of the teeth as well as to the surface of the model contained in part A of the flask (Fig 9-12d). Heat was applied to ensure that all the rubber was softened and uniformly distributed. After the packing of the rubber compound was finished, the flask was reassembled and was ready for the vulcanizer (Fig 9-12e). The completed denture was trimmed and brought to a high polish before presentation to the patient (Fig 9-13).

The process of vulcanizing or hardening of the rubber compound was accomplished by subjecting the flasks to high heat under steam pressure in special machines called *vulcanizers*.[9] Dental rubber com-

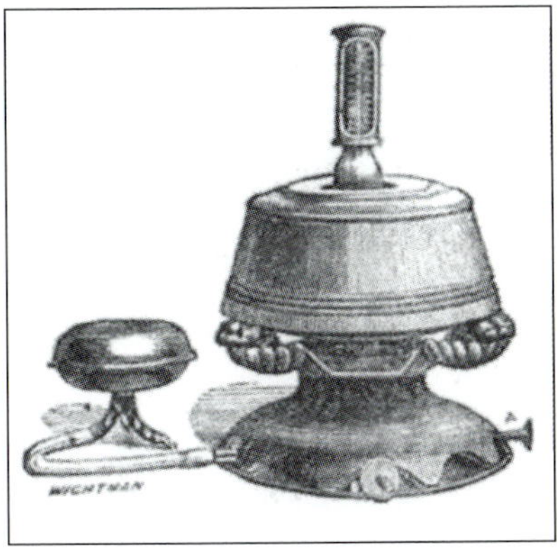

Fig 9-14 Single-flask, ironclad oven vulcanizer. The heat is supplied by an alcohol lamp. (From Richardson.[8])

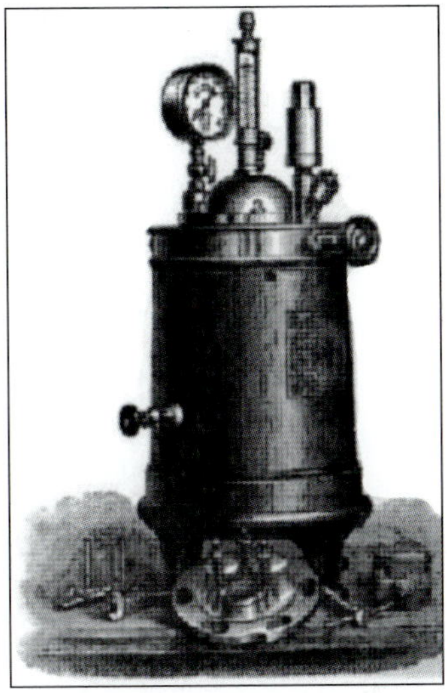

Fig 9-15 Seabury vulcanizer. (From Beale.[9])

pound sold by dental supply companies already contained the sulfur needed for the hardening process. The vulcanization was completed within 40 minutes at a temperature of 320 degrees from an alcohol lamp in the machine depicted in Fig 9-14. A variety of designs were manufactured, from the simple vulcanizer (as shown in Fig 9-14) to larger and more sophisticated models, such as the Seabury vulcanizer that could accommodate several flasks at a time (Fig 9-15). Early models were not the safest to use, and the literature contained numerous reports of exploding vulcanizers. Alfred Welch, reporting in *Dental Cosmos* in 1865, recounts the following accident:

> *I must confess to having felt a little afraid from the first, every time I have used these thin thermometer vulcanizers, especially so, since the bursting of one of Whitney's in our office at Wenona not long since. A slight oversight only was the occasion of that terrible explosion. Lucky, indeed, that my brother, and a lady patient in the chair at the time, were not both sent "kiting through the air, taking an aerial journey," as Dr. L. has it, "at the expense of all earthly ties." Fortunately no one was hurt, though the top of the vulcanizer was blown through the ceiling, knocking off the shingles of the roof above. The flask was blown to splinters, part of which, with the plate of teeth, was sent through the wall, and probably fell down between the joists. One thing is certain, we never could find a vestige of the teeth afterward. The intention of this writing is to contribute a little influence toward an overwhelming demand for safe vulcanizers. The makers would probably make money*

by the change; for what dentist would not gladly throw away his unsafe one and buy a new and safe vulcanizer?[9]

More often than not, accidents occurred because of inattention to the dangers of steam boilers and carelessness of dentists. As Dr W. H. Trueman reported in an 1869 issue of *Dental Cosmos*:

There is a lamentable degree of ignorance among those who are using vulcanizers as regards the character and expansive power of steam, and the strength of metals, as well as recklessness in their use. From the fact of their being steam-tight, and making no fuss like a whizzing, noisy engine, no danger is apprehended, though they may be subjected to many times the pressure of the boiler of any engine. The fact is, that at the ordinary temperature of vulcanizing, the pressure is fully up to the ordinary pressure of steam boilers, and the recklessness with which dentists subject their vulcanizers to three, four, or even five times this pressure, is sufficient to cause alarm in the mind of any person cognizant of the fact. From this cause there has been many amusing incidents, when the mind disconnects them from any thought of the danger incurred. Ideas of economy and convenience induce country and traveling dentists to use a cook-stove as a heating apparatus for vulcanizing. Several accidents have occurred from this cause. One man set his vulcanizer on the boiler-hole of the cook-stove while his wife was getting breakfast, and stepping outside to attend to some household duties, forgot it; an explosion eventually ensued, filling the kitchen with the fire, ashes, and fragments of the stove, fortunately without doing injury to anyone. Others have been known to place their vulcanizers in a hard-coal fire, and even to bank the coal up clear to the top of the machine. A more foolhardy or reprehensible practice can scarcely be imagined. But generally the accidents occur by the operator leaving the machine to attend to a patient, or to some other business in which the mind becomes engaged, and the vulcanizer is forgotten. A dentist in Canada once told his student to 'watch the vulcanizer,' without giving him any further instruction, although the young man had never been inside a laboratory before. He did 'watch it,'—until it blew up, and placed him in a position to 'see stars' in broad daylight.[9]

Many of the older dentists who had established a reputation for their expertise in gold plate denture technique, such as Dr M. L. Rhein of New York City, decried the deteriorating state of mechanical dentistry resulting from the introduction of vulcanite dental plates:

Every student of dental history recognizes the detriment that was wrought to the mechanical skill of the profession by the introduction of vulcanite. In an incredibly short time the number of gold-plate workers had become so few that they were easily counted. The prosthetic specialty of our calling had become so degraded that most of our best men intrusted this work to ordinary laboratory mechanics, whose compensation was on a par with the quality of their work.[10]

Vulcanite dentures were exploited by advertising dentists who promoted cheap products and gimmicks to attract customers. Dr L. H. Delange, writing in the *Proceedings of the New Jersey Dental Society*, recounted the following stories:

> *A lady, an acquaintance of my own, passing one of these cheap John's, entered the trap through curiosity, and inquired about a three dollar set of teeth. John hem'd and haw'd, and advised her in a friendly way to try a more expensive set; but finding her persistent, informed her that he did not think they would suit her, as he was compelled to use second-hand teeth for that price. Their advertisement has lately taken another form, they make presents to their patrons, as car tickets, chromos, etc. Persons calling with this advertisement clipped from the paper will find it good for one dollar. Teeth. teeth! Three dollars a set, warranted, etc.*[11]

With the discovery of inhalation anesthesia in 1844, patients were now more likely to undergo extractions in preparation for dentures. In the early 20th century, a tsunami of extraction and denture fabrication occurred when the theory of focal infection reached wide acceptance among the medical and dental professions. Dentists were rightly accused of placing less emphasis on restoring teeth and having wholeheartedly embraced the money-making denture business.

Unlike gold or silver dentures, vulcanite dentures were cheap to produce and could be fabricated by anyone after just a few weeks of training. Despite the difference in costs to the dentist, some practitioners felt justified in charging the same amount for vulcanite denture as for a gold denture:

> *One professional friend whom I asked what difference he made in his fees between gold and vulcanite work, replied, "Very little; I do not charge for the material of my work, any more than an artist does when he sells a picture; my fee is for my taste in suiting the expression of the countenance, and skill in overcoming the engineering difficulties which are met with in attaining the desired end."*[12]

The history of vulcanite dentures illuminates a particularly troublesome period in the development of dentistry, a time when constraints were imposed on practitioners by the enforcement of patents. As the use of dentures became more widespread, in part following the introduction of general anesthesia and the cheapness of the rubber compound and artificial teeth, the potential lucrative aspects of licensing fees for use of vulcanite became apparent. Some years later in 1858, Charles Goodyear, Nelson's brother, was awarded a United States patent for the use of the vulcanization process in the fabrication of dentures. In the 1850s, the Goodyear Company sold rubber compound and right-to-use licenses to dentists, collecting royalties for each denture fabricated by the vulcanization process.[7] Forced by threats of prosecution, the dentists of New York formed the New York Dental Protection Union.

The Goodyear Company did not take dentists to court over the illegal use of vulcanization because all transgressions were settled out of court. Many dentists simply ignored the restrictions of the patent and were never caught. But in 1862, the American Hard Rubber Company (Goodyear) sued the New York Tooth Manufacturing Company for infringement of their patent for the vulcanization of rubber. In that same year, the New York Dental Protection Union was informed that "H. B. Goodyear was flooding the country with circulars threatening to prosecute all dentists who vulcanize hard-rubber plates for teeth, unless they pay tribute to him."[13] The American Hard Rubber Company was employing spies and collectors to get as much money as possible out of the dental profession. The battle took a turn for the worse in 1866, when Josiah Bacon, a Boston businessman and treasurer of the Goodyear Dental Vulcanite Company, obtained sole possession to the patent rights.[7]

Bacon began a campaign of vigorously enforcing the collection of royalties and the initiation of court proceedings against dentists who were not licensed to use the vulcanization process in fabricating dentures. Dentists who had purchased licenses were told to maintain a log of all vulcanite denture cases, made ready to be inspected by Bacon or his representative at the time of collection of royalties. Over the next decade, the Goodyear Dental Vulcanite Company under Bacon's leadership successfully prosecuted dentists and threatened hundreds of others across America. In 1877, the US Supreme Court ruled against an organized dentistry petition (led by Dr S. S. White) in favor of Josiah Bacon's legal rights to the process of vulcanization and the products of that process (ie, the actual manufacture of dentures). The dental profession was hounded by Bacon for nearly 15 years, until Easter Sunday morning in San Francisco in 1879, when Bacon was shot dead by Dr Samuel Chalfant, a local dentist who had been pursued for several years for collection of royalties.[7,14] Chalfant served 10 years in San Quentin State Prison before taking up the practice of dentistry once more in San Francisco. With Bacon dead and the expiration of the patent rights in 1881, the dental profession was finally freed from the pressures of court enforcement of patent rights for vulcanized dentures.

As technology advanced over the latter half of the 19th century, dental practice continued to be plagued by the protectionism of the patent system. Every new instrument, modification of an existing one, or introduction of a new technique was seen as an opportunity to make a fortune. Encouraged by patent lawyers, dentists were quick to take advantage of the system. Dr J. D. White, in an editorial on patents, wrote critically of mechanical dentists (patentees) who associated on equal terms with the more liberal operative dentists:

> *But as it is, there are conflicting interests; one portion (operative dentists) are anxious to teach all they have learned by study and experience from liberal sentiments, to enlarge and extend the basis of their profession, and elevate its standing; but another set (mechanical dentists) are non-committals; they have a good deal to say, but nothing definite to communicate; they learn all they can for selfish purposes, and as soon as an idea has assumed a tangible form, whether it has been helped forward by the liberal portion or not, it is patented, and brought into the society or offered to the profession for sale. We do not object to dental patents of mechanical matters, any more than we do to patents generally, but we do hold that patentees and liberal dentists can never associate on the same grounds in the same society.*[15]

Delegates to the American Dental Convention of 1862 were asked to support a resolution condemning:

> *The practice of forcing upon us the use of certain patent-rights, sometimes by threats, until tribute is paid, and sometimes upon influential members by presentation patents upon articles either worthless in themselves, or by right or prior invention, belonging to the profession, or patents in themselves otherwise invalid.... We are obliged to rise in our might to protest against it.*[16]

Further consideration of the controversy over patents is presented in chapter 13.

Summary

Restoration of missing teeth, the work of the "mechanical dentist," was mainly a craft or, as some would argue, an art concerned with metallurgy and esthetics and less with the biology of living tissue. Dentists who were skilled in creating masterpiece dentures out of precious metals were also likely to pride themselves in the use of the gold foil technique in operative dentistry. These men came to resist change introduced by the use of "plastic" materials such as amalgam and vulcanite. They were less likely to appreciate the importance of research and science in the advancement of the profession. But with time, these prejudices would fade and mechanical dentistry would evolve into a true clinical science during the latter half of the 20th century, with the introduction of new impression materials, better metal alloys, and computer-driven fabrication techniques. Coupled with advances in endodontics and implant dentistry, the specialty practice of prosthodontics flourishes today. For the wealthy patient, a highly functional and esthetic full restoration of the dentition is possible.

References

1. Delabarre CF. Traite de la partie mecanique de l'art du chirurgien-dentiste. Ouvrage orne de 42 planches. Paris: Croullebois, Gabon et Mequignon-Marvis, 1820.
2. Fauchard P. The Surgeon Dentist; Or, Treatise on the Teeth, ed 2. Paris: P. J. Mariette, 1746.
3. Guerini V. A History of Dentistry from the Most Ancient Times until the End of the Eighteenth Century. Philadelphia: Lea & Febiger, 1909:188–199.
4. Fox J. The History and Treatment of the Diseases of the Teeth, the Gums, and the Alveolar Processes, with the Operations Which They Respectively Require. London: Thomas Cox, 1806.
5. Harris CA. The Principles and Practice of Dental Surgery, ed 8. Philadelphia: Lindsay & Blakiston, 1863.
6. Le dentier de Paganini. Revue et Archives Suisses D'Odontologie 1887;1: 319–340.
7. Prioli C. Rubber Dentures for the Masses. Invention and Technology Magazine 1991;7:28–31,34–37.
8. Richardson J. A Practical Treatise on Mechanical Dentistry. Philadelphia: P. Blakiston, Son, & Co, 1888.
9. Beale AP. The American System of Dentistry. Philadelphia: Lea Brothers, 1887.

10. Rhein ML. Ideal bridge work. Dent Cosmos 1894;36:97–110.
11. Delange LH. Dental rat traps. In: Condensed Proceedings of the NJ State Dental Society for the Years 1875, 1876, and 1877. Newark: LJ Hardham, 1878:45–48.
12. Balkwill FH. Mechanical Dentistry in Gold and Vulcanite. London: J. & A. Churchill, 1880.
13. McQuillen JH. Review of dental literature and art. Dent Cosmos 1862;4:211–216.
14. White SS. Obituary: The death of Josiah Bacon. Dent Cosmos 1879;21:350.
15. White JD. Division of labor. Dent Cosmos 1859;1:90–91.
16. Ellis GW. Proceedings of the American Dental Convention. Dent Cosmos 1862;4:77–98.

10

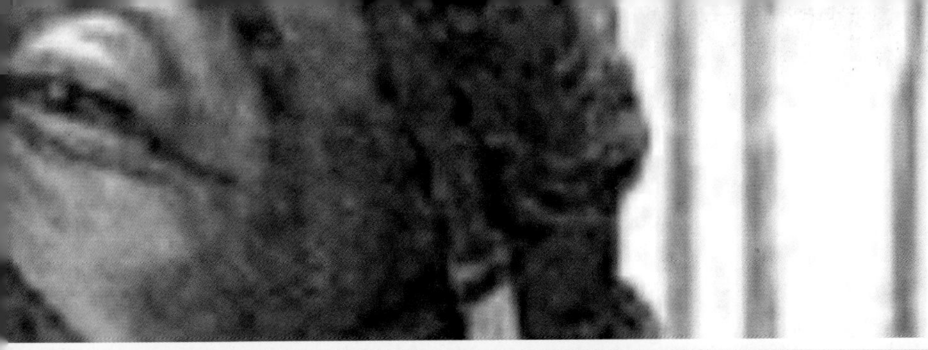

Operative Dentistry

Dental decay and the toothache it causes are among the oldest of man's afflictions. Various approaches to the treatment of toothache have been attempted from the earliest days of medical practice. Rhazes, an Arabian physician of the 9th century, recommended filling cavities with resin and herbal medicines (see chapter 1). Later, Guy de Chauliac, in his treatise on surgery written in the 14th century, advised that decayed teeth should be cleansed of all rotten matter and the cavity filled with wax or mastic containing opium, camphor, and other medicinal herbs (see chapter 2). Tooth operations for the removal of dental caries and the filling of cavities with lead or gold began in earnest during the late Middle Ages. The Italian Renaissance surgeons Giovanni d'Arcoli and Giovanni de Vigo described the use of drills for the removal of decay and the introduction of lead and/or gold fillings[1] (see chapter 3). Gold fillings were meant to serve as permanent restorations of tooth substance as opposed to a mere temporary relief of pain with herbal-based remedies.

Fauchard noted that there were an innumerable number of people who made false claims to have found remedies for toothache. In Paris, there were charlatans who boasted of killing tooth worms and others who cured toothache by simply touching the aching tooth "with their fingers dipped or washed in rare and mysterious liquor." Some were followers of the Italian physician M. Valsalva, who treated toothache by "scarifying the ears with a lancet or cauterization with a red hot iron." They assumed that in this process they were blocking the blood supply to the tooth. Fauchard recalled that he knew of "a Turkish clockmaker of this persuasion who was renowned for this way of curing toothache. I know also that in spite of these pretensions that most of those who put themselves in his hands were afterwards obliged to come to me to relieve them of their sufferings." Fauchard suggested that any cure that may have resulted from such methods had to be attributed to the force of imagination, of a strong belief in the mysterious remedy, akin to the "animal faculty" by which men wounded in battle feel no pain.[2]

Caries

Fauchard was of the opinion that caries that had not yet reached the pulp of the tooth was curable by four remedies: the first by filing away the decay, the second by inserting lead, the third by oils (cinnamon and cloves), and the fourth by cautery with a hot iron. Another method, favored by the Paris surgeon Dionis, was to cauterize the lesion with vitriol (sulfuric acid). But Fauchard cautioned that vitriol could increase the pain and render it long-lasting by its ability to penetrate and injure the healthy parts of the tooth, instead advocating his preferred method:

> *When a tooth is slightly carious it is enough to remove the caries by instruments and to fill the cavity with lead. When the caries penetrates further and causes pain after removal put into the cavity every day a ball of cotton dipped in oil of cinnamon or cloves. Continue this for a sufficient time adjusting and pressing down the cotton by degrees to accustom the sensitive parts to pressure. Four or five days later remove the carious matter left in the cavity. This prevents the return of pain. It produces in the osseous fibers of the tooth a slight exfoliation which suffices. It prevents sometimes further progress of the caries and the pain. If enough time had elapsed and the pain does not cease, the actual cautery must be applied and several months later fill the cavity if the condition of the carious cavity permits, because sometimes there are cavities which it is impossible to fill.*[2]

For removal of the carious portion of a tooth, Fauchard employed several types of instruments, such as drills (like those used by clockmakers), chisels, and scrapers (Fig 10-1). The drills, used in enlarging the openings of the lesions, were "turned between the thumb and first finger from left to right and right to left." Fauchard went to great length to describe the best positioning of the dentist and the patient, the method of stabilizing the patient's chin and lips, and the

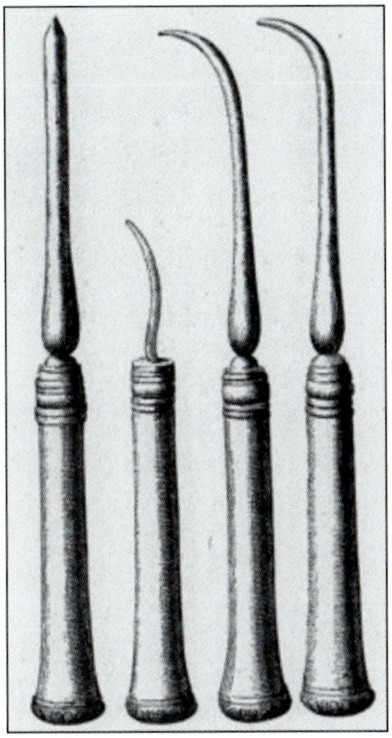

Fig 10-1 Fauchard's instruments for excavating dental decay.

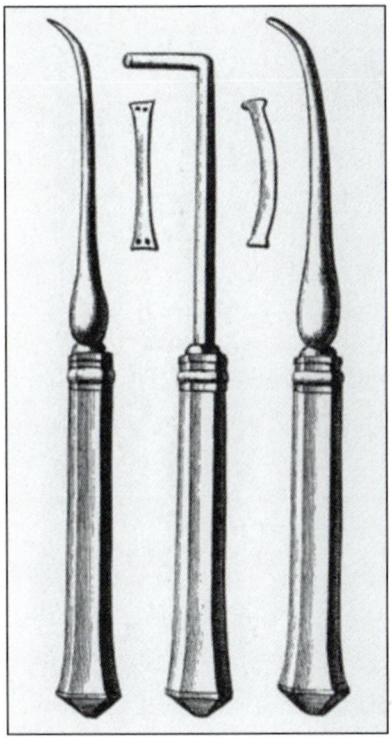

Fig 10-2 Fauchard's instruments for plugging cavities.

correct manner of holding the instruments when doing fillings in all areas of the mouth. Several types of instruments with round or curved ends, called *pluggers*, were used to fill or plug cavities. Instruments for condensing had rounded ends bent at a right angle to the shaft of the instrument (Fig 10-2). Both types of instruments were securely fastened to handles made of ivory or wood.

Tin, lead, and gold were hammered into thin foils approximating the thickness of paper. Thin strips of the foil were placed into the cavity and compressed down with condensers. Upon filling the cavity, the surface of the metal was pierced several times with a sharp-pointed instrument and further condensed to ensure full compaction of the metal. Lastly, the surface of the filling was smoothed and polished. Although several operators preferred to fill cavities with gold, Fauchard preferred lead and tin. According to Fauchard, tin and lead were more pliable and adaptable than gold and less expensive for the patient, although some patients, believing that gold had special virtues, were willing to accept the higher cost. Fauchard cautioned that

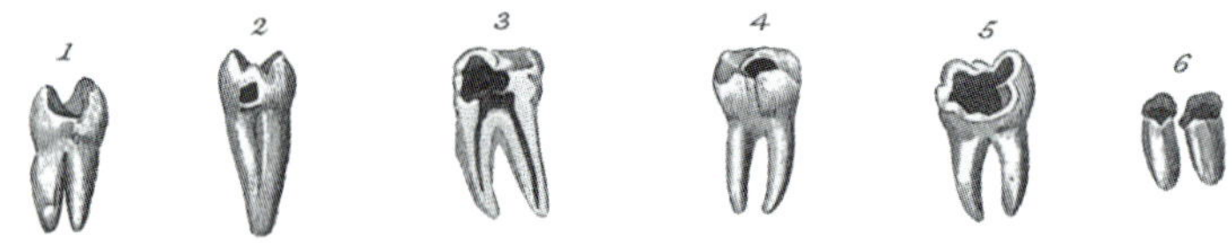

Fig 10-3 Progress of dental caries from a dark spot (2) to large cavities in molars (3 to 6) to destruction of the entire crown (6). (From Fox.[3])

some were fooled by the fraudulent practice of coloring leaves of tin or lead with a saffron-based dye.[2]

Cautery was applied in treating carious teeth that caused great pain. Fauchard used brass knitting needles, curved at their end, for cauterizing caries lesions. After the decayed substance and the burnt cauterized matter had been removed, the cavity was medicated with a cotton ball steeped in oil of cinnamon before being plugged with metal. It was sometimes necessary to apply cauterization repeatedly before eliminating the pain of toothache. Often the lesions were so sensitive that it was necessary to leave a medicated cotton ball in the cavity for an extended period of time before attempting to plug the tooth. When caries had penetrated into the pulp, causing an abscess, it became necessary to probe the cavity to create an exit for the pus. After several months, the tooth would be filled to prevent any further decay.[2]

In his book *The History and Treatment of the Diseases of the Teeth, the Gums, and the Alveolar Processes, with the Operations Which they Respectively Require*, published in London in 1806, Joseph Fox provided the earliest illustrations of dental caries (Fig 10-3). For his description of the process, see pages 85–86.

The pain of toothache, according to Fox, was one of the most excruciating to which man is liable. He noted that it was caused by inflammation of the highly vascular and innervated membrane of the internal cavity of the tooth. Swelling of the tissues, caused by inflammation, being resisted by the confining hard parts of the tooth, amplified the pain. Relief was almost always achieved with a tincture of opium, camphor, and cloves applied to the affected part, but more permanent relief required filling or plugging the cavity. Like Fauchard, Fox recommended the use of gold foil or pure tin beaten into

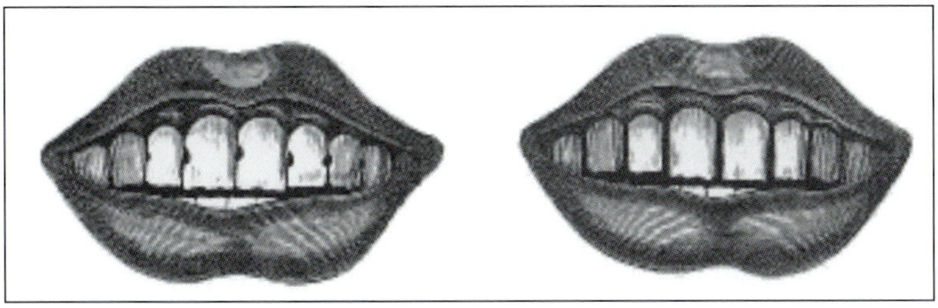

Fig 10-4 Interdental decay *(left)* and its removal by filing tooth structure *(right)*. (From Fox.[3])

leaves as the most favorable filling materials. Lead was considered to be deleterious because it was corroded by the saliva and caused stomach problems. Fox described how the progress of caries seemed to be retarded after the crown had been completely destroyed in that the decay scarcely ever attacked the roots. In such cases, the roots could be made useful as sites for the insertion of pivot teeth.

Filing of Teeth

A technique for removal of decayed tissue that was used before the art of plugging teeth was perfected was to file the tooth, removing sound tissue along with the decayed area. This method was applied only in relatively small cavities, especially in the incisors (Fig 10-4), where the cavities could be eliminated and the enlarged interdental areas more easily cleaned. Thin, flat, and rounded files were used. The obvious drawbacks to filing were that a considerable amount of good tooth structure was sacrificed and the operation was painful. This method continued to be used sparingly well into the 19th century.

In 1871, Dr Robert Arthur, the man who had played a key role in discovering and promoting adhesive gold fillings, shocked the profession when he admitted that he had made significant use of files for treating dental caries in his practice. In his book *The Treatment and Prevention of Decay of the Teeth*, he asked the profession to reexamine its love affair with gold fillings and to consider filing teeth as an economical and effective treatment modality.[4] According to Arthur, dental authorities had taken the view that filling or plugging the teeth was the only remedy for decay. Contemporary textbooks of dentistry hardly gave any consideration to the treatment of decay by filing tooth structure. He explained that decay usually attacks the teeth at such places where the teeth are in contact, places that favor the lodgment and retention of food particles. Decay would not occur if the teeth stood apart from each other.

In exhibiting a drawing of the teeth of a 76-year-old lady filed at 12 years of age, Arthur established the fact that it was a reliable practice. He argued that filing fell into disfavor because of the imperfect manner in which his successors attempted to carry it out, noting that in his time, "it was almost impossible to obtain proper instruction, and many men assumed the responsibilities of the dental profession who were entirely incompetent." If incipient caries was properly removed by filing, the disease was not likely to recur. To emphasize his point, Arthur recalled:

> *A gentleman for whom I was operating asked my opinion of his front teeth. My answer was, "They have been pretty severely filed." "Yes," he replied, "and I did it myself. Twenty-two years ago my front teeth were very badly decayed. I went to one of the most celebrated dentists in Philadelphia to have them filled. To my horror and disgust, he said, 'They are too far gone to fill and save. I would advise you to let them alone, and when they commence paining have them extracted and artificial ones substituted.' I went down into Market Street and purchasing a broad, flat file, I went home, placed myself in front of a glass, and, though it hurt almost beyond expression or bearing, filed a broad space between each of my front teeth."*[4]

Arthur observed that "the spaces were enormous, but every tooth was in its place, and likely to remain; the decayed portions yet remained by slight concavities, and others by discolored but not entirely decomposed bone."[4]

Although one might fear that the removal of enamel by filing would lead to a greater chance of decay, Arthur argued to the contrary:

> *There is abundant reason for believing that the exposed surface of the dentine from which the enamel has been cut away, provided it can be kept perfectly cleansed, undergoes the conservative alteration described. The contents of the exposed tubuli become changed into a hard ivory-like substance, and it is quite probable that in the intertubular substance there is an exchange of particles of lime for animal matter. The new formation differs from normal dentine in being always denser and generally slightly or considerably discolored. It has been termed "eburnated," from the ivory-like character, in the consistency at least, of its surface. It can readily be detected by anyone who has once examined it.*[4]

Filling of Teeth

Notwithstanding the potential usefulness of filing enamel to remove incipient caries and to create more easily maintained sites, Arthur admitted that, by far, the commonest method of treating dental caries was the removal of decayed tissue by instrumentation followed by the insertion of a filling material to restore the original occlusal surface and contact points. He acknowledged the fact that the daily routine of most dentists of his day consisted "almost exclusively of plugging and extracting carious and, by no means infrequently, sound teeth and inserting artificial teeth."[5]

Chapin Harris, author of the first American textbook on dentistry, stated that filling teeth was one of the most difficult operations the dentist was called upon to perform: "It is the only certain remedy that can be applied for arresting the progress of deep-seated caries; but to be effective it must be executed in the most thorough and perfect manner."[6] Dr E. Parmly stated that the operation of filling teeth "is imperfectly and improperly performed more frequently than any other operation on the teeth."

According to Harris, the following considerations were essential to success in operative dentistry:

> *First, the instruments used must be of the proper construction and variety; second, the metal employed must be properly prepared as well as properly introduced; third, the cavity which receives the metal must be so shaped as to retain it in such a manner as to exclude not only solids, but all fluids, and even the atmosphere itself; fourth, the surface of the metal must be left in such condition as to place it beyond the reach of injury from food and any mechanical agents with which it necessarily comes in contact; fifth, the tooth thus stopped should be free from pain, and every known cause of internal inflammation.*[6]

Dr Thomas Fillebrown, professor at the Harvard Dental School, defined *operative dentistry* as all work dependent on the natural teeth for support, done at the operating chair, and most with the patient present.[7] Dr Louis Jack, in *The American System of Dentistry* (1887), provided the following description of the process of filling teeth:

> *A stopping process may be defined as any method of treatment of dental caries which effects the removal of the carious matter and substitutes therefore some material possessing such inherent physical properties as render it capable of introduction into all parts of the resultant cavity and of protecting its margins and inner surface from further destructive influences. The most important properties such materials should possess are adaptability, immunity from oxidization at*

> *ordinary temperatures, and incapability of solution in the fluids of the mouth. This process is with propriety divided into two distinct parts—the surgical treatment, and the mechanical treatment. The first comprises every preliminary effort which has to do with the preparation of any given case for the succeeding mechanical processes, such as the separation of the teeth, the relief of sensibility, the removal of caries, the definition of the boundaries of the healthy structures, the careful and exact formation of the cavity to facilitate the insertion of the stopping and to enable the stopping, of whatever material it may be composed, to be retained. The subjective consideration of the ultimate form of the filling with reference to its usefulness, its appearance, and its relation to the other teeth has also from the beginning of the case to be clearly kept in the mind of the operator. The mechanical treatment includes the preparation of the stopping material, the insertion of it, the formation and finishing of the external surface of the inserted material and of the adjacent dental margins in such manner as to ensure the purposes of the stopping. This involves a knowledge of the chemical and physical properties of the materials, a general knowledge of physics, a correct eye for good forms, a clear judgment, and, moreover, a sensitive and well-trained hand.*[8]

Materials used in plugging teeth were gold, platinum, silver, tin, lead, fusible alloys, amalgams, gutta-percha, oxychloride of zinc, and gum resins. Harris noted that none of the above met all the requirements of a perfect filling material, which were:

> *1, resistance to the mechanical action of mastication; 2, resistance to the chemical agencies of the mouth; 3, facility of introduction and consolidation; 4, harmony of color; 5, absence of all galvanic, chemical or vital action upon the teeth or the general system; 6, absence of all heat-conducting property.*[6]

Harris made it clear that gold was the only material that could be used for permanent filling of teeth. Of the six characteristics of the perfect filling material, it met conditions 1, 2, 3, and 5 but was deficient in harmony of color and absence of heat conductivity. The introduction in 1855 of crystalline or sponge gold foil, a highly adhesive metal, made the filling of large cavities possible because the gold was more easily welded into a solid restoration by pressure with special plugging instruments.

For a long time, dentists were obliged to make their own instruments, but by the mid 19th century, a wide number of commercially available instruments had been developed for accomplishing every step in the process of preparing and filling teeth. Simple dental drills equipped with steel burs were employed to gain access to the cavity (Figs 10-5 and 10-6). Spoon-shaped excavators were then employed to remove soft, decayed dentin (Fig 10-7). Other instruments in the

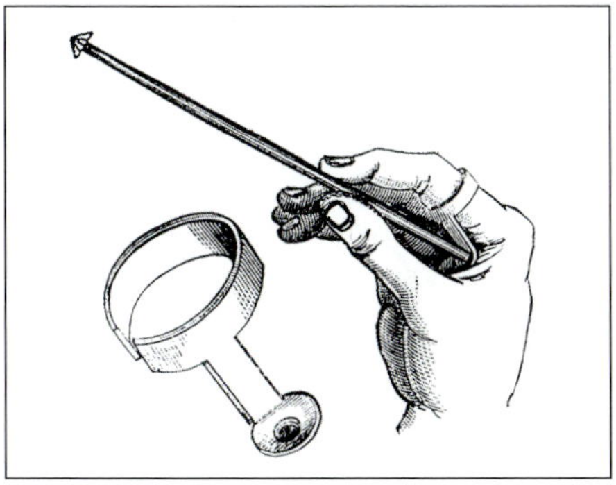

Fig 10-5 Finger drill with ring for index or middle finger and a socket for stabilizing the drill. The drill is rotated with the thumb and fingers. (From Taft.[9])

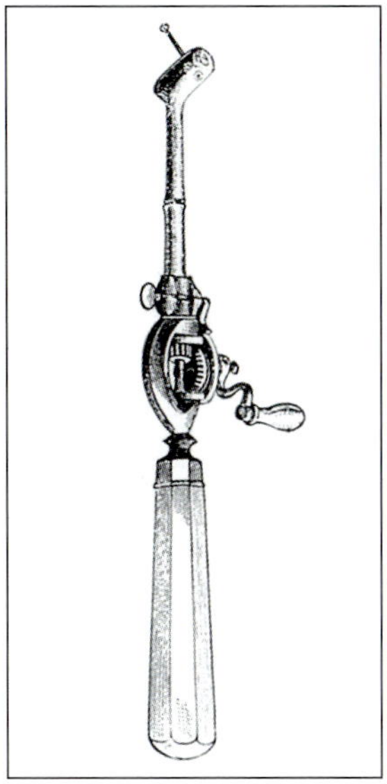

Fig 10-6 Chevalier's drill provided more power and possibility of directing the drill bit in various directions. (From Taft.[9])

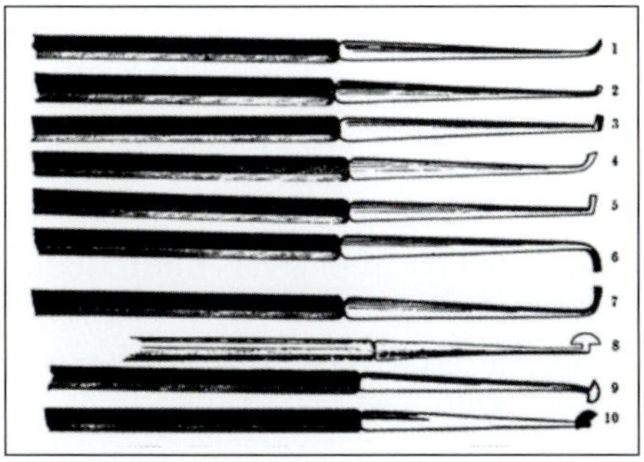

Fig 10-7 Various types of excavator instruments. Each style from 1 to 7 was made in up to six sizes. (From Taft.[9])

form of hatchets, hoes, and chisels of many different angles were used to remove unsupported enamel and to obtain a retentive form within sound dentin to receive the filling material. To reach all aspects of caries lesions in all types of anterior and posterior teeth, a wide spectrum of instruments were developed.[7] Burs were fabricated in a wide variety of styles for use as handheld drills or in machine-driven engines. The dental armamentarium also included broaches and reamers for removing the pulpal tissues of the root canal. Pliers, mirrors, and pluggers were needed for stopping the cavities with metal and/or gutta-percha. The proliferation of instruments designed to meet every possible function of operative dentistry led to the commercial

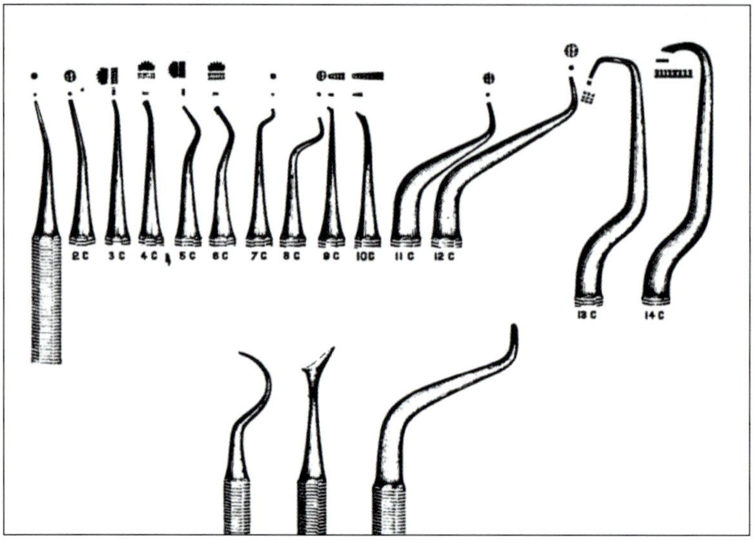

Fig 10-8 Set of Woodbury-Crandall gold pluggers for cohesive gold fillings. They were used in conjunction with a hand mallet in the hands of an assistant. (From Ward.[10])

production of complex sets, such as the set of pluggers illustrated in Ward's textbook[10] (Fig 10-8).

In preparing cavities for filling, the orifice of the lesion was enlarged by cutting down the enamel walls with chisels and burs and the decalcified carious dentin removed with excavators and burs. A thin floor of hard dentin was retained to protect the underlying pulp. Great detail was applied in creating a cavity with sound walls and with slight undercuts to retain the filling material.[9] Foot drills, introduced in 1871, and motorized dental drills, introduced in the late 18th century, facilitated cavity preparation.[11] Toward the end of the 19th century, the ultimate concepts of cavity preparation were defined by Dr G. V. Black in his classic textbook of operative dentistry.[12]

Gold

Of the many filling materials, gold was considered the material of choice.[6] In his textbook, Harris stated that gold foil manufactured in sponge form (also known as *crystalline gold*) was "so adhesive, that any number of pieces may be welded one to another; thus a part, or even the whole of the crown of a tooth, may be built up with it."[6] Harris noted that the most skillful operators in the United States used it almost exclusively in their practice. He had "seen fillings made by some of these gentlemen, which for beauty and solidity [I do] not think could be surpassed."[6] Harris was of the opinion that tin was second best to gold:

> *In consequence of its greater softness, it can oftentimes be employed for filling a badly-shaped and large cavity where gold cannot be used. If skillfully introduced, it will prevent the recurrence of caries. But if the fluids of the mouth are vitiated, it soon oxidizes and turns black; and then, instead of preventing, it rather promotes a recurrence of the disease.*[6]

Tin was employed when patients were not able to afford gold. Harris made it clear that, as far as he was concerned,

> *if a tooth is worth filling at all, it is worth filling in a proper manner, and with a suitable material (gold), and it would be more creditable to the operator to divide the expense with his poor patient, than to use an article that may never benefit him.*[6]

Gold foil operators took great pride in their skill. Dr E. Parmly Brown, in reply to an assertion that to learn mechanical dentistry takes ten times as long as it does to fill teeth with gold, stated that he was diametrically opposed to that view:

> *I have been watching the progress of dentistry in the United States, and especially in New York, for thirty years, and I can remember a hundred capable mechanical dentists where I can count ten who were as capable relatively of making good gold fillings. At the age of sixteen, after one or two years of instruction, I could produce finely finished partial gold plates, but it has required twenty years' study and labor to accomplish as good work comparatively in filling. I will venture the assertion, that of ten students taken at random from any dental college in the land, eight can be made expert workmen in the laboratory, where but one of them could be made to do as well in the operative department. The making of gold plates is to a large extent imitative, while filling requires innovation, almost every case being a new problem. In one case the work is upon inanimate metal; in the other it is upon the sensitive tissue of an animate being.*

In his textbook *A Practical Treatise on Operative Dentistry*, in stating that "A tooth that can be filled at all, can be filled with gold," Dr Jonathan Taft explained how this had been made possible by the development of adhesive (crystalline) gold:

> *This assertion was made a number of years ago; and if it was true then, it is much more true now; for then the adhesive property of gold was not employed at all, or even recognized as available; but now this property has been rendered efficient and practicable. Then, our best*

operators did not aim to unite the different portions of gold of which the fillings were composed. The idea that such consolidation could be effected seemed never to have entered their mind. Indeed, with the instrument and the method of manipulation then employed, this adhesive property could not have been made available; but when it came to be recognized, the instruments and the manipulation were adapted to the purpose. Formerly, an ordinary gold plug when removed from a cavity would be separated into as many pieces as originally composed it; but now, when adhesive gold is skillfully used, the mass comprising a filling cannot be divided into its original parts, but may be wrought into plate, wire, or foil. Non-adhesive gold—the modification in which till recently, it was always employed—would not weld, even under great pressure; but, in the mode in which it is now prepared, it will weld readily and thoroughly.[9]

In speaking on the subject of gold restorations before the Maryland Association of Dentists in 1867, Dr G. S. Fouke stated that gold foil should be used in small portions, heated to a "dull red heat" before being introduced into the cavity, and then condensed thoroughly with sharply serrated instruments. It was the remarkable and peculiar property of gold to "weld" or to adhere, when cold, after being annealed. Condensation of the gold with manual or automatic mallets was essential to form a solid restoration (Figs 10-9 and 10-10). Fouke said that the stroke of the mallet upon gold, with the property of malleability unimpaired, was far more effective than the force of simple pressure and produced more reliable work. The electric mallet was both a labor- and time-saving invention[13] (see Fig 10-10).

Gold fillings were time-consuming, expensive, and stressful for the patient, who sat in the dental chair for several hours, with mouth wide open, taking the punishment of hammer blows delivered by a mallet as innumerable pieces of gold foil were placed and condensed into the tooth cavity. The filling was then polished to a bright finish equal to any valuable piece of jewelry. Wealthy patients were willing to make this sacrifice, because they believed that they were receiving first-class dentistry. They were being treated by the elite members of the profession. But gold fillings, especially when placed by less skilled dentists, did not last a lifetime. The gold did, but not the restoration. Often the margins between the filling and the walls of the cavity began to leak, and the process of decay resumed, mostly undetected, until the tooth became painful and infected.

In the mid 19th century, the gold foil filling represented the best in dentistry. It was considered to be the only material that could be used to create permanent restorations. Dr Marshall Webb, writing in the *American Journal of Dental Sciences* in 1878, stated the following:

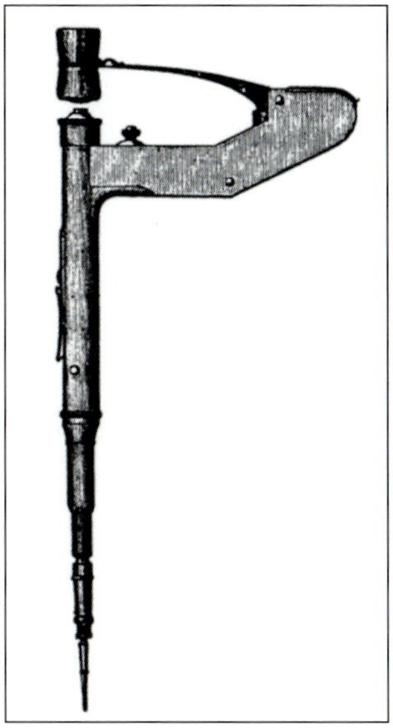

Fig 10-9 Hand mallet adapted with a spring-operated hammer attachment. (From Taft.[9])

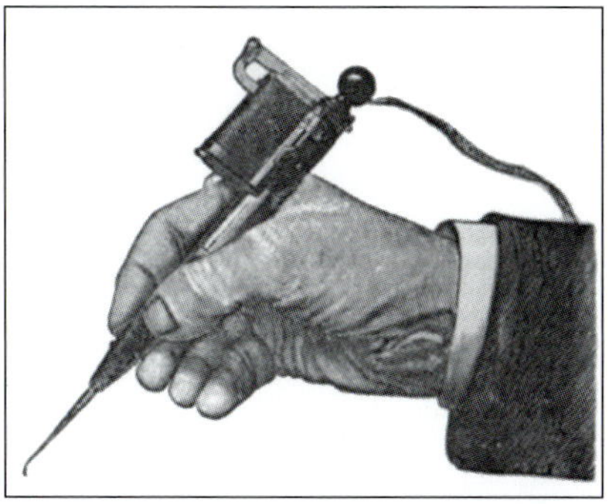

Fig 10-10 Electric mallet used in condensing gold fillings. (From Fillebrown.[7])

In the hands of a qualified and skillful operator, it (gold) can be so manipulated as to make operations permanent. Permanent signifies continuing in the same state, or without any change that destroys form or character, remaining unaltered or unremoved, continuance in the same state or place, duration, fixedness. So far as the materials used in the performance of dental operations are concerned, therefore, gold is the only material that can be made to answer all these requirements.[14]

Rapid advances in operative dentistry were made in the United States during the last half of the 19th century. This was a period in which the inventive spirit of the new profession engendered a steady increase in the development and commercialization of dental equipment and supplies. Operative dentistry reached a new high when cohesive gold was introduced by Dr Robert Arthur in 1855. The invention of the rubber dam (Fig 10-11) in 1864, along with the introduction of the automatic saliva ejector to create a dry operative field and the development of the foot-driven Morrison dental engine in

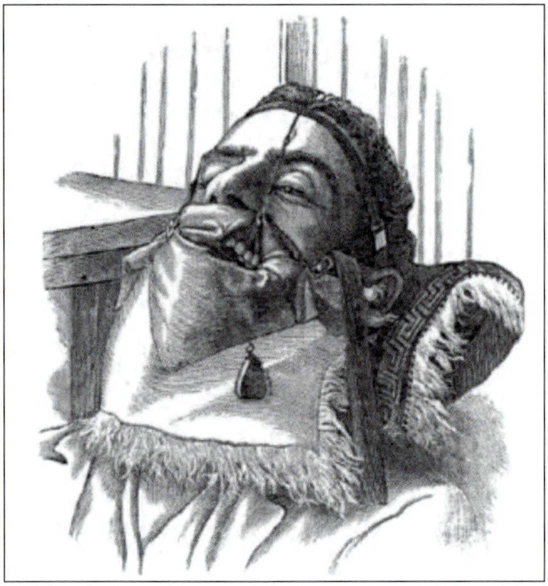

Fig 10-11 Isolation of the operative field by rubber dam.

1871, gave the dentist an effective system for restoring teeth.[15] Of special merit was the invention of the flexible cable and the handpiece drill. A typical dental operatory of the mid 19th century is depicted in Fig 10-12.

The first-class dentist, skilled in gold work, possessed, in the words of Dr Webb, "the genius of the artist, and the knowledge of the anatomist, histologist, physiologist, pathologist, etiologist and therapeutists" and the ability to "intelligently apply remedial agents for the removal of abnormal functions and abnormal growths, that the physiological energies may hold normal sway in the production and maintenance of the elements of the tissues and organs."[14] It was as if the champions of gold fillings were naturally superior in intellect to those lesser dentists who employed pernicious materials for filling teeth. In the florid prose of the 19th century, Dr Webb expressed his idea of the dentist as an artist:

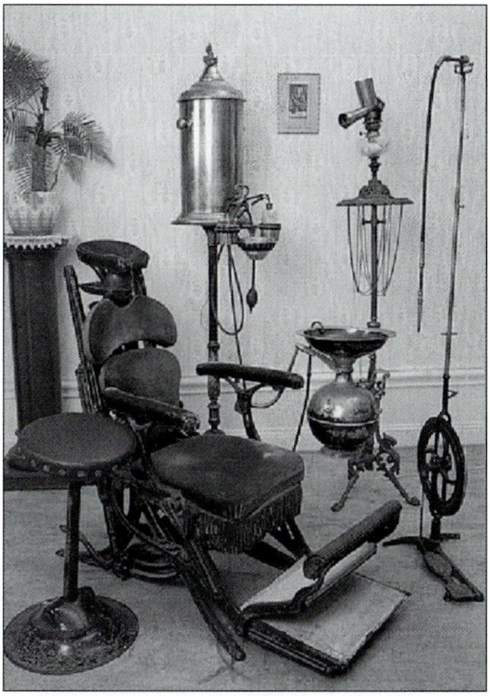

Fig 10-12 Dental operatory in the mid 19th century.

> *When we are governed by the "nobler sentiments of the human mind," as other artists are, and do all in our power to perform first-class operations, and make each and every operation a specimen of "fine art," then will we deserve and have brotherhood with the painters and sculptors (which latter we ought to be) and also to be the "architects" not only of fine work but of our own fame and that of our calling.*[14]

Amalgam

As early as 1840, American dentists who attempted to produce permanent dental restorations with anything less than gold were regarded by the leaders of the profession as doing an injustice to their patients and essentially practicing shoddy dentistry. The use of amalgam for filling teeth was viewed with disfavor ever since it had been introduced by the Crawcour brothers in New York City in 1833. The Crawcour brothers, described as "adventurers, without skill or experience, or any claim to the title of dentist" announced their arrival in New York with "a shower of advertisements, a profusion of display and a metaphorical flourish of trumpets" to the indignation of the dental establishment. Before long, patients were opting for the cheaper and quicker amalgam restorations.

Members of the American Society of Dental Surgeons, meeting in New York City in 1841, formed a committee to investigate the use of amalgam. The members of this committee included Chapin Harris, E. Parmly, J. Parmly, S. Brown, and E. Baker, all highly respected members of the profession (see chapter 5). Their report concluded that amalgam was "hurtful to the teeth and every part of the mouth." There was reason to suspect that their conclusions were not entirely based on scientific fact, considering that they, the elitist branch of the profession, were losing patients and income to the growing number of dentists who provided to the public a cheaper and less painful alternative to filling teeth with gold.[16]

The amalgam question continued to dominate the discussion until 1843, when Chapin Harris introduced a motion declaring the use of amalgam as malpractice. The American Society of Dental Surgeons went on to pass a resolution stating "that any member of this society who shall hereafter refuse to sign a certificate pledging himself not to use any amalgam, and, moreover, (not) protesting against its use, under any circumstances, in dental practice, shall be expelled from this society." Failure to sign the pledge was grounds for dismissal from the society. When the membership was finally polled in 1845, 78 members signed the pledge, 53 failed to respond, and 3 refused outright.[16] Dr Benjamin Brown, a highly regarded physician and dentist from St Louis, Missouri, was one of the three who challenged the legality and professional nature of this attempt to enforce specific modes of practice. Brown wrote: "Every formula, which requires the members of a learned profession to be pledged, like lost drunkards at a temperance meeting, is in my humble opinion, an outrage upon the profession itself, and revolting, in the highest degree, to the personal dignity of the gentleman and the scholar." Over the next several years, 21 members (including Dr Brown) were expelled, and many members resigned. The controversy had so shattered the membership that the American Society of Dental Surgeons was dissolved in 1856.[16]

Gradually, dentists and the public came to accept the fact that gold was not all that it had been held out to be. Amalgam was increasingly viewed as a material that could perform as well as gold and was in many cases a superior material.

In 1806, Joseph Fox had described a new method of filling teeth with metal:

> *A new method of stopping the teeth has been recommended to me by some chemical gentlemen, which promises to be very successful in all cases where the tooth is not tender, and the caries is situated in the center. A composition has been made by a union of several metals, which, from the very moderate degree of heat required to melt it, is called the fusible metal: it becomes fluid at the temperature of boiling water. The cavity in the tooth, being wiped perfectly dry, may be stopped by pouring a drop of this metal into it, when it instantly becomes solid, and as, in cooling, it strikes into all the irregularities of the carious part, it is a most perfect mode of filling it up.*[3]

Fox was likely referring to an alloy of bismuth, lead, and tin proposed by J. Darcet, a Parisian chemist. In 1818, the Parisian dentist L. Regnart described a method for using this metal for filling cavities. He had improved the alloy by adding mercury, thereby reducing its melting point.[15] In 1826, Auguste Taveau introduced his "pate d'argent," an alloy comprised of silver and mercury.[14] Lefoulon gave it the name *amalgam* in 1841.

The acceptance of amalgam as a substitute for gold was due in large measure to the forceful promotion of Dr Josiah Foster Flagg. He initiated a campaign called the "New Departure," which attacked the use of gold while demonstrating the superior value of plastic filling materials such as gutta-percha and amalgam. His views were based on a long clinical experience with plastic fillings. In the *American Journal of Dental Science*, Flagg noted that "so long as the filling of teeth with gold remains a tedious and painful operation, the public generally, since they have to bear the pain, will naturally prefer the employment of plastic fillings, if such fillings can be made to do reasonable service."[17] On that point the profession was deeply divided, one school holding that nothing was better than gold, the other that cheaper and more easily inserted fillings were better than gold. The history of the American Society of Dental Surgeons had demonstrated how bitter opinions on the subject could become destructive of collegiality.

Josiah Foster Flagg came from a long line of dentists. His grandfather, Josiah Flagg, was a prominent dentist in colonial America. To demonstrate the longevity of plastic fillings, Flagg recounted the following story of one of his father's patients:

> *Twenty-six years ago Dr. G., of Philadelphia, came to my father, desiring his services. My father introduced eleven gold fillings-good, old-fashioned, solid, "straight from the shoulder" fillings. Besides these cavities, there were four enormous places in the four wisdom teeth (poor teeth, according to accepted views,) and these were filled, " experimentally," three with amalgam and one (the buccal face of the right lower wisdom) with gutta-percha, with the idea that they might "last for a year or two." The last one of the eleven gold fillings was*

renewed a few months since, and the three amalgam fillings, and the gutta-percha filling, are still preserving their forlorn and worthless wisdom teeth, as they have done for more than a quarter of a century. These are not isolated cases. They are, far more, typical cases. I have, in the mouths of my patients, hundreds upon hundreds of gutta-percha fillings, which have been doing service for from five to fifteen years, and bid fair to continue so doing for years to come.[17]

Flagg admitted that amalgam fillings were produced with greater ease to the operator but not done out of "laziness," as the opponents of amalgam were prone to accuse. On the contrary:

> *It is from a desire to lay aside the forceps. It is from a desire that our patients shall eat upon the roots of which, at least, are in their jaws. It is from a desire that they shall be exempt from the infliction of artificial work. It is from a desire to extend the blessings which the hand of our profession holds to bestow. It is that we may be sought rather than avoided, that we may be extolled rather than decried, that we may be esteemed rather than censured, that rather than feared, we may be loved and respected.*[17]

In 1878 in the *American Journal of Dental Science*, Flagg outlined the basic principles of the "New Departure" system. He hammered home the many points that made plastic fillings superior to gold fillings. Aroused by the constant criticisms that amalgam filling material was "pernicious and poisonous" and the choice of less skillful dentists, Flagg called on his considerable oratorical talents:

> *Now, gentlemen, I want to tell you one thing more which has grown out of our long work on plastic fillings—that we have not come before you prepared for only a small struggle. We are ready for the fight. We have opened our batteries against the accepted dentistry of the day. We are an aggressive party, and we purpose insisting that our "basal principles" shall be thoroughly discussed. We purpose making it respectable that teeth shall be filled with materials which experience has shown to be able to save them; and we purpose making it not respectable to fill teeth with materials which experience proves daily to be unequal to the emergency.*[17]

In an address delivered before the American Dental Association in 1878, Flagg spoke with his usual conviction, based on 30 years of practice, of the basic principles that should govern practice, the aim of which was to save teeth:

> *If I can say to you that with the gradual abandonment of gold, I have also equally come to the abandonment of artificial dentures, it behooves you to look to it and see the connection which exists, if there be any, between the two. Is gold the easiest material with which to fill? Is it*

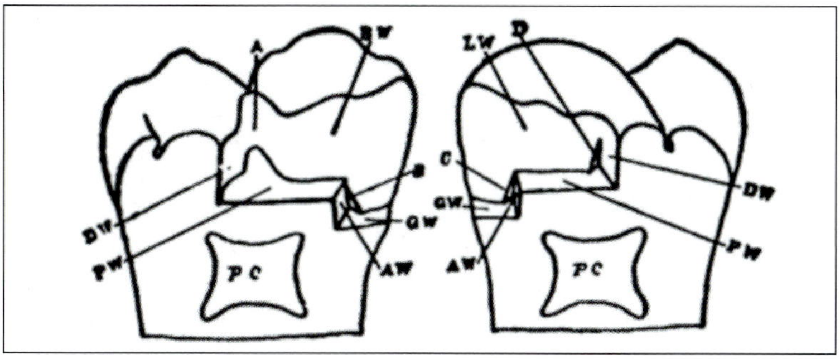

Fig 10-13 Two halves of a molar tooth with cavity preparation according to Black's outline form. The cavity walls are lettered (axial, buccal, distal, lingual, mesial, pulpal, etc. D and C represent convenient points to start the insertion of gold foil). (From Black.[12])

> *not the most difficult? Is gold the quickest material with which to fill? Is it not the greatest consumer of time? Is gold the most comfortable material with which to fill? Is its use not usually attended with more discomfort than any other filling? Is gold the most economical material with which to fill? Is it not, by far, the most expensive? Is gold the most durable material with which to fill? I ask you, gentlemen, is it possible that your experience is so adverse to mine as that you can say that in the teeth which most need saving, gold is the most durable of all your fillings? Then, if gold is the most difficult, the most tedious, the most uncomfortable, the most expensive and not the most durable material with which to fill teeth, is it not a reasonable deduction that its almost exclusive use, and its constant adulation, its upholding as the test for dental ability, and its universal acceptation as the best of filling materials, has much to do with all this flood of pulpless teeth, of alveolar abscesses, discolored crowns, and jagged roots, of toothless jaws and plates of India-rubber?*[18]

Due in large measure to the experience of Dr Flagg and other members of the "New Departure" movement, the use of amalgam continued to gain acceptance. However, it was not until the research of Dr G. V. Black had produced new amalgam formulations that made the material less prone to shrinkage and corrosion over time that it became adopted almost universally. Now, based on the type of lesion and the needs of the patient, the eclectic operator could choose between gold, amalgam, and gutta-percha without sacrificing the quality of his work or his reputation.

Black described the various classes of caries lesions and taught the appropriate protocol for their restoration using a standardized nomenclature. Each type of lesion demanded a specific cavity outline preparation (Fig 10-13) designed to maximize retention of the filling material and minimize recurrence of decay. His concept of "extension for prevention" dictated placing the margins of restorations in self-cleansing surfaces even if that meant cutting away sound tooth structure. Every aspect of the cavity outline was formed with specific instruments (eg, chisels, hoes, and burs). To obtain efficiency, dentists "should learn to systematize the preparation of each cavity so that each step will be performed in its proper order and the cutting to be done by each instrument will be completed while that instrument is in the hand."[11] Black's classic textbook of operative dentistry, with its highly detailed approach to tooth restoration, served numerous generations of dentists, and his precepts were only modified or replaced with the modern introduction of adhesive composites.

It is of interest to note that well into the latter half of the 20th century, the gold foil restoration was still regarded as the epitome of fine dentistry and a prominent component of state licensure examinations.

Summary

Operative dentistry started in Italy during the 16th century when surgeons reported the removal of decay and the use of lead and gold to plug cavities. Herbal remedies, in use for centuries, continued to be used to reduce pain and to promote healing. Better instruments were in use during the rise of the surgeon dentist, but rapid progress was not made until the 19th century when new cutting instruments and improved filling materials were developed. By the end of the 19th century, the gold foil restoration had been perfected as an art form and was claimed to be the symbol of excellence in dentistry. Rebelling against the preeminence of gold, Josiah F. Flagg campaigned for wider use of amalgam through his "New Departure" philosophy. As a result of improvements in amalgam and other plastic materials, they were increasingly used to restore large cavities and were advocated for general use in patients of limited means. Local anesthetics and motor-driven drills increased efficiency and minimized patient discomfort during long operative procedures. Textbooks of 500 or more pages in length spelled out the step-by-step procedures for excavating teeth and placing a variety of restorations. G. V. Black set standards in operative dentistry technique that would shape dental practice for at least two to three generations of American dentists. The majority of dentists performed operative dentistry to the exclusion of all other services. At the turn of the 20th century, operative dentistry dominated the dental curriculum, and competency in that area alone determined whether one would become licensed to practice dentistry.

References

1. Guerini V. A History of Dentistry from the Most Ancient Times Until the End of the Eighteenth Century. Philadelphia: Lea & Febiger, 1909;188–199.
2. Fauchard P. The Surgeon Dentist; Or, Treatise on the Teeth, ed 2. Paris: P. J. Mariette, 1746.
3. Fox J. The History and Treatment of the Diseases of the Teeth, the Gums, and the Alveolar Processes, with the Operations Which They Respectively Require. London: Thomas Cox, 1806.
4. Arthur R. Treatment and Prevention of Decay of the Teeth. Philadelphia: Lippincott, 1871.
5. Arthur R. Opening address, sixth annual meeting of the Southern Dental Association. Dent Cosmos 1875;17:57–72.
6. Harris CA. The Principles and Practice of Dental Surgery, ed 8. Philadelphia: Lindsay & Blakiston, 1863.
7. Fillebrown T. A Textbook of Operative Dentistry. Philadelphia: P. Blakiston, Son, & Co, 1889.
8. Jack L. The stopping process with gold and the related procedures. In: Litch WF (ed). The American System of Dentistry. Philadelphia: Lea Brothers, 1887.
9. Taft J. A Practical Treatise on Operative Dentistry, ed 4. Philadelphia: P. Blakiston, Son, & Co, 1883.
10. Ward ML. American Text-Book of Operative Dentistry. Philadelphia: Lea & Febiger, 1920.
11. Gelber S. 125 years of developments in dentistry, 1800-2005, part 3: Dental equipment and materials. Br Dent J 2005;199:536–539.
12. Black GV. A Work on Operative Dentistry. Chicago: Medico-Dental, 1908.
13. Fouke GS. Annealed gold. Dent Cosmos 1867;8:652–654.
14. Webb MH. Gold can be so manipulated as to make operations permanent. Am J Dent Sci 1878;12:268–272.
15. Hoffmann-Axthelm W. History of Dentistry. Chicago: Quintessence, 1981.
16. Meyerhof PJ. Early struggles to identify ethical standards in dentistry: Dr. Benjamin Brown and the amalgam war of the 1840s. J Hist Dent 2007;55:139–149.
17. Flagg JF. Plastic filling, and the basal principles of the new departure. Am J Dent Sci 1878;12:1–18.
18. Flagg JF. Plastic filling as a power in dentistry. Am J Dent Sci 1878;12:347–357.

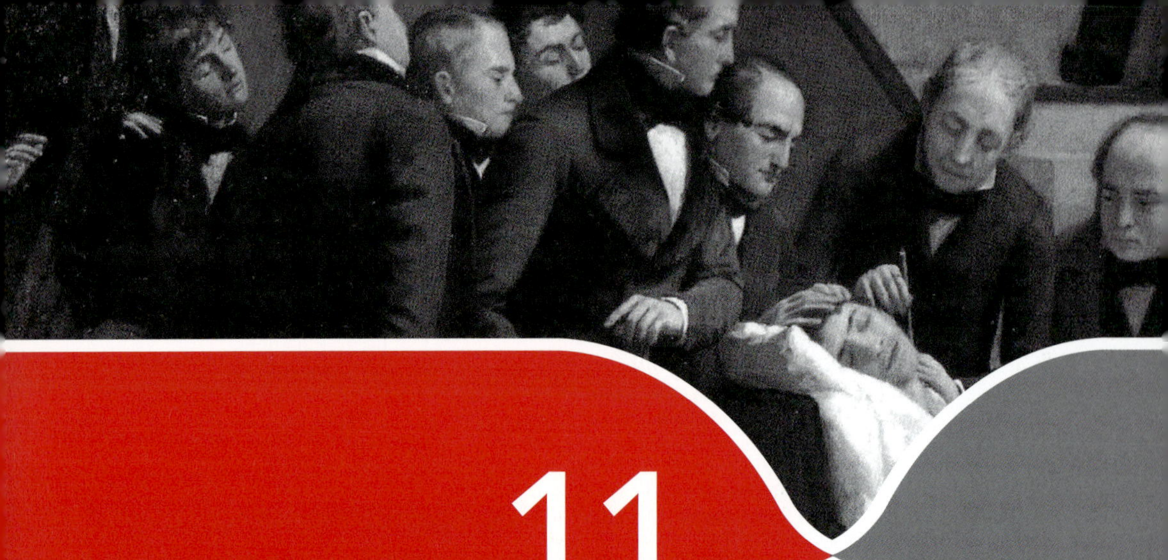

11

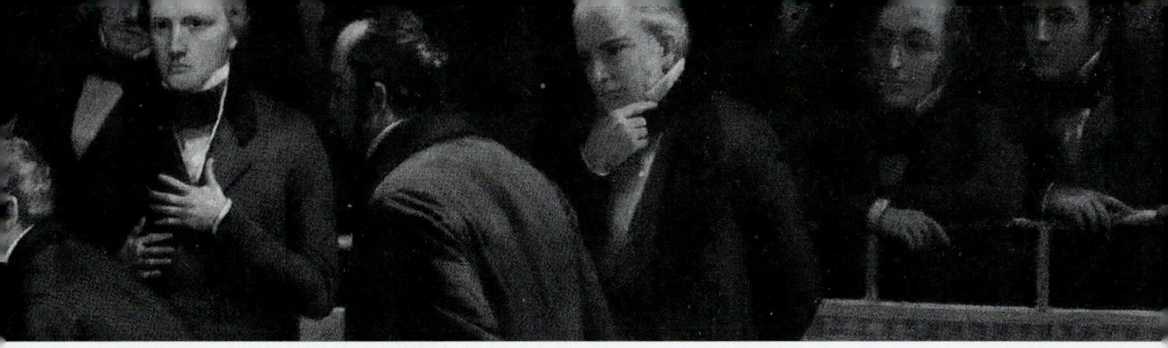

The Discovery of Inhalation Anesthesia

Over the course of history, man has attempted to eliminate pain through the use of herbal drugs, alcoholic drinks, and hypnotism. From antiquity, henbane, poppy, and mandragora (mandrake) have been used to induce insensibility in preparing patients for surgery. These methods were largely unsuccessful because they could not be counted on to act similarly and effectively in every patient and were often dangerous to life.[1] Thus, surgery remained akin to the worst kind of torture. Surgeons had to work quickly, with little time to perfect their technique or to develop new approaches. Thus, it is not surprising that surgeons had to possess courage, skill, and enormous self-confidence. The physical pain and mental anguish endured in major surgery is told in the New York Herald of July 21, 1841 and recounted in H. R. Raper's book *Man Against Pain*:

> *The patient was a youth of about fifteen, pale, thin, but calm and firm. One professor felt for the femoral artery, had the leg held up for a few moments to insure the saving of blood, the compress part of the tourniquet was placed upon the artery and the leg held up by an assistant. The white swelling was fearful—frightful. A little wine was given the lad; he was pale but resolute; his father supported his head and left hand. A second professor took the long glittering knife, felt for the bone, thrust in the knife carefully but rapidly. The boy screamed terribly; the tears went down the father's cheeks. The first cut from the inside was completed, and the bloody blade of the knife issued from the quivering wound, the blood flowed by the pint, the sight was*

> *sickening; the screams terrific; the operator calm. Again the knife was thrust under the bone, the terrific screaming was renewed; one or two picked up their hats to leave; scream upon scream and again the bloody blade of the knife issued from the wound and was laid aside. The flesh quivered and the boy cried agonizingly. The flesh was thrust back with a small piece of wet linen; the divided ends of the quivering muscles were stopped from blood with a sponge; the saw glistened in the hands of the operator, the father turned pale as death; the boy's eyes fastened on the instrument with glazed agony; grate—crush—once, twice, and the useless limb from the toes to the center of the thigh, was quickly dropped into the tub under the table.*[2]

Certainly one of the most significant events in the history of medicine and dentistry was the discovery of inhalation anesthesia. For centuries dentists had dreamed of extracting teeth without pain, and thus it is fitting that two dentists played a key role in the momentous discovery of general anesthesia. Two New England dentists, Horace Wells and William Morton, acting separately over the short span of 2 years (1844–1846), discovered that the inhalation of nitrous oxide (Wells) and ether (Morton) could eliminate the pain associated with dental surgery. Morton's discovery was soon adopted by the foremost general surgeons of the Massachusetts General Hospital (MGH) and became the preferred method of inducing insensibility during major surgery. The story of this discovery and the rivalry between the main characters has been told many times over. Several recent full-length studies include the books by Julie M. Fenster[3] and Richard J. Wolfe.[4]

The term *anesthesia* was suggested to Dr William Morton by Dr Oliver Wendell Holmes, professor of anatomy at the Harvard Medical School and famed Autocrat of the Breakfast Table. Holmes recounts that "after trying two or three words, aesthetic occurred to me as meaning sensitive, and in consequence anesthetic as being insensitive easily followed."

Ether and Nitrous Oxide

The first account of the synthesis of ether was published by Valerius Cordus in 1561.[5] He gave a clear description of its preparation from sulfuric acid and alcohol. In describing some of its properties, Cordus noted that it had an "agreeable taste" and "that even chickens would eat it, whereupon they sleep for a moderately long time, and reawake without having been injured."[5]

In 1823, an English physician, Henry H. Hickman, while investigating methods of producing "suspended animation" by depriving

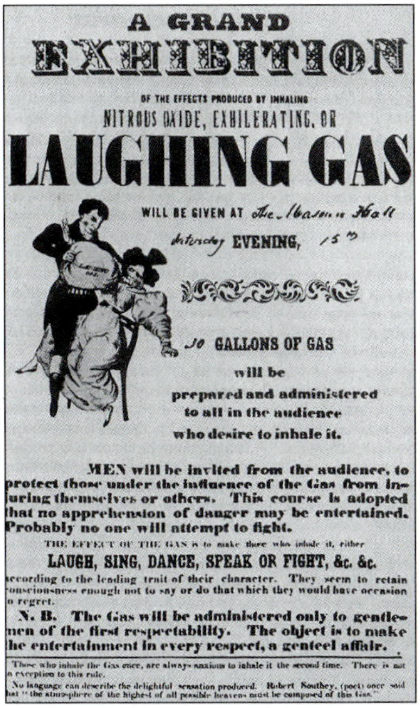

Fig 11-1 Poster advertising a nitrous oxide laughing gas exhibition.

animals of air and letting them breathe carbon dioxide gas, found that during the state of suspended animation, animals showed no pain when undergoing surgeries. Hickman apologized for his use of living animals and for risking accusation of self-adulation in publishing his observations. Because suspended animation was the equivalent of asphyxiation by oxygen deprivation, it did not gain much favor in contemporary medical circles.[2]

Joseph Priestly discovered nitrous oxide in 1772, but it was Sir Humphries Davy (1778–1829) who reported that nitrous oxide induced a state of exhilaration when inhaled. Davy also discovered that nitrous oxide could dull the pain of toothache and suggested that it might be useful in surgeries.[2,6] Although the medical applications of these discoveries remained unexplored, the induced exhilaration caught on for its entertainment value.

Exhilaration created by the inhalation of nitrous oxide captured the attention of the public, and soon breathing it was popularized as a source of entertainment at "Laughing Gas Parties" (Fig 11-1). The *Western Dental Journal* reprinted an editorial recounting an episode of the exhilarating effect of breathing ether:

> *When a mere boy, with others, the most of whom were a little older, on a number of occasions he visited the village drug store, where we all contributed our pennies to a common fund for the purchase of ether, to be administered to anyone who would take it. He also recollects that the usual way to give it was to pour it into a wide saucer, and invert over that a funnel, the boy who took it placing his mouth to the nozzle and sucking in the vapor until intoxication was reached. There was one young fellow, now long since dead, who gave great exhibitions whenever he could be prevailed upon to take ether—and it did not usually require much coaxing to get his assent—for he became extremely hilarious. There is a clear recollection of one instance in which he got away from the rest of us, and rushed on a canal boat lying at the adjacent dock, where he seized the tiller and broke it off, at the same time quite seriously injuring one of his fingers. The efforts to recover him are yet fresh in memory, with his bewildered exclamations regarding the hurt finger, and his wondering curiosity as to how he could have so injured himself, clearly indicating that there was no consciousness of pain until he had passed out from the influence of drug.*[7]

From 1842 to 1844, Phineas T. Barnum, showman and circus promoter, looking to find new modes of entertaining the public, encouraged "Professor" G. Q. Colton to feature laughing gas parties in his chemistry road shows. The *Hartford Courant* of December 10, 1844 announced a "Grand Exhibition of the effects produced by inhaling nitrous oxide or Laughing Gas...The gas is reported to cause those who inhale it to laugh, sing, cry, dance, speak or fight," or in other words, to act foolishly in ways sure to entertain all in attendance. Despite the comedic nature of these events, they were billed as scientific experiments because Professor Colton preceded his demonstrations with a lecture of the properties and history of nitrous oxide. In 1844, Dr Horace Wells (Fig 11-2), a young dentist of Hartford, Connecticut, attended the exhibition, inhaled the gas, and, according to Mrs Wells, "made a spectacle of himself."[2]

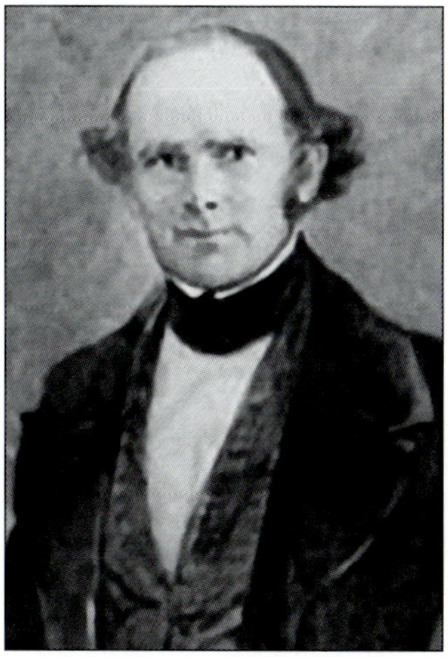

Fig 11-2 Horace Wells.

Horace Wells and the Discovery of Nitrous Oxide Anesthesia

During the laughing gas demonstration, Wells observed that Sam Cooley, his volunteer patient, fell and cut his leg while under the influence of nitrous oxide. Impressed by Cooley's lack of pain, Wells visualized the possibility of painless dental surgery. In his practice of mechanical dentistry, Wells was hampered by the fear his patients had for dental extractions. If he could find a way to extract teeth without inflicting pain, his practice would grow because more patients would be receptive to artificial dentures. With this objective in mind, on the very next day he arranged to have Colton bring laughing gas to his office for an experimental surgery. The patient was none other than Dr Wells himself, and the surgeon was Dr John Riggs, a former student apprentice of his. In this private demonstration, Wells inhaled nitrous oxide administered by Colton while Dr Riggs extracted a painful third molar.[8] Some years later, Wells recalled how Sam Cooley's experience had led to his discovery:

> *I was led to inquire if the same result would not follow by the inhalation of exhilarating gas, the effects of which would pass off immediately, leaving the system none the worse for its use. I accordingly procured some nitrous oxide gas, resolving to make the first experiment on myself, by having a tooth extracted, which was done without any painful sensations. I then performed the same operation for twelve or fifteen others, with the like results.*[9]

Riggs recalled that they had agreed to administer the gas to a point that had never been attempted before:

> *We knew not whether death or success confronted us. It was a terra incognita we were bound to explore. The result is known to the world. No one but Wells and myself knew to what point the inhalation was to be carried. The result was painfully problematic to us. But the great law of nature, hitherto unknown, was kind to us and a great discovery was born into the world.*[9]

During the winter of 1844, Wells and Riggs used nitrous oxide to extract teeth on numerous patients.[6] In December of 1844, Wells visited Boston to communicate his success with nitrous oxide to Dr William Morton, a former dental partner, and to Dr Charles Jackson of the Harvard Medical School.[6] Wells recounted how he had come to know Drs Morton and Jackson:

> *Dr. Morton, who is a dentist in Boston, was instructed in his profession by myself, about five years since, and I subsequently assisted in establishing him in the city of Boston, and after I had made the above discovery, I had frequent interviews with him; and he, being aware that I had relinquished my professional business in consequences of a protracted indisposition, requested me to instruct him how to prepare the gas which I had been giving so successfully in Hartford, stating that he wished to make a trial of it in Boston. As this interview was in Hartford, I told him to request Dr. Charles T. Jackson (with whom we were both acquainted) to prepare him some of it, as he was a chemist. Accordingly, Dr. Morton went to Dr. Jackson for the gas, who gave him ether, as being attended with the least trouble.*[9]

Morton and Jackson "expressed themselves in the disbelief that surgical operations could be performed without pain, both admitting that this modus operandi was entirely new to them."[9] Encouraged by success and a growing conviction that nitrous oxide could be used in major surgery, Wells arranged to demonstrate its use to the medical faculty and students at Harvard Medical School. In January 1845, in an amphitheater classroom, before the assembled medical faculty and students, Wells applied the gas and began to extract the patient's tooth. When the young patient cried out during the extraction, laughter and accusations of fraud erupted from the benches. Wells related that he had removed the gas bag too soon. Although the patient subsequently asserted that he had felt no pain, the event was viewed as a total fiasco.

In his big moment before Dr John Warren and his medical students, Wells suffered severe embarrassment. He became regarded as an imposter, and no one would assist him in further experiments with nitrous oxide. Dr Henry J. Bigelow later wrote that Wells failed because he had used an inadequate volume of nitrous oxide to produce deep anesthesia and thus "narrowly missed a great invention."[1] Wells said that the disappointment and embarrassment of this misadventure brought on an illness lasting several months, causing him to relinquish his dental practice.[9] Dr Riggs took over the practice and continued to apply nitrous oxide for dental extractions.[2] On December 7, 1846, Wells finally made a formal announcement of his discovery in a letter to the *Hartford Courant*, but it came 2 months after Dr William Morton's demonstration of ether anesthesia in Boston.[10]

After the disappointing demonstration at Harvard, Wells, deeply depressed, ceased to make any further experiments with nitrous oxide from 1844 to 1847.[1] During that interval, Wells traveled to Europe in the bizarre hope that he could purchase cheap paintings that could fetch a profit in the United States. Notwithstanding his failure at Harvard, the news of his results in Hartford had spread to Paris, where the medical establishment was eager to learn of his experiments. He received numerous invitations to speak of his discovery, and he was widely celebrated for his achievement. Meanwhile, the news of the successful demonstration of ether anesthesia in major surgeries at the MGH had also reached Europe. Seeing his work diminished by the news of Morton's success and his claim of priority of discovery challenged, Wells returned to Connecticut determined to resume his experimentation with nitrous oxide and defend his claim of priority in discovery of inhalation anesthesia. In March 1847, Wells reported that he had conducted 50 or more surgeries not only with nitrous oxide anesthesia but also with ether anesthesia, reasserting his claim of priority of invention.[10]

Also in March 1847, Wells, in writing a brief account of his discovery of nitrous oxide anesthesia, described his disappointment over the attempt by Morton and Jackson to claim primacy of discovery and to commercialize the use of ether. Wells stated:

> *On making the discovery, I was so much elated respecting it, that I expended my money freely, and devoted my whole time for several weeks, in order to present it to those who were best qualified to*

> *investigate and decide upon its merits, not asking or expecting anything for my services, well assured that it was a valuable discovery. I was desirous that it should be as free as the air we breathe; but judge of my surprise, after the lapse of many months, when I was informed that two individuals (Drs. Jackson and Morton) had claimed that discovery, and had made application for a patent in their own names.*[9]

Wells had the support of many dentists in the Hartford community who had been quick to adopt the use of nitrous oxide in their practices. One of his most ardent supporters, Dr E. E. Marcy, argued that:

> *The man who first discovered the fact that the inhalation of a gaseous substance would render the body insensible to pain under surgical operations, should be entitled to all the credit or emolument which may accrue from the use of any substance of this nature. This is the principle; this is the discovery. The mere substitution of ether-vapor, or any other article for gas, no more entitles one to the claim of a discovery than the substitution of coal for wood, in generating steam, would entitle one to be called the discoverer of steam.*[10]

Subsequent to Wells's experimentation with nitrous oxide, Colton (of laughing gas fame) went on to prosper by anesthetizing patients in several dental offices in Connecticut and New York.[10] Colton administered nitrous oxide for Drs Dunham and Smith of New Haven, Connecticut, the latter of whom extracted 3,000 teeth in a period of 23 days.[11] In 1863, Colton, along with John Allen, a New York City dentist, established the Colton Dental Association, whose only mission was the painless extraction of teeth by nitrous oxide anesthesia. By 1866, Colton had opened branches in Philadelphia, Baltimore, St Louis, Brooklyn, Boston, and Cincinnati and had administered nitrous oxide over 25,000 times.[10]

In 1847, Wells moved to New York City, where he established a dental practice, promoting his experience with nitrous oxide, Letheon (ether), and the newly discovered chloroform.[2] On August 17, 1847, Wells anesthetized a patient during the removal of a large growth by Dr E. Marcy.[6] Other cases in which Wells administered nitrous oxide involved amputation of a thigh and the excision of a fatty tumor. However, in that same year, at a demonstration of nitrous oxide anesthesia before a group of physicians at the New York Hospital, Wells once again met with failure.[10] From that point on, he entered a spiraling path of destruction. He began to experiment with chloroform and may have become addicted to its use. Living away from his family in New York City's worst sections, he was arrested and jailed, accused of having thrown acid on two prostitutes. Shortly thereafter in January 1848, Wells committed suicide in his jail cell by severing his femo-

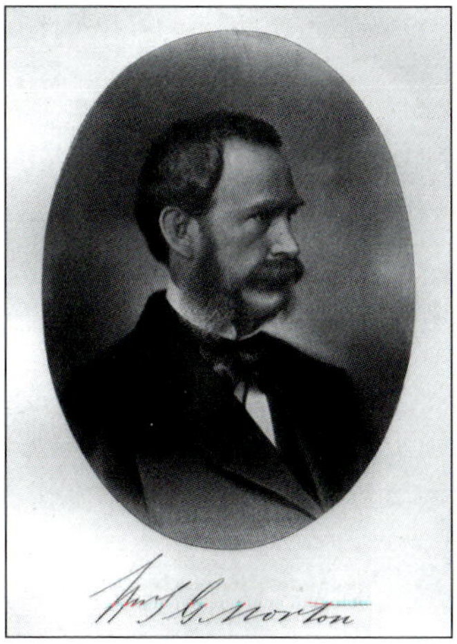

Fig 11-3 William Morton.

ral artery.[2] Wells's family and supporters in the Hartford community criticized the New York City Police for not recognizing Wells for a sick man in need of medical and psychiatric care. They reasoned that repeated exposure to chloroform coupled with the stress of recent events had driven him insane.[2]

On April 27, 1848, several months after the death of Horace Wells, Dr Henry Bigelow, in an effort to prove to himself the usefulness of nitrous oxide in major surgery, removed a cancerous breast from a 45-year-old woman at the MGH. In that operation, Bigelow made sure that the patient inhaled a sufficient supply of gas (60 gallons) through a double mouthpiece.[10] During this successful operation, the patient had been placed in a dangerous state of asphyxia, causing those present to conclude that nitrous oxide should be reserved for minor surgical operations.

William Morton and the Discovery of Ether Anesthesia

William Morton (Fig 11-3) was born in Charlton, Massachusetts, in 1819. His formal education ended when he was 17 years old, whereupon he entered upon a career in business. Failing in business, he decided to enroll in the first class of the newly established Baltimore College of Dental Surgery under the tutelage of Dr Chapin Harris.[8]

Although there is some doubt as to whether he did attend dental college, it is known that he studied dentistry with Horace Wells in Boston and for a brief period of time was in dental partnership with him.[12] It was during this time that he, Wells, and John Riggs (another student of Wells) were involved in developing a new process for soldering artificial teeth to gold denture baseplates.[12]

As a practicing dentist, Morton spent much of his time with the mechanical aspects of tooth repair and denture fabrication. In making dentures, the first step was to fabricate a gold or tin baseplate that was closely adapted to the surface contours of the jaw. Removal of all roots and root fragments from the area being treated was highly recommended. When roots were retained under the finished denture, the underlying tissues were less compressible and less comfortable for the patient. More important, leaving roots in a denture-bearing surface created potential sites of infection. But most patients were unwilling to undergo the painful extractions. Morton was keenly aware that if he could find a method to induce insensibility long enough to extract teeth, he would build his practice to a new level and in the process relieve the suffering of his patients.[13]

With the knowledge that Wells (his former partner) had already made some progress with the use of nitrous oxide to induce insensibility during tooth extraction, Morton realized that even though Wells's demonstration at Harvard had failed, he had better move rapidly if he wished to make a name for himself in this potentially lucrative clinical area. Wells recalled how Morton had paid him a visit in Hartford to enquire on the best method of preparing nitrous oxide, stating "that he wished to make a trial of it in Boston."[9]

Morton was now enrolled in the Massachusetts Medical College. After completing two courses of lectures, Morton returned to dental practice with Dr Nathan Keep.[13] While in medical school, he became acquainted with Dr Charles T. Jackson, professor of chemistry. Jackson learned of Morton's interest in agents capable of deadening pain and encouraged him to experiment with sulfuric ether. In fact, Jackson advised him to use pure sulfuric ether and explained how to go about getting it.[14] Jackson knew of Sir Humphrey Davy's early experiments with nitrous oxide and was of the opinion that the respiration of gases deserved further investigation.[15] Jackson also knew that breathing ether induced insensibility but that it was dangerous and sometimes fatal. Jackson had inhaled ether to treat accidental inhalation of chlorine gas, and on one occasion he attained a "state of complete general insensibility."

Morton embarked on a series of experiments on animals and himself. Realizing that he was on the cusp of a potentially momentous discovery, he became increasingly protective of his experiments. Although Morton was indebted to Jackson for recommending that pure ether would work best, he admitted that in getting information from Jackson he was careful to keep him from gaining full knowledge of his progress. In Morton's words:

> *I went to Dr. Jackson, therefore to procure a gas bag, also with the intention of ascertaining something more accurately as to the different preparations of ether, if I should find I could do so without setting him on the same track of experiment with myself. I am aware, that by this admission I may show myself not to have been possessed by the most disinterested spirit of philosophic enthusiasm, clear of all regard for personal rights or benefits; but it is enough for me to say, that I felt I had made sacrifices and run risks for this object; that I believed myself to be close upon it, yet where another, with better opportunities for experimenting, avail himself of my hints and labors, might take the prize from my grasp.*[15]

Additional evidence of his deception is seen in his attempt to trick his professional colleagues as well as the public into believing that he had discovered a new substance, which he called *Letheon*. To disguise the fact that Letheon was only sulfuric ether, he shielded its telltale odor by the addition of scented oils. This fraud was also necessary in order to obtain a patent for the discovery of a new substance, because ether was readily available from any apothecary shop.

Finally, on September 30, 1846, Morton administered ether via a handkerchief to a patient in his office and successfully extracted a tooth without causing any pain. Well aware of the power of publicity, Morton did not waste any time in bringing his success before the public. The *Boston Daily Journal* of October 1, 1846 reported that a dentist had found a way to perform painless dental extractions[8]:

> *Last evening, as we were informed by a gentleman who witnessed the operation, an ulcerated tooth was extracted from the mouth of an individual without giving him the slightest pain. He was put into a kind of sleep, by inhaling a preparation, the effects of which lasted for about three quarters of a minute, just long enough to extract the tooth.*

Morton's practice was already very successful, but the rapid spread of the news of his discovery generated enormous personal gains in prestige and income. The increased number of patients that came to his practice led him to hire additional clinical associates. Morton was now generating approximately $20,000 per year in gross income.[16]

Surprisingly, Morton's success aroused the anger of jealous dentists led by Dr J. F. Flagg. In organizing a movement to suppress the use of anesthesia, Flagg also attacked Morton's character.[13] Rumors were spread in the Boston papers of the serious risk involved in submitting to anesthesia. It was reported that several young ladies suffered bleeding lungs and melancholy following inhalation of ether at Dr Morton's dental office.[16]

Although Morton may have been exposed to human anatomy, physiology, and some chemistry while attending lectures at the medical college, he gave no evidence in his writings that he had any interest in the biologic effects of ether inhalation other than to produce insensibility. According to Bowditch, Morton was no scientist and learned what little he knew of ether from discussions with Jackson.[15] Dr McQuillen, editor of *Dental Cosmos*, upon attending a presentation by Dr Morton on his discovery of the anesthetic properties of ether, had become convinced by what he heard that "the speaker had very little, if anything, to do with the discovery."[17] This conviction was further confirmed by several subsequent interviews that he had with Morton:

> *There was such a manifest want of familiarity with the most ordinary relations of the subject, that it is a matter of surprise that anyone who has once heard him could for a moment credit him with being the kind of man that would be likely to institute a series of careful and long-continued experiments, with the view of ascertaining the relative anesthetic properties of various substances.*[17]

Mr Theodore Metcalf, the apothecary that had sold Morton a small amount of sulfuric ether, recalled a discussion of the substitution of ether for nitrous oxide and warning Morton that excessive inhalation of ether would "produce dangerous, if not fatal consequences." It was the belief of most physicians that the inhalation of ether was injurious and a highly risky activity. Was Morton acting recklessly in going against the best opinion of the times?

Dr Henry J. Bigelow, eminent Boston surgeon and professor at the Harvard Medical School, upon learning of these painless extractions, came to visit Dr Morton to see for himself the potential of this new discovery. After witnessing three painless dental extractions, Dr Bigelow was convinced that Morton's chemical preparation, Letheon, had potential application in general surgery.[18] Dr Bigelow knew the history of ether as an internal medication for several intestinal diseases and of its inhalation as a remedy for asthma and other lung disorders. He was also very much aware of its potential danger, yet it had not prevented him from experimenting on himself. He reported that it produced exhilaration similar to that produced by nitrous oxide but "less pleasurable."[18] To learn more, he administered ether to three or four volunteers, reporting that some subjects became uncontrollable

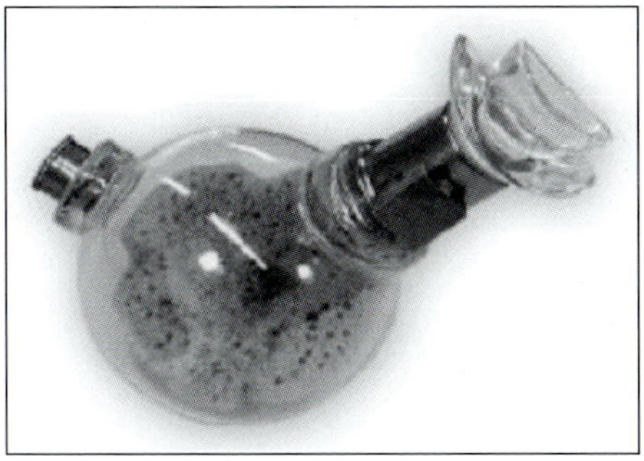

Fig 11-4 Glass ether inhaler.

while others fell into a state of partial paralysis.[18] Overexposure to the vapor of sulfuric ether had been reported as the cause of death in several cases.

Convinced of its successful use in dental surgery, Bigelow, with the approval of Morton, encouraged Dr John Warren, chief of surgery at the MGH, to experiment with its use in major surgeries. Buoyed by his success and with the encouragement of Dr Bigelow, Morton approached Dr Warren and convinced him to permit a demonstration of the anesthetic properties of Letheon before a group of Harvard medical students and physicians at the MGH. The fact that Morton, while a student at the Harvard Medical School, had become known to professors Warren, Bigelow, and Jackson made it easier for the surgeons of the MGH to accept his credibility and to risk their reputation and the survival of their patients in these demonstrations.[16]

On October 16, 1846, Dr Warren and his assistants, along with the apprehensive patient, awaited the arrival of Dr Morton past the scheduled time for the operation. Had Morton, a dentist and still a medical student, lost his courage and decided not to show? Morton was clearly nervous, terrified according to Mrs Morton. She described:

> *The night before the operation, my husband worked until one or two o'clock in the morning upon his inhaler [Fig 11-4]. I assisted him, nearly beside myself with anxiety, for the strongest influences had been brought to bear upon me to discourage him from making this attempt. I had been told that one or two things was sure to happen. Either the test would fail and my husband would be ruined by the world's ridicule, or he would kill the patient and be tried for manslaughter.*[19]

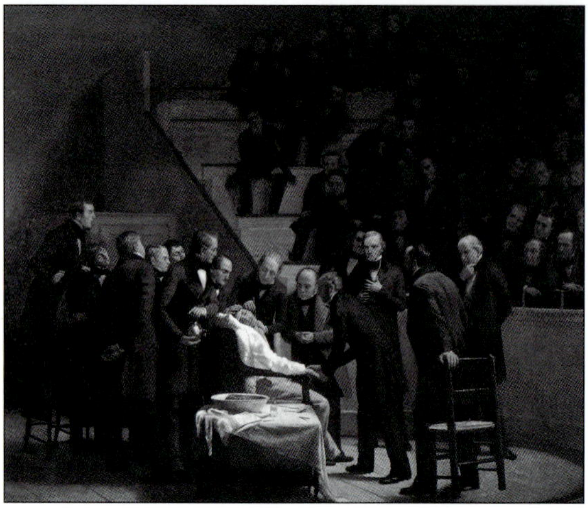

Fig 11-5 Robert C. Hinkley's painting depicting the first use of ether inhalation anesthesia in a surgical operation at the MGH.

Morton did finally arrive, and in the surgical amphitheater under the famous Bulfinch dome of the nation's most prestigious hospital, began to administer Letheon to Dr Warren's patient (Fig 11-5). Dr Jackson, knowing that Morton was going to administer ether and fearing that Morton was about to recklessly do some mischief, was conspicuously absent.[15]

As Warren completed the removal of a tumor from the neck of the completely insensible patient, he turned to the assembled doctors and made his now famous exclamation: "Gentlemen, this is no humbug." Dr Bigelow, present during the operation, stated: "I have seen something to-day that will go around the world."[8] Indeed it did; with exceptional speed the message spread from the Boston papers to all major cities of America and Europe. Dr Oliver Wendell Holmes, a member of the faculty of Harvard Medical School, suggested to Morton that he use the word *anesthesia* to describe the state of unconsciousness produced by ether.[8] Because medical ethics at that time prohibited the use of medicines that were of a secret composition, the surgeons at the MGH ultimately demanded that Morton reveal the composition of Letheon in order to continue its administration at the MGH (Fig 11-6).

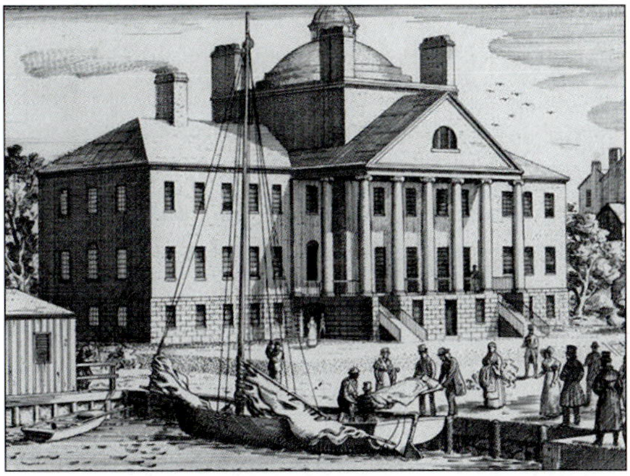

Fig 11-6 Massachusetts General Hospital.

Dr Bigelow noted that during the operation, Morton had continued to administer ether to the patient "long after insensibility was manifested." The patient's pulse was very feeble. It was Bigelow's opinion that the patient had been etherized almost beyond recovery.[1] Morton and the team of MGH surgeons had been lucky; they had just barely avoided disaster. Bigelow noted that ether could be administered safely if attention was paid to the pulse, which gave warning "between harmless inebriation and fatal narcotism."

Dr Henry Bowditch, professor of physiology at Harvard Medical School, in his *History of the Massachusetts General Hospital*, reported that by 1848, some 132 surgical operations had been performed safely under ether anesthesia.[15] He noted that ether's ability to diminish muscular and nervous resistance extended the domain of surgery. The trustees of the hospital, in recognizing that the discovery of ether anesthesia was the most important advance ever made by the MGH, praised the medical and surgical staff for their early appreciation of the validity of Morton's discovery and for their courage in promptly demonstrating its successful application.

Dr Bowditch stated that if the medical and surgical staff had used excessive caution in the use of ether, "its application might have been restricted to the comparatively unimportant operations of the dentist."

The worldwide prestige of the MGH raised Morton's discovery from potential obscurity to acclaim within the medical world. Statistics published in 1892 showed that in 109,196 cases of surgery under general anesthesia, only 39 deaths were recorded, none associated with 8,431 cases of ether anesthesia.[20]

Morton should have been praised to high heaven for his discovery, yet the opposite happened. Morton was attacked by religious fanatics, who believed that man gained redemption from original sin by suffering pain and thus it was immoral to intervene in God's will.[13] A group of prominent Boston dentists led by Dr J. F. Flagg petitioned in the *Daily Advertiser* against the use of ether as a dangerous substance capable of inducing a wide range of maladies.[8] Dr Robert Huston, editor of the *Philadelphia Medical Examiner*, wrote:

> *A certain Dr. Morton, a practicing dentist in Boston, is advertising, in the newspapers of this city, that he has received a patent for what he calls "his improvement, whereby pain may be prevented in dental and surgical operations;" and he now offers to sell licenses to use said improvement to dentists, surgeons, and other suitable persons. Looking upon this as nothing more no less than a new scheme to tax the pockets of the enlightened public, we should not consider it entitled to the least notice, but that we perceive, by the Boston Medical and Surgical Journal, that prominent members of the profession in that city have been caught in its meshes.... If such things are to be sanctioned by the profession, there is little need of reform conventions, or any other efforts to elevate the professional character; physicians and quacks will soon constitute one fraternity.*[13]

Dr Charles A. Lee, editor of the *New York Journal of Medicine*, writing in opposition to Morton's discovery, stated:

> *We are sorry to see so many of our brethren, at home and abroad, stooping from the exalted position they occupy in the profession, to hold intercourse with, and to become abettors of, quackery in any form. Such doings are certainly contrary to the ethics of the profession, and should not be tolerated for a moment in any one.*[13]

Drs Chapin Harris, Amos Westcott, and Edwin Dunning, editors of the *American Journal and Library of Dental Science*, warned against Morton's anesthetic:

> *The effects resulting from, or at least liable to result from, the inhalation of the vapor of sulphuric ether, are, in our opinion, more to be dreaded than the pain of almost any surgical operation. We would, therefore, caution our professional brethren against the use of an article capable of producing such sudden, powerful, and dangerous effects.*[13]

The Patent

In the 19th century, the medical profession considered the patenting of medicines as unethical and detrimental to their image. Dentists, in general, exhibited fewer restrictions in this area. In fact, patents were awarded in high numbers for inventions of new dental instruments and for technical procedures in mechanical dentistry throughout the latter half of the 19th century. Morton executed a patent application on October 27, 1846. His initial intention was to name himself as the sole discoverer and inventor of the method of application of sulfuric ether anesthesia; however, on the advice of his attorney (R. H. Eddy), Morton included Jackson as a co-discoverer. The patent, number 4848, was granted on November 12, 1846, less than 3 weeks from the filing date.[10]

Dr Henry Bigelow advised Morton against seeking a patent on the use of ether; viewing it as an invention "like Whitney's cotton gin… so valuable that the world would combine…to take possession of it,"[1] Bigelow felt that the public would contribute to honor Morton. He later supported Morton's petition to Congress for a monetary award of $100,000.

According to Dr W. H. Potter, speaking at the Pan-American Medical Congress of 1893, Morton had made a mistake in seeking a patent for his discovery: "Morton would have been better received by the medical profession if he had given his discovery to the public. In seeking to patent his discovery Morton faced the charge of quackery from physicians and the anger of dentists who hoped to use it without hindrance."[14]

Dr Jackson was reluctant to have his name connected with the patenting of a medical substance, fearing being accused of quackery by the Massachusetts Medical Society and the opprobrium of his close medical colleagues. Nevertheless, following discussions with Mr Eddy, Morton's attorney, Jackson agreed to place his name on the patent as co-discoverer but to cede his claims to patent rights in return for $500, receiving a 10% return on the sale of licenses until the $500 had been paid.[13] It was Eddy's belief that the chances of a successful application would be greatly improved by having Jackson, a respected scientist, listed as co-discoverer. Of his conversations with Jackson, Eddy wrote:

> *I would here remark, that I found Dr. Jackson tinctured with old and exploded prejudices against patents, and I labored to remove them. So successful was I, that he subsequently informed me, that, after a consultation with a distinguished chemist at the south, he had resolved to secure every invention he might hereafter make; and, in accordance*

> *with such views, he sent me the specification of an alleged improvement in preparing a certain article for dentistry purposes, with the view of filing a caveat and taking out a patent on the same.*[13]

Morton sold licenses for the use of Letheon to dentists on the following terms: $50 for 5 years in towns with less than 10,000 persons and up to $200 in larger cities. Surgeons were contracted at 25% of fees charged for surgeries. Drs D. S. Blake and A. Blaisdale, acting as agents of Morton, sold licenses in parts of Massachusetts, New York, New Jersey, Virginia, and in several southern and western states.[21] Both dentists and surgeons were required to remit records and payments on a quarterly basis.[10] In his sales promotions, Morton would always assure his clients of the safety of sulfuric ether by emphasizing that the eminent chemist Charles Jackson, professor at Harvard, had been instrumental in the discovery and in the experimental demonstration of its safe application. By appropriating the mantle of Harvard and the reputation of Jackson, Morton hoped to quell criticism of his commercialism and lack of scientific expertise.[21] In the view of the medical establishment, Morton's patent "was obtained for the purposes of gain."[22] Although Morton gave free license to the use of his discovery to numerous hospitals, he attempted to reap high profits by patenting the ether anesthetic under the name Letheon. Despite the fact that Jackson removed himself from the patent, he shared some income from the sale of licenses and was aggressive in his fight against Morton and Wells for a potential monetary award of $100,000 being considered by the United States Congress.

Wells, in contrast, had made no effort to patent his use of nitrous oxide in anesthesia (see block quote on pages 275–276). However, Wells was not adverse to the idea of a patent, for he had advised Morton to use a proper method to "dispose of his rights" and thereby gain a fortune.[13]

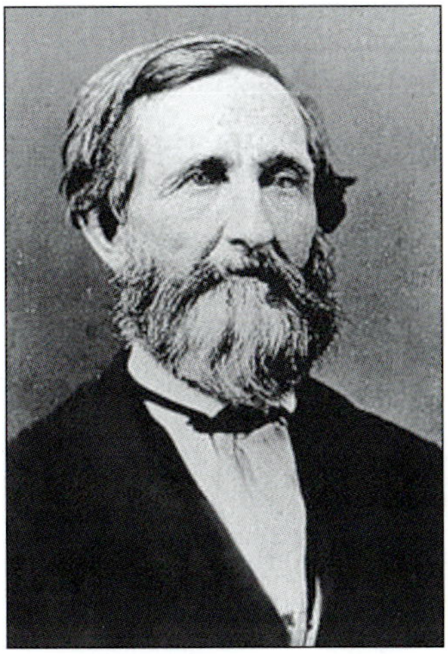

Fig 11-7 Crawford W. Long.

Crawford W. Long

Crawford W. Long (1815–1878) (Fig 11-7), a country doctor in rural Georgia, may have been the first person to induce insensibility by administering ether gas. Long is believed to have been put on the trail of ether from reports that a young Negro boy had been placed in a deep narcosis during a local "ether frolic."[2] In 1842, Crawford Long removed a tumor from the back of the neck of James Venable, who had been anesthetized by ether inhalation. He used ether anesthesia some four of five times during the ensuing 4 years but did not publish his experiences or communicate them to any local medical association. It was only after Morton had demonstrated the usefulness of ether in Massachusetts that Long was stirred to action. However, by that point, the recognition given to Morton as the discoverer of ether anesthesia was too great to overcome.

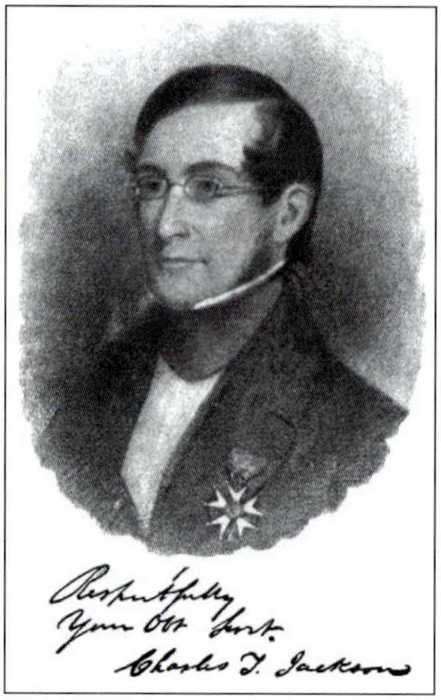

Fig 11-8 Charles T. Jackson.

Charles T. Jackson and His Claims of Discovery

Dr Charles T. Jackson, a graduate of Harvard Medical School, was not only a physician but also a well-known geologist and chemist (Fig 11-8). He was characterized as brilliant and tremendously ambitious.[2] Jackson had distinguished himself as a geologist by his mining explorations in Nova Scotia and New England. He held an international reputation as an expert in this field. During the course of his career, he made several controversial and unfounded claims of being a co-discoverer of major inventions. He told Morton that while on a return trip from Europe in the company of Samuel B. Morse, he had given Morse the idea for the telegraph during long conversations on the potential ability of electrical currents to carry information.[13] He had made similar unfounded claims to the invention of guncotton. This tendency to falsely associate himself with the work of others arose again during his campaign to wrest the glory of discovery from Morton.

Jackson had prior knowledge of the effects of ether, and he directed Morton to experiment with ether to induce insensibility in dental operations, yet he was not present at the first application of ether at the MGH, and furthermore he declined an invitation from Dr Warren to attend and administer ether in the hospital's first capital operation.[10] How could Jackson, a scientist and physician, stay away from such a significant event? The best answer is that Jackson was highly concerned of the potential danger of the inhalation of ether and felt that it was in his best interest to be positioned at a distance from these initial ventures. Jackson had expressed his fears that Morton was a "reckless man" and would likely "kill somebody yet."[10] Despite his early association with Morton, Jackson feared being labeled a quack and kept himself at a distance from Morton.

Jackson considered himself to be the brains behind anesthesia. That Morton, an "ignoramus" when it came to scientific matters, and Wells, a mere dentist, were being acclaimed as the discoverers of inhalation anesthesia, a discovery second only to vaccination, while he was being ignored, did not sit right with him.[12] When the success of the initial operations at the MGH were announced and Boston's medical establishment recognized the safety of ether anesthesia, Jackson felt it was time to gain some of the fame, as well as some of the potential profits, by declaring himself an equal partner with Morton in the invention of ether anesthesia.

Jackson made a formal claim to priority of discovery by recruiting international scientists to his cause. He wrote to the French Academy of Sciences in November 1846, in a letter to L. Elie de Beaumont, a fellow geologist, stating how he had made the discovery of the anesthetic properties of sulfuric ether.[10] In that letter, Jackson informed de Beaumont that he had enticed a dentist to administer the vapor to persons who were to have teeth extracted. Jackson also affirmed his right as the discoverer of inhalation anesthesia in a paper submitted in 1847 to the American Academy of Arts and Sciences. Jackson mailed this paper to scientific colleagues in London before it was formally accepted by the Academy. In this duplicitous maneuver, he hoped to convince the scientific communities of Britain and Europe that he had obtained the Academy's recognition of his priority to discovery and thereby undercut any movement to proclaim Morton or Wells as the discoverer.[13] In neither communication to the scientific academies did Jackson mention the names of Morton or Wells.[10]

Years later, in a statement to the French Academy, Morton recalled how he had learned of the potential benefits of ether in quelling pain. In acknowledgment of Jackson's role in the discovery of the power of ether to produce insensibility, Morton made it clear that Jackson had a limited and indirect role:

> *I am ready to acknowledge my indebtedness to men and to books for all my information on this subject. I have got there a little and there a little. I learned from Dr. Jackson, in 1844, the effect of ether directly applied to a sensitive tooth, and proved by experiment that it would gradually render the nerve insensible. I learned from Dr. Jackson, also in 1844, the effect of ether when inhaled by students at college, which was corroborated by Spear's account, and by what I read. I knew of Dr. Wells' attempt to apply nitrous-oxide gas for destroying pain under surgical operations. I had great motive to destroy or alleviate pain under my operations, and endeavored to produce such a result by means of inhaling ether; inferring that if it would render a nerve insensible when directly applied, it might, when inhaled, destroy, or greatly alleviate sensibility to pain generally. Had the ether I tried on August 5 been pure, I should have made the demonstration then. I further acknowledge that I was subsequently indebted to Dr. Jackson for valuable information as to the kinds and preparations of ether, and for the recommendation of the highly rectified article from Burnett's, as to the most safe and efficient. But my obligation to him hath this extent, no more.*[10]

The battle over priority of discovery escalated over the next few years, as appeals were made to the president and the Congress of the United States for an award of $100,000 to the discoverer of anesthesia.

The Controversy over Priority

Soon after his successful demonstration at the MGH, Morton started a campaign to ensure for himself the priority of discovery of anesthesia. In this he was confronted with the counterclaims of Wells and Jackson. Wells received strong support from his dental colleagues in the Hartford community and especially from Senator Smith of Connecticut. Senator Smith published a lengthy account of his investigation of the discovery of anesthesia in the *Medical and Surgical Reporter* of 1864. Smith's report, appearing as a 10-part series, supported the merits of Horace Wells while challenging and discrediting Morton's and Jackson's attempt to appropriate to themselves the discovery of inhalation anesthesia. The editors of the *Reporter* concluded, "It has been shown beyond the possibility of cavil, that Morton was not, and that Horace Wells was the discoverer of the application of anesthetics to surgical uses."[2]

Wells made his case for discovery in a short pamphlet entitled *A History of the Discovery of the Application of Nitrous Oxide Gas, Ether, and Other Vapors to Surgical Operations*. Wells attacked the honesty of Jackson's claim to be the sole discoverer of ether anesthesia before the scientific communities of London and Paris, underscoring the fact that Jackson never mentioned the role that he and Morton had played in the events leading to the demonstration at the MGH. In response to Jackson's and Morton's arguments against the use of nitrous oxide, Wells stated that it was not a matter of which gas was used to induce insensibility but of which gas was less likely to harm the patient.[9] On this question, he and Dr Marcy, who had administered both nitrous oxide and ether in surgical cases, were of the opinion that nitrous oxide was safer, and it was for this reason that he had abandoned the use of ether. The fact that Morton had chosen to administer ether gave him no right to usurp Wells's priority of discovery.

Opponents argued that Wells's experiments with nitrous oxide were minimized by the fact that nitrous oxide had not been administered in a major surgical operation. Furthermore, Wells had been unsuccessful in efforts to convince Boston's medical elite of nitrous oxide's potential. To diminish Wells's importance, it was pointed out that Sir Humphrey Davy had first discovered that inhalation of nitrous oxide could remove the pain of headache and toothache and that Davy had suggested that it could be used to advantage in surgical operations.[13]

The medical staff of the MGH was eager to claim the prize for Morton and Boston. Dr Henry Bigelow, a giant among Boston's medical establishment, made forceful arguments in support of Dr Morton.[1] Bigelow recalled that although a resection of a cancerous breast under nitrous oxide gas had been performed in 1848 at the MGH (2 years after Morton's demonstration of ether anesthesia), nitrous oxide anesthesia for surgical cases had been subsequently abandoned in favor of ether because nitrous oxide caused an asphyxiation of the tissues and rigidity of the musculature. Furthermore, the need to prepare large amounts of the gas and the bulky apparatus needed for its administration made its use inconvenient. However, Bigelow noted that dentists might favor the use of nitrous oxide in view of the lingering odor of ether.[23]

Although Bigelow characterized Morton as "scientifically ignorant" and, in the view of the scientific community, reckless and perhaps culpable in subjecting "every patient he could procure to this danger," Bigelow concluded that Morton had proved the scientifically learned world to be wrong.[23] Dr Bigelow, who was present at the demonstration, recalled that he had been invited by Morton "for the purpose of aiding him in emergency with professional advice...but I assumed no responsibility. Had the patient died in a stupor, as he might well have done, Morton was liable; and as the patient did not die, his was the credit." In further support of Morton's claim, Bigelow stated:

> *Thousands of people had been made insensible, many by inhalation, some by ether. But until 1846 neither ether nor gas was known to produce at will an anesthesia that was complete, sure to occur in every individual, and safe. On the contrary, all previous insensibility was either uncertain to occur when wanted; or it was incomplete, as against the severer forms of pain; or it was considered to be of doubtful safety. Morton's discovery consisted in his proof that ether insensibility was possible to everybody, that it could always be made complete when the operator desired it, and that it was safe. It detracts nothing from his discovery that, like every discoverer that ever lived, he availed himself of all previously existing knowledge, written or oral.*[1,23]

The facts are that Morton made the first clinical application of ether's anesthetic properties and proved that its administration was safe and of sufficient duration to permit the completion of major surgical operations.[10] According to John C. Warren, the surgeon of the first ether operation, the experimental question originated in Morton's mind; he asked the question and provided the nerve, and recklessness too, to do the experiment that Jackson was unwilling to risk.[13] Furthermore, Morton had assumed all of the risks and consequences of potential failure. Morton's wife recalled those days as "so full of anxiety and, to me, of absolute terror, waiting for the disaster which everybody assured me would come."[10]

Jackson did not enter the battle for priority until he recognized the safety of ether anesthesia and the possibility that the US Congress was about to award a large monetary prize to the person deemed to have been the discoverer of anesthesia. Jackson hired the legal firm of Lord and Lord to compile evidence supporting his claim to discovery of anesthesia by etherization. This pamphlet, *A Defense of Dr. Charles T. Jackson's Claims to the Discovery of Etherization*, accused Morton of many falsehoods, including his assertion that he had made many experiments with ether prior to September 30, 1846, the date that Jackson had first informed him of ether's ability to induce insensibility.[21]

Jackson's critics also argued that if Jackson knew of ether's ability to induce insensibility in 1842, why hadn't he approached his medical colleagues at the Harvard Medical School, or at the MGH, to suggest experiments with ether in surgeries? Why did he wait 4 years to propose its use to a dentist?[13] Jackson's claim to knowledge of the ability of ether to produce insensibility in 1842 was challenged by pointing out that Jackson did not advise Morton to administer ether when he brought two members of his family to Morton's office for dental extractions in 1844.[10] This appears odd, considering that Jackson claimed to have inhaled ether and experienced its anesthetic properties in 1842.

In regard to the numerous counterclaims and accusations of dishonesty surrounding the question of discovery, Dr Gould, in frustration, said: "The subject of the discovery of etherization has become so offensive to us all in this vicinity, that I would gladly avoid ever alluding to it again in any shape."[10] MGH surgeons fled at the sight of Morton, and just the word *ether* led to an end to conversation.[10]

The Subsequent Events

In the hearings in Washington DC, Congress was unable to come to any decision as to who merited the honor of discovery and the associated $100,000 prize. In the opinion of Dr Bigelow, the result of a tribunal not "accustomed to estimate the weight and quality of scientific evidence…was, that every new discussion began and ended like the preceding, and to as little purpose."[1]

The controversy took a severe toll on the health of all three men. Wells, in failing to convince the medical profession that he was the rightful discoverer of inhalation anesthesia, became depressed and addicted to chloroform inhalation. Arrested and jailed in New York City for intoxication and confrontation with prostitutes, Wells committed suicide in his jail cell.

Dr Bigelow stated that Morton, amid mounting criticism, lived his last years in "poverty, privation, and discouragement." Morton's widow wrote that her husband's "life for twenty-two years was one long and bitter contest, and to which in the prime of his life he succumbed, leaving his family penniless."[10] Morton died on July 15, 1868 from a massive stroke while in Central Park, New York. A publication at that time supporting Jackson's claim to priority of discovery may have added to his mental stress and contributed to his death.[10] Dr Jacob Bigelow, Morton's staunch supporter, wrote the following epitaph inscribed on Morton's tomb: "Inventor and revealer of anesthetic inhalation. By whom pain in surgery was averted and annulled. Before whom in all times surgery was agony. Since whom science has control of pain."

This fight took such a toll on Jackson's mind that he ended up spending his last years in an insane asylum. A monument in Mount Auburn Cemetery, Cambridge, Massachusetts, commemorating his life contains the following inscription: "Through his observations of the peculiar effects of sulphuric ether on the nerves of sensation, and

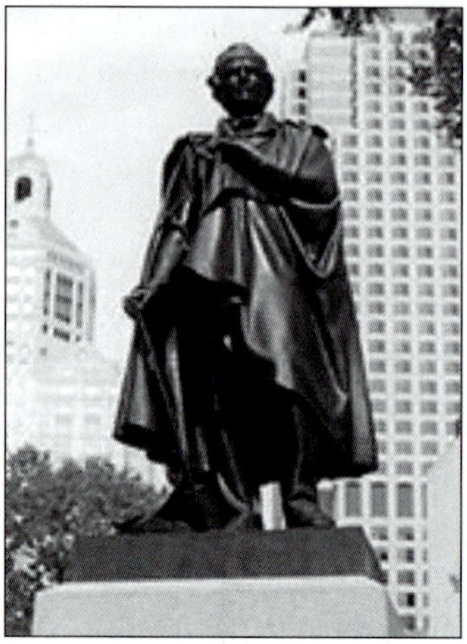

Fig 11-9 Statue of Horace Wells in Bushnell Park, Hartford, Connecticut.

his bold deduction therefrom, the benign discovery of painless surgery was made."

In 1870, the Connecticut Medical Society, upon its investigation of who rightly should claim to be the discoverer of anesthesia, concluded that the honor belonged to Horace Wells.[24] The decision was endorsed by the Boston Gynecological Society and by Sir James Y. Simpson, Edinburgh's physician who introduced chloroform for the relief of pain in childbirth. Joint support from the Connecticut Dental Association, the Connecticut Medical Association, and the American Medical Association moved the Hartford City Government and the Connecticut State Legislature to appropriate $5,000 each for the dedication of a bronze statue of Dr Wells, erected in Bushnell Park, Hartford, Connecticut[24] (Fig 11-9).

Summary

The story of the discovery of anesthesia has been romanticized as the quest of altruistic men to rid the world of pain. The unfortunate truth is that any great desire to benefit mankind was mixed with a heavy dose of greed. The men involved in the quest for painless dentistry suffered much self-inflicted pain. Although it may be unfair to judge them by today's ethical standards, their actions speak clearly that financial gain was a powerful motivator. In attempting to do what had not been done before, they accepted personal risk, not to mention the safety of their patients. In this respect, it can be suggested that they were reckless and not all that rational. It is evident that both Wells and Morton had the inventive and entrepreneurial spirit that was common among many who opted to make dentistry a business, if not an honorable profession. Had they been less concerned with profit and fame, and more with the public's welfare, Wells's and Morton's roles in the discovery of inhalation anesthesia could have marked dentistry's finest hour.

References

1. Bigelow HJ. A history of the discovery of modern anesthesia. Am J Med Sci 1876;71:164–184.
2. Raper HR. Man Against Pain. New York: Prentice-Hall, 1945.
3. Fenster JM. Ether Day: The Strange Tale of America's Greatest Medical Discovery and the Haunted Men Who Made It. New York: HarperCollins, 2001.
4. Wolfe RJ. Tarnished Idol: William T. G. Morton and the Introduction of Surgical Anesthesia. San Anselmo, CA: Norman, 2001.
5. Leake CD. Valerius Cordus and the discovery of ether. Isis 1925;7:14–24.
6. Prinz H. Dental Materia Medica and Therapeutics. St Louis: Mosby, 1909.
7. What was the discovery of anesthesia? (editorial). West Dent J 1897;11:329–330.
8. Smith CA. The discovery of anesthesia. Sci Monthly 1927;24:64–70.
9. Wells H. A History of the Discovery of the Application of Nitrous Oxide Gas, Ether, and Other Vapors, to Surgical Operations. Hartford: J. Gaylord Wells, 1847.
10. Hodges RM. A Narrative of Events Connected with the Introduction of Sulphuric Ether into Surgical Use. Boston: Little, Brown, 1891.
11. Latimer JS. Gleanings from proceedings of the Society of Dental Surgeons of the City of New York. Dent Cosmos 1864;5:303–306.
12. Robinson JB. William T. G. Morton and ether. J Am Dent Assoc 1946;33:1572–1576.
13. Warren E. Some Account of the Letheon: Or, Who Is the Discoverer? Boston: Dutton and Wentworth, 1847.
14. Potter WH. The discovery of the anesthetic power of ether. Dent Cosmos 1893;35:1157–1163.
15. Bowditch NI. A History of the Massachusetts General Hospital. Boston: Bowditch Fund, 1872.
16. Rice NP. Trials of a Public Benefactor, as Illustrated in the Discovery of Etherization. New York: Pudney and Russell, 1859.
17. Tees A. Anesthesia. Dent Cosmos 1863;5:202–210.
18. Bigelow HJ. Insensibility during surgical operations produced by inhalation. Boston Med Surg J 1846;35:309–317.
19. Ash HL. Anesthesia's dental heritage. Anesth Prog 1985;32:25–29.
20. Gurlt E. Deaths under anesthetics. Dent Cosmos 1893;35:489.
21. Lord JL, Lord HC. A Defence of Dr. Charles T. Jackson's Claims to the Discovery of Etherization. Boston: Littell's Living Age, 1848.
22. Smith E. The ether patent. Am Med Times 1862;4:83–84.
23. Bigelow HJ. Surgical Anesthesia: Addresses and Other Papers. Boston: Little, Brown, 1900.
24. Report of the Committee of the Connecticut Medical Society on the discovery of anesthesia. Proc Conn Med Soc 1897:50–51.

12

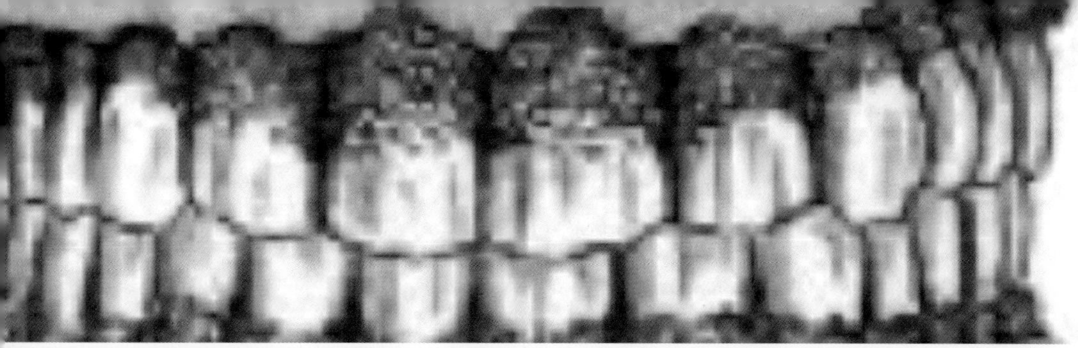

Diseases of the Periodontium

Diseases of the gingivae and the periodontal supporting tissues appear to have been common in ancient times. Evidence of periodontal bone loss was found in the jawbones of Neanderthal skulls.[1] The Ebers Papyrus describes gumboils and alveolar abscesses, and Egyptian and Phoenician skeletal remains contain evidence of advanced periodontal bone loss.[2,3] Elliot Smith reported that among 500 Egyptian skeletons, "tartar-formation, dental caries and alveolar abscesses were at least as common as they are in modern Europe today."[4] References to diseased gums and loose teeth are contained in the writings of Hippocrates and Galen.[4–6] Treatment consisted of scraping away tartar from around the teeth, applying astringent compounds to the tissues, and removing tissue by cautery with red-hot oil or iron.[4,5] Special instruments for scraping tartar and for cauterizing gingival tissue were described and illustrated (see Fig 1-10) by Albucasis in the 10th century.[1,4;1]

Notable surgeons of the Middle Ages, such as Mondeville and Chauliac, repeated the advice of the Arabian physicians in treating gingival and alveolar bone abscesses with cautery, excisional drainage, and astringent mouth rinses and/or herbal plasters.[1,4,5] Paré in the 16th century continued this approach to treatment while attempting to identify the causes of gingival and alveolar pathology.[1] The accumulation of faulty humors, the consumption of unhealthy foods, and

---

[1] For an in-depth review of the development of periodontology, see Arthur-Jean Held's *Periodontology from Its Origins up to 1980: A Survey.*[1]

the use of cosmetics containing mercury were some of the popular explanations for gingival suppuration and the resulting loosening of teeth.

Urbain Hémard, author of the first book in the French language dealing with dental health, wrote that the teeth are subject to encrustations that with time become as hard as stone. These substances cause the gingivae to separate from the teeth, rendering the teeth mobile and stinking. He attributed the encrustation to precipitates in the exhalations from the stomach, "which attach themselves like smoke on the walls of the chimney."[7] He advised scraping away the encrustations with a "burin," a tool similar to those used by engravers. Pierre Dionis, First Surgeon to the dauphine of France, instructed operators for the teeth to use special care in cleaning the teeth of women. To minimize trauma to their delicate mouths, the operator should use a soft touch by wrapping the hand used for isolating the lips and cheeks with a soft white linen cloth and similarly wrap the noncutting parts of his instruments.[8]

Fauchard

Pierre Fauchard considered diseases of the gums as being "the ones which destroy the teeth most frequently and cause them infinity of troublesome accidents." Fauchard described the most common form of gingival disease:

> *The gums become so flabby, so spongy, so tender, so delicate that even a light touch or if the patient sucks out his saliva, blood flows. The teeth react sometimes to the extent of getting loose, and are lost for this reason, if remedies are not speedily applied. The cause of this is most commonly tartar which accumulates on the teeth and insinuates between them and the gums, which gives rise to compression of the vessels and obstruction to the passage of fluids.*[9]

Fauchard's treatment of this condition consisted of "removal of tartar with every care, scarification of the gums with a lancet fixed and covered with a small bandage up to its point, or with a sharp gum lancet, and cut the excessive gum with the scissors" (Fig 12-1). Ulcerations of the gums were to be feared as progressing to "gangrene or necrosis, very lively and violent pain, insomnia, even delirium." Ulcers were treated by syringing the lesions with a caustic tincture made from various herbs, including myrrh, colcothar, and red vitriol.

Fauchard also described a disease affecting the gums, the teeth, and their alveoli, caused by "a destructive scorbutic humour" that pene-

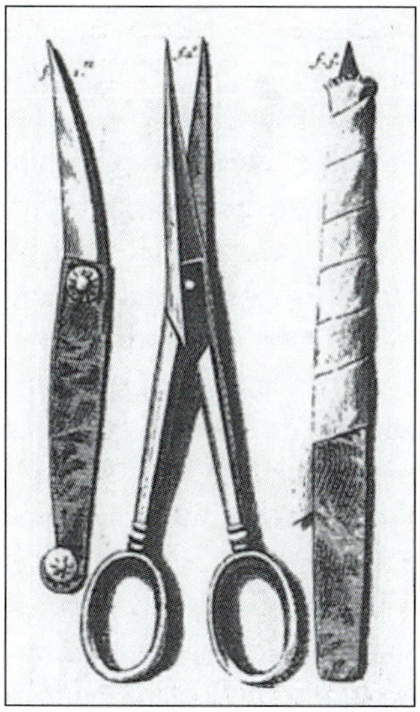

Fig 12-1 Fauchard's instruments for excision and scarification of the gums. (From Fauchard.[9])

trates and destroys the walls of the bony alveolus, ultimately resulting in loss of the teeth. This form of scorbutic disease was accompanied "by a whitish, slightly glutinous pus which can be expressed from the gums by application of the finger pressing pretty hard from below upwards in the lower jaw and from above downwards in the upper jaw." Fauchard made the astute observation that "those who have been treated for this complaint by internal remedies, whether they are anti-scorbutic, or otherwise, have not been cured, which makes me believe that there is no internal source or general cause, but that it has a local or accidental origin occasioned by the teeth." For treatment of this disease, he described that when the gums are

> *swollen and engorged with blood or a scorbutic humour it is necessary to perform scarifications often with well-sharpened lance or gum lancet. When the gums are so inflamed or tumified as to exceed their natural level, as nearly as possible all that which is detached from the teeth or alveoli is removed with scissors straight or curved but very sharp.*[9]

The surgical wound is then dressed with a linen bandage steeped in a special lotion formulated by Fauchard. In recognizing the local nature of the disease, and in attributing its cause to the accumulation of calculus, Fauchard emphasized the singular importance of professional scaling and the practice of oral hygiene.[1] This local scorbutic disease of the gums and alveoli would in the next century be identified as *pyorrhea alveolaris* and later as *chronic periodontitis* in the 20th century.

Bourdet

According to Etienne Bourdet, Parisian dentist of the 18th century, the major cause of gingival disease was tartar. Bourdet spoke of the many remedies (eg, elixirs, drogues) touted by dentists and street vendors for treatment of dental and gingival disorders. None of these preparations, he said, were successful unless accompanied by the work of the dentist in removing tartar and superfluous and stagnant blood.[10] He placed great emphasis on preserving gingival health, stating that "the preservation of the alveolar bone depended on the duration of the gingivae."

Bourdet applied scarification, excision, and cautery in treating gingival diseases. Because swollen gums were thought to result from congestion of blood vessels, scarification and lancing of the tissues, accompanied by pressure application with a linen cloth to express large amounts of blood, were the first steps in treatment. Astringent mouthwashes, some containing opium, were administered daily. When these treatments failed to reduce the size of the gums, excision was indicated. Cognizant of an esthetically pleasing mouth, Bourdet cautioned that in performing gingival surgery, one needed to guard against disfiguring the patient. He was critical of dentists who removed gingival tissue without regard for the esthetic outcome of the operations. In performing gingival resection, Bourdet used scissors to cut away swollen tissue in a manner to preserve pointed interdental contours. When the thickness of the swollen gingiva was excessive, he used a small, very sharp knife to create a beveled incision so as to remove excess tissue without exposing too much root surface[10] (Fig 12-2).

Bourdet postulated that suppuration around the teeth was caused by minute ulcerations of the gingival wall facing the tooth surface, a condition he cured by inserting thin, flat cauterizing instruments into the space between the gingiva and the tooth.[10,11] He hypothesized that gingival ulcerations were a source of corrosive exudations that were capable of destroying the alveolar bone. Bourdet recommended gingival resection in cases that were not resolved by cauterization. Gerauldy, a contemporary of Fauchard and Bourdet, described four types of gingival lesions: inflammatory tumors, gingival outgrowths, ulcerations, and fistulas. He viewed stagnation of blood flow within gingival blood vessels as a primary causative factor, which he proposed to cure by bloodletting and scarification of the tissues.[12; 2]

[2] Stagnation of blood flow as the cause of periodontal tissue damage would remain a key element of most attempts to understand periodontal diseases, influencing treatment protocols well into the mid 20th century.

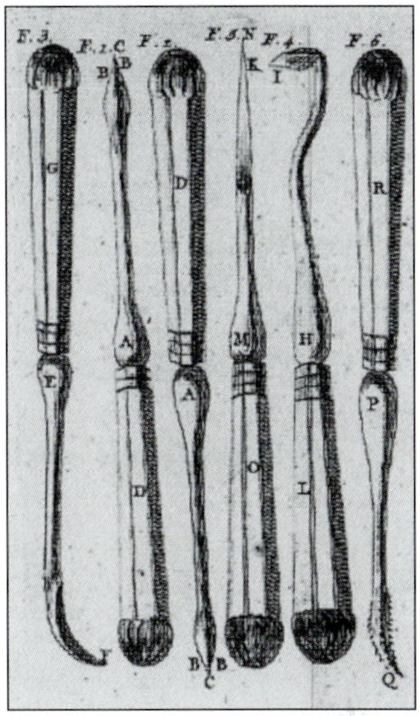

Fig 12-2 Bourdet's instruments for gingival surgery. (From Bourdet.[10])

Role of Tartar

By the beginning of the 19th century, it was the general opinion that gingival lesions and the more severe suppurating alveolar bone lesions were caused by tartar (calculus) and the soft deposits that accumulated on teeth. Joseph Fox explained in the early 19th century that "Excepting the disease of caries, nothing is so destructive of the healthy condition of the mouth, or of the duration of the teeth, as the accumulation of tartar. This is an earthy substance held in solution by the saliva, and is deposited upon the teeth, as the saliva undergoes decomposition." Fox sent a sample of tartar to the chemist W. H. Pepys, whose analysis revealed that 70% was "phosphate of lime," 18% "fibrin or cartilage," 6% "animal fat," and 6% "loss."[13] Fox observed that tartar "accumulates in greater quantity about those teeth situated near to the openings of the salivary ducts."[13] Fox emphasized that by practicing optimal dental hygiene, the buildup of calculus could be avoided and the teeth preserved into old age.

Despite the clear significance of local factors in most cases of gingival and alveolar bone diseases, there were cases where calculus was not evident and for which systemic abnormalities, mainly of a humoral nature, were invoked to explain the diseases.

Nothing had changed for 1,000 years; the cause of gingival and alveolar bone diseases were still unknown, and the methods employed in the treatment of these diseases had remained the same (ie, scraping tartar from the teeth, scarifying the gums, bloodletting, and excising overgrown tissue). But from the middle of the 18th century, increasing numbers of theories were put forth as causes of gingival and periodontal diseases. Although tartar continued to be viewed as a key inflammatory irritant by many, some practitioners believed it to be a secondary factor operating upon a primary constitutional (systemic) condition. Diseases such as syphilis, diabetes, gout, and scurvy were considered to potentiate the damaging effects of local irritants, whether they were calculus deposits or the malocclusion of teeth.[4]

The origin of tartar (dental calculus) was a subject of much speculation. Fauchard proposed three causes of the development of tartar: *(1)* degeneration of food retained about the teeth, *(2)* precipitations of substances in the exhaled breath, and *(3)* precipitation of saliva. Unless removed by daily tooth cleaning with a dentifrice, these substances accumulated in a solidified form, and by impinging on the gingival tissues and inserting themselves into the space between the gums and the teeth, they caused suppuration and ulceration of the gingivae.[9] Edward Cameron Kirk's theory of the origin of dental calculus, proposed in 1911, is believed to have been the first modern explanation:

> *As the saliva contains carbon dioxid in solution, it has been assumed, with some justification, that the escape of the carbon dioxid, which was the solvent of the calcium carbonate and tricalcic phosphate, causes a precipitation of those salts in the presence of the colloid mucin, in combination with which it deposits as tartar upon the teeth.*[14]

Kirk also proposed that ammonia exhaled in the breath could cause the precipitation of calcium phosphate from saliva. The contrary notion that calculus was a result of disease derived from an inflammatory exudate, not an inciting primary cause, was also proposed.[15,16] John Deans Patterson, in departing from the currently held idea that calculus was a precipitate of saliva, stated that subgingival (pocket) calculus deposits developed from "purulent matter and are the consequence of irritation and inflammation from the various causes referred to. They are not precedent to a lesion, but invariably are subsequent to irritation and exudation."[15] Seepage from inflamed blood vessels adjacent to the root surface was viewed as a source for the formation of serumal calculus.[17]

Distinctions were made between purely gingival lesions and deterioration of the periodontal membrane and cementum. As greater emphasis was placed on the health of the cementum and periodontal membrane, special terms were used to describe pathologic changes in those tissues: *alveolodental suppuration*, *pericementitis*, and *pyorrhea alveolaris* were among the most common terms used.

The French surgeon E. Magitot, in 1867, described periodontal disease as "osteo-periostite alveolo-dentaire," a complex disease originating in the periodontal membrane and cementum traced to deficiencies in systemic physiology and nutrition (ie, a constitutional origin). Magitot reported that periodontal disease was common in patients suffering from diabetes, gout, rheumatism, and albuminuria (too much protein in the urine). He considered calculus deposits to be a secondary, not a primary, cause of the pathology.[14] The notion that pyorrhea alveolaris was caused by an underlying systemic disorder remained most favored by the European schools of stomatology.

Pyorrhea

The first dentist in the United States to devote full attention to treating periodontal disease was John Riggs of Connecticut. He called this disease *alveolar pyorrhea* and defined it as a suppurated inflammation of the gums complicated by absorption of the gums and the alveolar process. The term *pyorrhea alveolaris*, used previously in France and Germany, was first used in the American dental literature by James Truman in 1875.[18] Riggs downplayed the idea that the disease had any constitutional origin. He claimed excellent success in treating pyorrhea by meticulous removal of all calculus with specially designed scalers followed by polishing of the root surface (a procedure called *oral prophylaxis*). George Mills described the use of Riggs's scalers to reach the remotest parts of all diseased teeth.[19] He claimed that thorough scaling, combined with the application of sulfuric acid to diseased root surfaces, was an excellent treatment for pyorrhea: "No operation performed by the dentist in the mouth is more appreciated by patients after they have seen the results. It is really a surgical operation, and is of vastly more importance than has been attached to it by the profession generally."

Shortly after Riggs brought increased attention to pyorrhea and its treatment, G. V. Black published a masterly account of this disease in 1886 (Figs 12-3 and 12-4). Black noted that the disease manifested itself in two forms: *(1)* calcic inflammation of the peridental membrane[3] and gums and *(2)* phagedenic pericementitis, or destructive inflammation of the peridental membrane.[20] The rationale for this classification was based on his clinical observations of differences in

[3] The connective tissue located between the alveolar bone and the root cementum, serving to attach the tooth to its alveolus. The term is synonymous with the modern term *periodontal ligament* and with the older term *pericementum*.

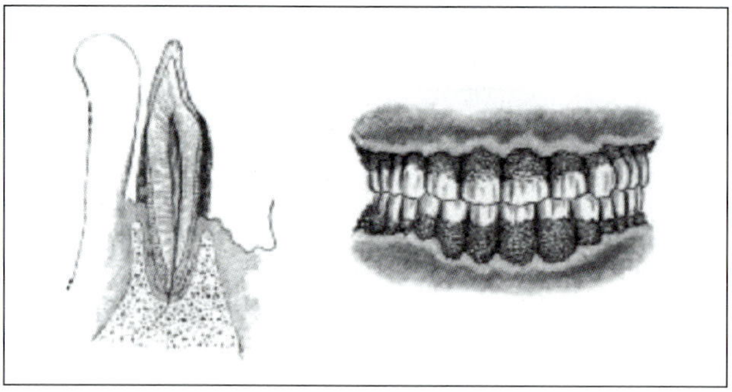

Fig 12-3 Heavy deposits of salivary calculus leading to gingival recession and alveolar bone resorption. (From Black.[20])

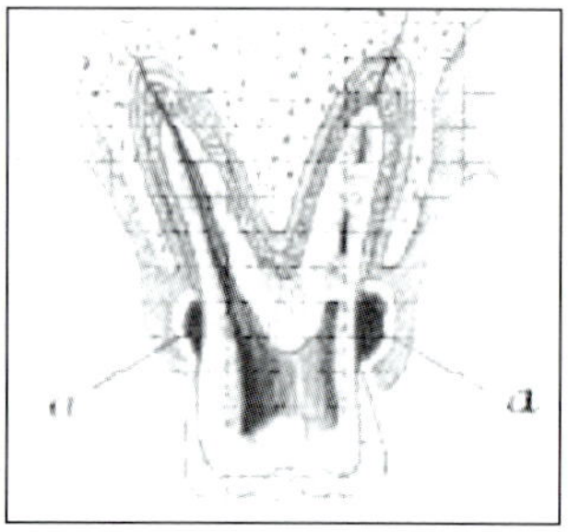

Fig 12-4 Serumal calculus deposited beneath the gingival margin causing pocket formation and resorption of the alveolar bone. (From Black.[20])

etiology, diagnosis, prognosis, and treatment protocols. Calcic inflammation of the peridental membrane and gums was

> *dependent directly upon the accumulation of calculus upon the necks of the teeth [Fig 12-5], and presents two forms that may appear distinct from each other or may be blended together in the most intimate way. This relates to the source of the calculus and the position of the deposit. One form is derived from the serum that exudes from the tissues in a state of disease, and is uniformly deposited under the free margin of the gum [see Fig 12-4]; the other is derived from the saliva and is deposited on the necks of the teeth close up against the free margin of the gum, but not beneath it.*

According to Black, *serumal calculus*, formed beneath the gum, led to an inflamed peridental membrane but not to its total destruction (an important distinction from phagedenic pericementitis). *Salivary calculus*, deposited above the gum line, was an irritant to the gingival tissues it contacted. Treatment consisted of "the removal of the concretions from the teeth, and next the arousing in the mind of the pa-

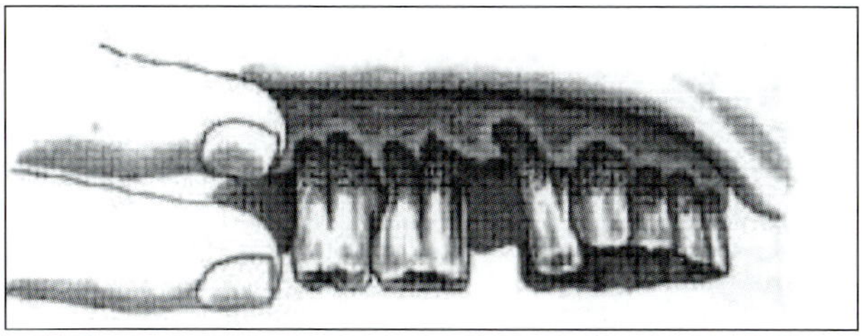

Fig 12-5 Advanced alveolar resorption in calcific pyorrhea. (From Black.[20])

tient an active determination to keep them clean in the future. These two measures are absolutely necessary to success; nothing can be accomplished unless they are scrupulously carried out." Black emphasized the difficulty involved with calculus removal:

> *The removal of these concretions in such a manner as to assure success is, however, one of the most difficult operations in dental surgery. Another very serious difficulty standing in the way of success is the very slack and inefficient notions that have been held in regard to it by the profession at large. When dentists learn to regard this operation as equal in importance to, and requiring as much thoroughness as, the filling of teeth, and when they apply themselves with the same diligence to acquiring the necessary dexterity in its performance, they will be rewarded with success; without this, success in the treatment of this disease cannot be attained.*[20]

Phagedenic pericementitis, according to Black, consisted of the following:

> *An inflammation of a peculiar character which results in the destruction of the peridental membrane. This destruction, also, is closely followed by the absorption of the walls of the alveolus; so that in the end both are destroyed. The disappearance of the two is so nearly synchronous that it is often difficult to say which has gone first; indeed, they seem to go together. In its least complicated form the disease is not accompanied with salivary calculus, or calculus of any kind. It seems to consist essentially in an inflammation—which may be acute or chronic—by which the peridental membrane is separated from the root of the tooth and destroyed fiber by fiber, cell by cell, very much as bone is destroyed molecule by molecule as in the disease known as caries.*[20]

Characteristic features of this disease were the formation of deep periodontal pockets with denudation of the root surface and absorption of the alveolar bone. Although the disease was predominately a chronic condition, acute episodes were common. Black noted that phagedenic pericementitis was often complicated by calculus deposits:

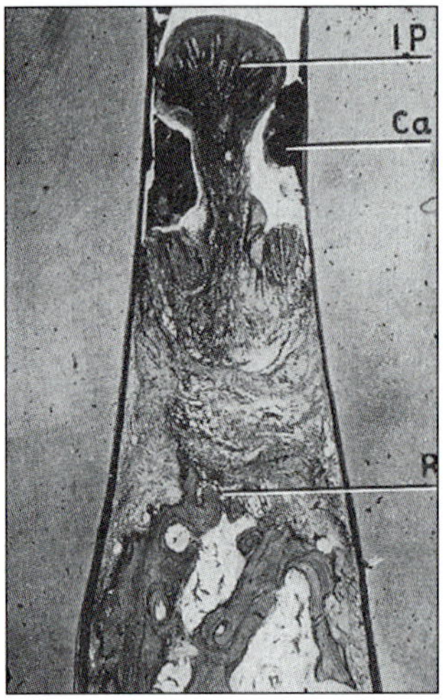

Fig 12-6 Inflamed interdental papilla (IP) compressed by subgingival calculus (Ca). Inflamed connective tissue and epithelium overlie the resorbing alveolar bone crest (R). (Adapted from Boyle P. Kornfeld's Histopathology of the Teeth. Philadelphia: Lea & Febiger, 1955.)

> *Here we have, in fact, two diseases existing together: calcic inflammation from the deposits of calculus [Fig 12-6], and phagedenic inflammation further up toward the apex. It is evidently this dual form so often presented by these affections that has so long delayed the recognition of the phagedenic variety as an independent disease.*[20]

Phagedenic pericementitis was "purely a local disease, and not dependent upon any poison circulating in the blood of the patient or upon any systemic disorder." This form of pericementitis later came to be known as *chronic periodontitis*.[4]

According to Black, phagedenic pericementitis was probably "caused and maintained by the presence of some peculiar fungus or form of microorganism." Although there was no direct proof of a microbial etiology, the fact that the disease responded favorably to germicides favored that idea. Black believed that this form of periodontal disease was infectious, warning that it could be spread from tooth to tooth within the mouth and from person to person through "inoculation," and warned of the danger of using contaminated instruments. The treatment of phagedenic pericementitis consisted of removal of all supragingival and subgingival calculus followed by the irrigation of all pockets with germicidal preparations. Black also advised conservative surgical access for localized excision of infected necrotic tissue and bone. In 1919, Black, with the accumulated knowledge of more than two decades of experience in treating the disease, put forth a very modern concept of the pathogenesis of pericementitis:

[4] The histopathology of periodontitis and periapical lesions are depicted in Figs 12-6, 12-9, and 12-10.

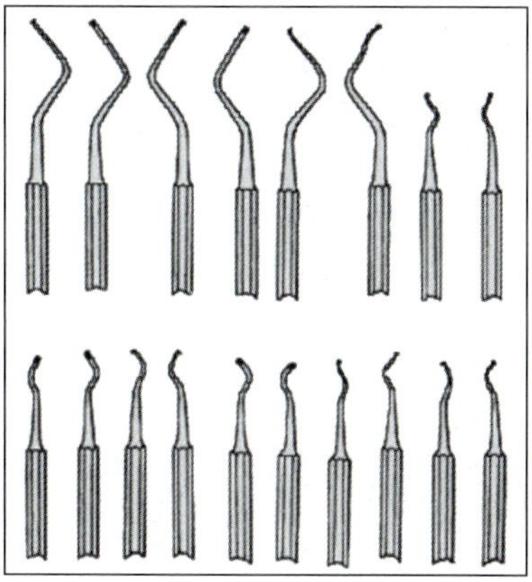

Fig 12-7 Example of some Carr scalers. (Adapted from Patterson.[15])

> *We may summarize succession of pathological changes as follows: There occurs an irritation of the gingivae which permits an invasion by micro-organisms. We are not unmindful of the fact that the systemic condition may have so reduced the resistance of the gingivae that infection may occur, apparently without a recognizable local irritation. The infection which penetrates the gingival tissue is taken up by the perivascular lymphatics and travels into the peridental membrane along the bloodvessel walls in a direction parallel to the long axis of the root. There occurs a thickening of the walls of the bloodvessels to resist infection, with final occlusion and obliteration of the vessel; there is an accumulation of round cells about the lymphatics, and the surrounding tissue is later broken down in the form of a circle, or tube, about the vessel. This may occur along several parallel vessels until an actual break in the tissue occurs—a pocket is formed.*[21]

Instruments for the treatment of pyorrhea pockets evolved from the early "scrapers" depicted in Albucasis's textbook (see Fig 1-10) to the better instruments used by Fauchard and Bourdet. Special sets of instruments for scraping teeth were designed, some made with precious metals to be used in treating royalty. Riggs, whose successful treatment of pyorrhea was based on a thorough removal of all calculus, used a special set of six instruments, which, according to Patterson, were "clumsy and impracticable."[15] As the importance of obtaining a thoroughly clean root surface became the basis of treatment, new instrument designs were introduced. Black emphasized the use of "pushing" instruments to plane the root surface, while most favored the "pulling" type of cutting instrument to remove all irritants from the root surface.[15] Large sets of instruments of many shapes to reach all root surfaces of each tooth type were marketed (Fig 12-7).

The subgingival use of these scalers to reach to the depth of the pockets was considered a surgical procedure requiring a delicate touch to discern a rough contaminated root surface from a polished treated surface.[19]

John Patterson, professor of operative dentistry in the Chicago College of Dental Surgery, noted that many dentists held the erroneous idea that pyorrhea alveolaris was a hopeless disease because they believed it had a systemic origin.[15] He supported the concept of a systemic, and in some families a hereditary, predisposition toward developing pyorrhea, but he noted that in all cases a local irritant was necessary:

> *Any irritant, of whatever nature, which impairs the integrity and continuity of the gingival gum margin, may cause pyorrhea; and without this impairment the condition will not be established.... Systemic conditions or a constitutional diathesis without local irritation do not destroy the integrity of the gingival border.*[15]

In 95% of all cases, calculus was present. Other common irritants were introduced by careless dentistry. G. V. Black blamed the profession when he stated that spaces created between adjacent teeth (open contacts) during the restoration of carious teeth caused 90% of pyorrhea cases.

After the classic research of Willoughby D. Miller on the bacteria of the mouth and their central role in dental caries, many dentists came to recognize that bacteria were also the cause of pyorrhea alveolaris. Microbes were known to be present in gingival pockets and were a constant component in suppurating lesions of the periodontium. G. V. Black had reported that oral bacteria produced poisons and showed that bacteria isolated from pyorrhea pockets were lethal when injected into experimental animals.[22] The beneficial use of germicides and antiseptics in the treatment of pyorrhea was admitted even by dentists who were not convinced of the pathogenicity of germs. When bacteria were found to be a constant component of calculus, it was proposed that they actively contributed to the mechanism of calculus formation.[23] In testing the effect of bacteria in calculus formation in an in vitro system, Bibby reported that "no calcareous deposits were formed from saliva unless bacteria were present."

Endamebas

In 1914, M. T. Barrett of the University of Pennsylvania and A. Chiavaro of the University of Rome reported that endamebas (Fig 12-8) were present in virtually all pyorrhea pockets.[24,25] Barrett was of the

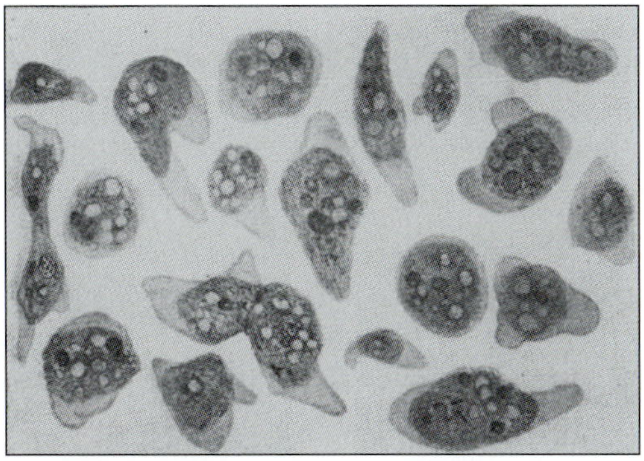

Fig 12-8 Common shapes of *Endameba buccalis*. (From Bass and Johns.[26])

opinion that endamebas were pathogenic organisms, but Chiavaro proposed that endamebas had an autodysinfectious action by virtue of their ability to ingest bacteria. In 1915, Bass and Johns reported that endamebas were found "in all of more than 300 cases" of pyorrhea, but never in normal gums.[26] The endamebas were identified by microscopic examination of suppurated materials removed from subgingival pockets. Bass and Johns reported that endamebas were more numerous in the deepest part of the pockets, "in the dying tissue in the bottom of the lesion, where bacteria and other agencies are few or entirely absent." Treatment of these lesions with the amebicide *emetin* produced favorable results, along with disappearance of the organisms, suggesting a causal relationship.[26] Bass and Johns hypothesized that infection by endamebas occurred through damaged gingival surfaces caused by tartar and possibly by "picking the teeth, cleaning with hard brushes, floss, rubbers, hard particles of food, and ill-fitting crowns."[26] It was proposed that microscopic examination of the contents of pyorrhea pockets (Figs 12-9 and 12-10) for the presence of endamebas was a useful method for monitoring the success of treatment of pyorrhea. According to Bass and Johns:

> *Practically all grown people have them (endamebas) in pyorrhea lesions in their mouths, and many younger people have them also. In fact, we think that almost all are infected before they are 20 years old. Any person who has pyorrhea is throwing off some endamebas in the saliva all the time. All our associates, including the immediate family, are a source of infection.*[26]

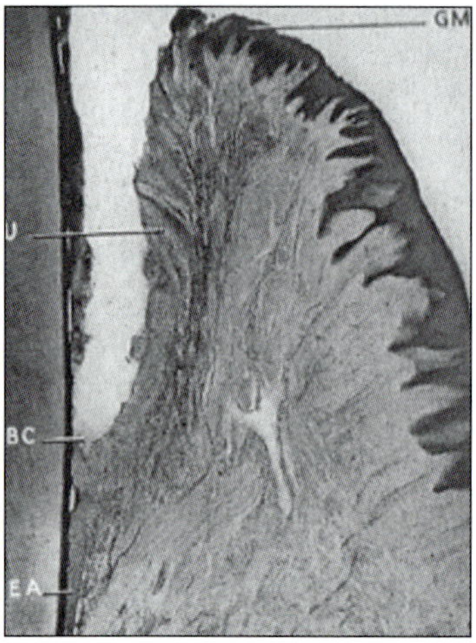

Fig 12-9 A gingival pyorrhea pocket characterized by an ulcerated wall (U). BC—bottom of the pocket; EA—epithelial attachment. (Adapted from Boyle P. Kornfeld's Histopathology of the Teeth. Philadelphia: Lea & Febiger, 1955.)

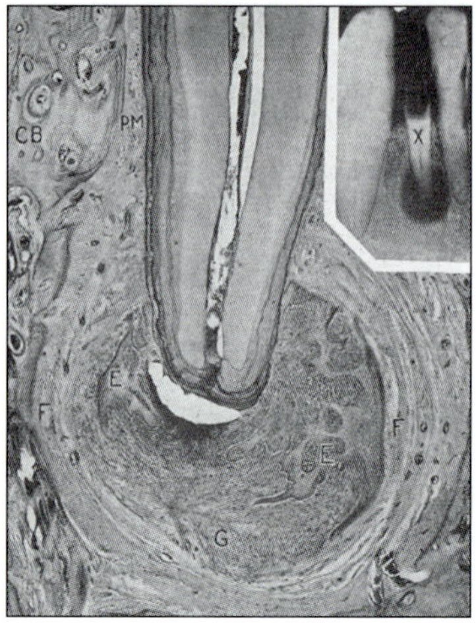

Fig 12-10 A periapical granuloma occupying an area of resorbed bone adjacent to a root tip. The inset depicts the lesions by radiograph. (Adapted from Boyle P. Kornfeld's Histopathology of the Teeth. Philadelphia: Lea & Febiger, 1955.)

Because there was no direct evidence that endamebas could cause direct tissue damage, Bass and Johns proposed that endamebas could transport pyogenic microbes and spirochetes and, through some form of symbiotic action, cause suppurated, destructive lesions.

Pyorrhea therapies

The germicidal effect of ultraviolet light (quartz light) was tried as a treatment for pyorrhea alveolaris by I. F. Folstein in 1925.[27] The ultraviolet rays generated from a "Kromayer" lamp were directed to the gingival tissue for several minutes; longer exposures caused burns and blistering of the gingivae. Because Folstein treated all pyorrhea patients with an initial deep scaling of root surfaces, it is possible that resolution of the disease was solely due to scaling. The limited penetrability of the rays to reach into the deepest pockets also raised doubts that germs were eliminated.

Quartz light therapy was not the only half-baked idea for curing pyorrhea. Dr Stevens of Atlantic City, New Jersey, reported that he restored the health of gingival tissues by passing a high-frequency current by "special vacuum electrodes directly upon the diseased tissue." He stated that the oscillating current promoted circulation, forced venous blood out of the diseased tissues, and thereby increased metabolism. But there was one key point in his therapy, and that was the precondition that "deposits and inflammation must necessarily be first removed."[28]

An additional pyorrhea therapy popularized in the early 20th century was the Dunlop vapor technique. Dr W. F. Dunlop of New York City created a machine for producing a volatile ethyl borate antiseptic gas, delivered under pressure via a hypodermic needle to the gums.[29] According to Dunlop, the gas "causes stimulation, and great quantities of blood are attracted to the parts, the blue color disappears and a beautiful pink results." Harold Box resurrected the Dunlop vapor system, creating a volatile compound of oxygen, oil of peppermint, alcohol, yeast, and boracic acid.[30] Box attributed an improved gingival and periodontal response to the oxygenation of anoxic tissues. Box conducted a limited experiment in sheep to compare insufflation of oxygen, Dunlop vapor, and nitrogen on tooth mobility. He demonstrated that both oxygen and Dunlop vapor gave a significantly better response than nitrogen. Nevertheless, vapor therapy was used only as an adjunct procedure to classical root scaling and tissue debridement.[30]

Pyorrhea vaccine

When it became evident that the efficacy of vaccination against smallpox, typhoid, cholera, and rabies was due to the body's production of circulating antibodies against the infecting organisms, it was a logical step to attempt to cure pyorrhea with vaccines.[31] Inoculation with combined stock vaccines to *Streptococcus-Staphylococcus-Pneumococcus* organisms was recommended for treatment of pyorrhea by Dr G. H. Sherman in his textbook *Vaccine Therapy in General Practice*.[32] Inoculations were made "about 4 or 5 days apart and continued at longer intervals for a month or more after the inflammatory condition has subsided in order to insure a permanency to the results." Sherman stated that appropriate local treatment should also be employed in conjunction with vaccines. T. D. Casto reported his use of a polyvalent vaccine injected into the gingiva submucosa of pyorrhea patients. The method consisted of 10 injections of minute amounts of vaccine given over several days to avoid an allergic reaction. He attested to short-term successful treatment of 25 patients but cautioned that "The vaccine treatment can only be effective as an adjunct to other remedial measures, such as corrected diet, removal of loose teeth, prophylactic treatment, correction of traumatic occlusion and the making and placing of suitable mechanical devices."[33]

Arthur H. Merritt raised several objections to vaccine therapy, noting that no one organism had been identified as the causative agent in pyorrhea and therefore no vaccines were specific. In fact, Merritt held the view that bacteria were purely secondary invaders, qualitatively similar to those that inhabited the normal mouth.[34] Furthermore, Merritt noted that "All writers have advocated careful local treatment along with vaccines. What part either played in the result no one has been able to say."[35] Unless appropriate controls were in place, there was no scientific support for the exuberant claims of vaccine therapy in the treatment of pyorrhea. Patients were being subjected to numerous injections of vaccine over several weeks of treatment with no scientific proof that the vaccines contributed to improvement of the condition.

Interstitial gingivitis

Many dentists were skeptical of the idea that pyorrhea was a single disease and that bacteria and amebas were the causative agents. Dr Eugene Talbot noted that until Koch's postulates had been proven, he would remain unconvinced of the pathogenicity of endameba in causing pyorrhea. He was one of many dentists who formed strong opinions in favor of a systemic or constitutional basis of periodontal diseases. Talbot divided gingivitis into those cases caused by local irritants and those caused by constitutional problems, such as malnutrition, anemia, and "auto-intoxication." His thesis centered on the notion that cementum and dentin were avascular tissues and thus dependent on the blood supply of adjacent tissues. Talbot considered these tissues and the alveolar process to be end-organs, supplied by looplike terminal arteries from the apical foramen and thus especially susceptible to "irritants, stasis and nutritional disturbances."[36] Constitutional stresses, whether from malnutrition or altered metabolism, caused local tissue deterioration that manifested itself in connective tissues of the gingiva and periodontium. He coined the term *interstitial gingivitis* to describe this condition,[37] in which stasis of the blood developed, leading to resorption of the alveolar process.

According to Talbot, pyogenic infection of interstitial gingivitis was a secondary phenomenon: "Pyorrhea alveolaris (pus infection) cannot be present without their first being an interstitial gingivitis."[38] Secondary infection of the interstitial lesion by "pus-germs" from around the necks of the teeth progressed to pocket formation with "inflammation extending into the peridental membrane along a blood-vessel or lymph stream."[39] The deposition of calculus on the root surface was secondary to the inflammatory destruction of periodontal tissue. In

Eugene S. Talbot

Eugene S. Talbot was a graduate of the Pennsylvania College of Dental Surgery (1872) and the Rush Medical College (1880). He was instrumental in establishing the Section on Stomatology of the American Medical Association, serving as its secretary for 33 years. His lifelong ambition was to improve dentistry by increasing medical sciences in the dental curriculum. He was well known on the international level for his expertise in stomatology, periodontal diseases, and orthodontics. Talbot was the author of 13 books and several hundred publications. He served as professor of stomatology at the Women's Medical School of Northwestern University.

accord with the concept of a primary constitutional cause for interstitial gingivitis, Talbot urged taking a medical history of all patients presenting with gingivitis and pyorrhea alveolaris, even going so far as to examination of the urine for evidence of a systemic disease. For decades, Talbot and others who supported the primacy of constitutional factors did so without any supporting experimental evidence. But this changed in the early 20th century with the discovery that vitamins and certain essential nutrients were important to the health of peridental supporting tissues. Evidence, primarily in animal experiments, showed that certain nutritional deficiencies (vitamins C and D) could lead to hemorrhage, connective tissue breakdown, and alveolar bone resorption. These results were embraced by the proponents of a constitutional origin for the alveolar and periodontal tissue destruction associated with pyorrhea alveolaris.[40]

Treatment of Gingivitis and Pyorrhea

During the latter half of the 19th century, approaches to the treatment of gingivitis and pyorrhea alveolaris fell into two camps: *(1)* a conservative protocol based on the initial ideas put forth by Riggs, involving thorough removal of calculus combined with astringent and antiseptic rinses, and *(2)* a radical protocol involving surgical excision of the inflamed tissue, along with calculus removal, bone contouring, and antiseptic rinses.

Conservative protocol

Arthur H. Merritt was influential in advocating the conservative treatment:

> *The most important factor in the treatment of pyorrhea and the most difficult to achieve is good root surgery. This requires the removal not only of all calcareous deposits upon the exposed surface of the cementum, but the complete removal of the necrotic pericementum, permitting thereby physiologic contact between the vital cells of the cementum and the overlying soft tissues.... When this is done reattachment takes place, pockets are obliterated, new bone is deposited about the roots, the teeth become firm, and health is re-established in these tissues, though complete restoration to previous conditions may not occur; in advanced cases there will probably be gum recession.*[34]

He asserted that despite the general assumption that reattachment was not possible, "such reattachment takes place, as a rule, in the hands of the skillful periodontist. No other result is regarded by him as a cure."[34]

Among the earliest microscopic studies of Riggs disease was a report that the cementum of the affected teeth was denser than normal.[41] The author of this study, Dr G. B. Clement, stated that the organic matter of cementum had been replaced by calcific matter and, in his view, "if the density of the cementum be carried beyond its physiological condition by hypercalcic deposit or infiltration the result is exfoliation of the tooth; because by a perverted nutrition we have an interference with those conditions by and through which only is there hope of vital union." Based on Clement's hypothesis, Stewart developed a treatment of the affected teeth that included scraping not only calculus but all cementum from the roots ("to scrape and chisel heroically"), roughening the scaled root surface with burs or other sharp instruments, treating the root surface with acid, and lacerating the gums to encourage a "violent" inflammation, all to create conditions for reunification to the periodontal membrane.[41] His claim that the operation was painless with local "eucain" infiltration anesthesia was not widely supported; few patients managed the courage to undergo the ordeal. Hartzell emphasized the complete removal of the outer surface of the cementum, which he considered to be a necrotic "culture bed for the propagation of both putrefactive and pus-forming bacteria."[17]

G. V. Black stated that Riggs's conservative approach was effective only in shallow pockets and only if repeated periodically. In more advanced cases, Black advised resection of the pockets:

> *The simplest method is to cut away the overlying tissue and thus eliminate the pocket. The operation is very simple. Novocaine is injected. The detached tissue is cut away with suitable knives, the edge of the process (alveolar) is cut away, not because there is any evidence that it is diseased, but because the peridental membrane is destroyed in advance of the bone and unless the edge of the bone is cut away the pocket will not be fully eliminated.*[21]

Black defended his excision of tissue by noting the ineffectiveness of the purely conservative scaling of root surfaces:

> *The treatment in vogue today has generally failed because all efforts have been centered on securing a reattachment of the tissue of the pocket to the dead cementum. We have persisted in attempting the impossible. Every imaginable medicament from the strongest acid, which we have dared to employ, to the mildest antiseptic, has been tried; soft tissues have been scarified and mistreated in every imaginable way; the cementum has been scraped until none remained; pulps have been removed with the belief that additional blood would flow into the peridental membrane and be of benefit; loose teeth have been held rigid with stay appliances; everything imaginable has been tried.*[21]

In the short term, inflammation was reduced, but the long-term success had proven less than satisfactory.

Radical protocol

Dr William Ziesel of Philadelphia viewed pyorrhea and local infection to be the most absorbing problem confronting the dental profession, and he urged his colleagues to confront this disease by extermination of pockets in a surgical approach he named "gingivo-ectomy." According to Ziesel, palliative treatment by instrumentation and antiseptic medication "though faithfully tried for fifty years was far from satisfactory, to say the least."[42] Ziesel noted that:

> *The tendency of the operator is generally toward too little cutting away of tissue rather than too much. The operator must always bear in mind in this connection the objective of utterly destroying all pockets, infected gingivae and necrosed process. When this technique is carried out faithfully success will follow as a matter of course, dentistry will be robbed of one of its most implacable foes, and at the same time, an additional remunerative field opened to the general practitioner.*

This radical surgical treatment for pyorrhea, involving the excision of the pocket wall and all tissues to the level of the alveolar crest as determined by probing and radiographic examination, was attacked by critics who pointed to the resulting denudation of the root surface, which led to subsequent sensitivity, and to the esthetic disfigurement of the patient.

Despite all the heated controversies regarding the causes of pyorrhea—local irritants versus constitutional factors, salivary versus serumal calculus, bacteria or endamebas—the treatment of pyorrhea alveolaris (or interstitial gingivitis, or whatever one wished to name the disease) was always basically the same. The essential elements of successful treatment were always calculus removal, antiseptic irrigation, massage of the gums, and the implementation of regular oral hygiene.

One of the earliest attempts to measure the incidence and cause of gingivitis was reported in 1913 by Dr Arthur D. Black, son of G. V. Black. Dr A. D. Black was dean and professor of operative dentistry at Northwestern University Dental School. In a study of 500 young adults from 20 to 35 years old, it was found that 19 out of every 20 had 8 or more regions of gingivitis.[43] Of all the gingivitis lesions, 31.6% were associated with salivary calculus, while 13.1% were associated with serumal calculus. The association of inflammation with calculus was expected, but the finding that 37% of all lesions were traced to "imperfect dental operations" was a glaring mark against the profession. Although Black generously attributed less-than-perfect dentistry to a lack of understanding of the physiology of the gingival tissues and the relationship between gingivitis and its potential progress to periodontal disease, it was evident that carelessness in operative procedures was leading to iatrogenic gingival disease. This fact had been observed in 1896 when E. Talbot cautioned that damage from rubber dam clamps, interdental wedges, protruding fillings, and open contacts could initiate gingivitis.[39] In his words: "Modern dentistry is producing more pyorrhea than any other one cause."

Focal Infection Theory

The significance of pyorrhea and other oral infections shot to the forefront of medical and dental literature in the late 19th century with the rise of the focal infection theory. The idea began in 1818 when Benjamin Rush, distinguished Philadelphia physician and patriot, wrote:

> *I have been made happy by discovering that I have only added to the observations of other physicians in pointing out a connection between the extraction of decayed and diseased teeth and the cure of general disease.... When we consider how often the teeth when decayed are exposed to irritation, from hot and cold drinks and ailments, from pressure by mastication, and from the cold air, and how intimate the connection of the mouth is with the whole system, I am disposed to*

believe they are often the unsuspected causes of general, and particularly of nervous diseases.... I cannot help thinking that our success in the treatment of all chronic diseases would be very much promoted by directing our inquiries into the state of the teeth in sick people and by advising their extraction in every case in which they are decayed. It is not necessary that they should be attended with pain in order to produce diseases.[44]

Rush's suspicion was in part confirmed by the research of W. D. Miller. Miller, the authoritative figure in oral microbiology, stated in his treatise *The Human Mouth as a Focus of Infection*:

It shall be my endeavor in the following pages to call attention to the various diseases, both local and general, which have been found to result from the action of micro-organisms which have collected in the mouth, and to the various channels through which these microorganisms or their waste products may obtain entrance to parts of the body adjacent to or remote from the mouth.[45]

Miller injected saliva (and its bacterial content) into the peritoneal cavity of mice and recorded that 90% of the animals died. He isolated four lethal types of cocci, which he named *micrococci of sputum septicemia*.

The realization that the mouth was an incubator for hundreds of different forms of bacteria and could become a focus of infection from which microbes and/or their products could spread to other organs of the body began to take hold during the latter half of the 19th century. Pyorrhea, deep dental caries, and apical root infections were implicated, without any direct scientific proof, as the cause of joint disease, liver disease, brain abscesses, etc. Dentists and physicians and the general public began to believe in this idea as if it had been irrefutably established.

In 1901, William Hunter, a London physician, published a small book, *Oral Sepsis as a Cause of Septic Gastritis, Toxic Neuritis and Other Septic Conditions*, containing clinical cases purported to show a vital relationship between oral sepsis and systemic disease. In this book, he excoriated the dental profession for its failure to recognize the danger of infected teeth and prosthetic appliances:

For every one case of gastric affection traceable to pyorrhea alveolaris, a hundred cases no less marked are daily met with associated with other septic inflammatory conditions of the gums so commonly met around necrosed carious teeth and roots. In short, they are produced by every form of oral trouble due to septic infection from diseased teeth, especially when that infection is aided, as it so often is, by such potent adjuncts as ill-fitting, neglected septic tooth plates, bridges, gold caps, metallic stoppings, and the like.[46]

At the 1914 convention of the American Medical Association, the Section on Stomatology held a symposium on mouth infection at which Dr Frank Billings of the Rush Medical Clinic of Chicago, Dr Charles Mayo of Rochester, Minnesota, and clinical microbiologist Dr E. C. Rosenow upheld the theory of oral sepsis. What these men had to report carried great weight, because they were the recognized authorities in this area of medical science. Dr Billings, dean of Rush Medical College, noted that alveolar focal infection was probably the dominant factor in the production of systemic diseases such as endocarditis, chronic arthritis, and myositis. He reported that sites of focal infection were created by lack of oral hygiene "intensified and prolonged by irrational dentistry—teeth with infected pulp crowned or improperly filled."[47] Dr Mayo called on better cooperation between dentists and physicians in combatting oral sepsis: "The physicians engaged in this line of observation require fully as much training in the rudiments of dentistry as the dentist does in the signs of infectious diseases."[48] The value of roentgenographic examination of the jaws for detection of periapical lesions was emphasized by several participants. In one study of 332 cases of chronic arthritis examined with oral radiographs at the Presbyterian Hospital of Chicago under Dr Billings, 89% were found to have evidence of alveolar abscesses.[49] In the discussion that followed the main papers, Dr G. V. Black, in support of the focal infection theory, expressed his opinion that pyorrhea pockets should be excised to prevent reinfection and alveolar abscesses should be treated by root resection or tooth extraction. Dr F. B. Moorehead, in stating the problem that dentists faced in deciding what teeth could be safely saved, opined that "It is far better to take out teeth than to sacrifice the comfort and usefulness of the patient."[50]

Rosenow's bacteriologic and animal experimentation, published widely during the early 20th century, were accepted as strong confirmation of the focal infection theory. He demonstrated that certain microorganisms (mainly streptococci) had special abilities to localize to specific tissues, where they caused inflammation and disease.[51] These same microorganisms were thought to reside in a relatively quiescent state in sites of focal infection, such as the tonsils, carious teeth, pyorrhea pockets, etc. Under conditions of stress, poor diet, and lowered body resistance, these bacteria were disseminated from the focal infection site through the blood or lymph to distant organs, where they caused disease. Thus, faced with patients suffering from chronic diseases such as arthritis, nephritis, cardiomyopathies, gastric disorders, and even central nervous conditions, dentists and physicians had to find and surgically remove sites of focal infection.

Rosenow advised that "A severe pyorrhea, if incurable by other means, calls for extraction of the affected teeth. Pulpless and abscessed teeth are to be regarded as a serious menace to continued health, and, with relatively few exceptions, should be extracted."[51]

Rosenow called for a closer affiliation between dentists and physicians:

> *The dentist of the future should not be isolated in a small office over a drug-store, his chief work being to devitalize and fill teeth without regard to the general health. Properly trained dentists should be part of the public school system and hospitals, in which instruction in the care of teeth should be given.*[51]

Subsequent research pointed to flaws in Rosenow's work, and retrospective findings showed that most cases of rheumatoid arthritis had no evidence of focal infection.[52]

Throughout the era of the acceptance of focal infection, there had been no clinical studies involving the examination of healthy control populations.[53] Unfortunately, an entire generation of young children underwent unwarranted tonsillectomy, and many adults were needlessly rendered edentulous during the focal infection scare. The business of exodontia and vulcanite denture production experienced a boom lasting until the middle of the 20th century. But the focal infection scare had one good outcome: It made the public especially conscious of the need for improved oral hygiene and of the potential danger of pyorrhea.

However, the public, always seeking quick and easy remedies to cure itself of disease, and in attempts to treat pyorrhea, was especially susceptible to fraudulent practices. Numerous mouthwashes and dentifrices were peddled by mail with extravagant claims to bring perfect success against pyorrhea, trench mouth, sore bleeding gums, and loose teeth (Fig 12-11). "Pyro-Kill," touted as a pyorrhea toothpaste at 50 cents a bottle, was attested to in fraudulent testimonials: "My teeth became loose, my gums bled and I could hardly eat.... Used 10 different kinds of treatment, with no relief until Pyro-Kill completely rid me of this distressing disease." Moore's Pyorrhea Remedy, obtainable at any drug store or through the mail, claimed to give "permanent relief from ulcerated gums and pus pockets."

"X-It" was a similar product sold with a rubber massage cup. X-It was "a liquid vegetable preparation worked out specifically for the prevention and treatment of pyorrhea and other germ diseases." According to its claims, X-It "is the product of long and careful scientific and practical research, and has proven most effective in accomplishing its purpose." Analysis by the chemists of the American Medical

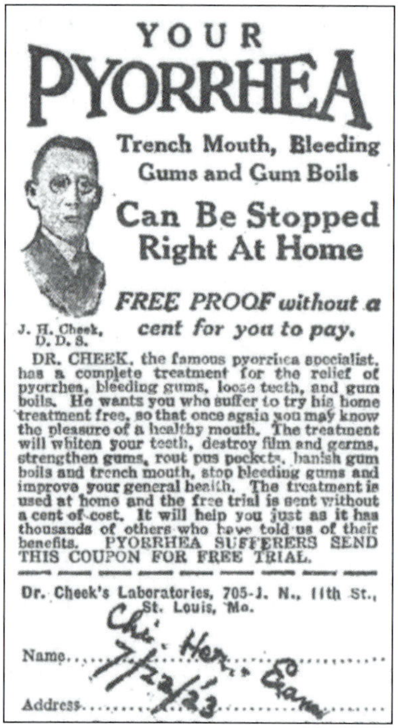

Fig 12-11 Alleged cure for pyorrhea closed down by postal authorities. (Adapted from JAMA.[56])

Association revealed it to be no more than a simple solution of benzoin, zinc chloride, and wintergreen.

Investigations by the American Medical Association and the American Dental Association in concert with the United States Postal Service eventually led to the successful prosecution of these practices.[54–56] More often than not, the men and women behind these schemes were not physicians, dentists, or chemists but simply dishonest persons who capitalized on the gullibility of the average person on the street.

Summary

In describing diseases of the gums and bony alveolar sockets, Fauchard, Bourdet, and Fox were in agreement in stating that these disorders were caused locally by calculus accumulation around the necks and roots of the teeth. Effective treatment consisted of thorough scaling to remove all calculus and the excision of inflamed hypertrophied tissue. Fox postulated that calculus was precipitated from saliva or blood and speculated that in the rare absence of calculus, a constitutional component was at work. The view that systemic diseases, such as diabetes, scurvy, or gout, were causal factors became increasingly popular in the 19th century. The French surgeon E. Magitot went so far as to suggest that calculus was a secondary component of periodontal disease. John Riggs downplayed constitutional causes in reporting that thorough scaling (prophylaxis) performed with specially designed instruments was the only certain remedy for treating pyorrhea. As knowledge of the microscopic anatomy and pathology of dental tissues grew in the last half of the 19th century, periodontal disease came to be described as a complex disease with numerous pathogenicities, all speculative and short of scientific proof. G. V. Black hypothesized that periodontal disease might have a microbial origin, warning that it might spread from tooth to tooth by inoculation. Germicides became widely employed as an adjunct to prophylaxis treatment. Black demonstrated courage in announcing that his research showed that 50% of periodontal disease was caused by slipshod operative dentistry.

In the early 20th century, the acceptance of focal infection theory by the medical and dental professions elevated periodontal therapy to new prominence. Emphasis on the eradication of dental infection led to aggressive surgical elimination of periodontal pockets. Dental schools were urged to expose their students to more pathology and general medicine. New pyorrhea therapies, such as ultraviolet light, Dunlop vapor, and vaccines, were promoted without scientific proof of their effectiveness. Over-the-counter, mail-order medications were popularized with false claims of curing pyorrhea.

Many readers of this chapter will no doubt be aware of the recent resurgence of a variation of the "focal infection" theory in the current emphasis on periodontal disease as a risk factor in cardiovascular disease and diabetes and for the revival of the call that dentists must be physicians of the mouth. H. N. Neuman, in reviewing current research relating oral infections to systemic diseases in the *Journal of Dental Research* stated that "The problem about the original discovery was the tenuous link between the putative oral foci of infection and related disease. And that is the warning to us: that for the hypothesis not to fall into disrepute for a second time, there must be no unsubstantiated attributions, no theories without evidence."[57]

References

1. Held AJ. Periodontology from Its Origins up to 1980: A Survey. Basel: Birkhauser, 1989.
2. Leek FF. The practice of dentistry in ancient Egypt. J Egypt Archaeol 1967; 53:51–58.
3. Forshaw RJ. Dental health and disease in ancient Egypt. Br Dent J 2009; 206:421–424.
4. Hoffmann-Axthelm W. History of Dentistry. Chicago: Quintessence, 1981.
5. Guerini V. A History of Dentistry from the Most Ancient Times Until the End of the Eighteenth Century. Philadelphia: Lea & Febiger, 1909:188–199.
6. Lufkin AW. A History of Dentistry. Philadelphia: Lea & Febiger, 1948.
7. Hémard U. Recherche de la vraye anathomie des dents, nature et propriete d'Icelles. Lyon: Rigaud, 1582.
8. Dionis P. Cours d'operations de chirurgie, demontrees au Jardin Royal. Bruxelles: Les Freres Serstevens and A. Claudinot, 1708.
9. Fauchard P. The Surgeon Dentist; Or, Treatise on the Teeth, ed 2. Paris: P. J. Mariette, 1746.
10. Bourdet E. Recherche et observations sur toutes les parties de l'art du dentiste. Paris: J. T. Herissant, 1757.
11. Garant PR. The contribution of Etienne Bourdet (1722–1789) to the diagnosis and treatment of periodontal disease. Bull Hist Dent 1993;41:69–72.
12. Gerauldy C. L'art de conserver les dents. Paris: Le Mercier, 1737.
13. Fox J. The History and Treatment of the Diseases of the Teeth, the Gums, and the Alveolar Processes, with the Operations Which They Respectively Require. London: Thomas Cox, 1806.
14. Kirk EC. The American Textbook of Operative Dentistry. Philadelphia: Lea & Febiger, 1911.
15. Patterson JD. Pyorrhea alveolaris. In: Johnson CN. Textbook of Operative Dentistry. Philadelphia: P. Blakiston, Son, & Co, 1909:451–470.
16. Prinz H. The origin of salivary calculus. Dent Cosmos 1921;68:231–238.
17. Hartzell TB. The practical surgery of the root surface in pyorrhea. Dent Cosmos 1911;53:513–521.
18. Benton GB. History of the diseases and treatment of the investing tissues of the teeth. In: Black AD (ed). G.V. Black's Work on Operative Dentistry with Which His Special Dental Pathology Is Combined. Chicago: Medico-Dental, 1936.
19. Mills GA. Directions as to the treatment of the so-called Riggs's disease with the instruments devised by Dr. Riggs. Dent Cosmos 1878;20:92–94.
20. Black GV. Diseases of the peridental membrane. In: Litch WF (ed). The American System of Dentistry. Philadelphia: Lea Brothers, 1886.
21. Black GV. The pathology and treatment of diseases of the peridental membrane. Dent Cosmos 1919;62:820–825.
22. Black GV. The formation of poisons by micro-organisms. A biological study of the germ theory of disease. Philadelphia: P. Blakiston, Son, & Co, 1884.
23. Bibby BG. The formation of salivary calculus. Dent Cosmos 1935;77:668–676.
24. Barrett MT. The protozoa of the mouth in relation to pyorrhea alveolaris. Dent Cosmos 1914;56:948–953,1345–1350.
25. Chiavaro A. Researches upon the *Endamoeba buccalis*. Dent Cosmos 1914; 56:1089–1091.
26. Bass CC, Johns FM. Alveolodental Pyorrhea. Philadelphia: W. B. Saunders, 1915.
27. Folstein IL. Quartz light in the treatment of pyorrhea. Dent Cosmos 1925;67:153–158.
28. Stevens M. Demonstrating the use of a high frequency current in the treatment of pyorrhea alveolaris and all congested conditions of the oral cavity. Dent Cosmos 1914;56:111.

29. Dunlop WF. Treating pyorrhea by the aid of ethyl borate gas. Dent Cosmos 1914;56:111–112.
30. Box HK. Twelve Periodontal Studies. Toronto: University of Toronto, 1940.
31. Bosanquet WC, Eyre JW. Serums, Vaccines and Toxins in Treatment and Diagnosis. London: Cassell, 1916.
32. Sherman GH. Vaccine Therapy in General Practice. Chicago: Successful Medicine, 1912.
33. Casto TD. The treatment of periodontoclasia with a polyvalent vaccine (Goldenberg's Inava Endocorps vaccine). Dent Cosmos 1925;67:689–691.
34. Merritt AH. The pathology, etiology, and treatment of pyorrhea. Dent Cosmos 1918;60:574–581.
35. Merritt AH. The irrationality of bacterial vaccines in the treatment of pyorrhea alveolaris. Dent Cosmos 1916;58:62–69.
36. Talbot ES. Histo-pathology of the jaws and apical dental tissues. No. XII. Dent Cosmos 1920;62:856–862.
37. Talbot ES. The treatment of interstitial gingivitis and pyorrhea alveolaris. Dent Cosmos 1915;57:485–491.
38. Talbot ES. Treatment of interstitial gingivitis. Dent Cosmos 1909;51:153–155.
39. Talbot ES. Pyorrhea alveolaris. Dent Cosmos 1896;38:310–321.
40. Talbot ES. Late researches on interstitial gingivitis. Dent Cosmos 1921;63:795–803.
41. Stewart HT. Partial removal of cementum and decalcification of tooth in the treatment of pyorrhea alveolaris. Dent Cosmos 1899;41:617–626.
42. Ziesel W. Pyorrhea extermination: Gingivo-ectomy. Dent Cosmos 1921;63: 352–368.
43. Black AD. Something of the etiology and early pathology of the diseases of the periodontal membrane, with suggestions as to treatment. Dent Cosmos 1913;55:1219–1226.
44. Rush B. Medical Inquiries and Observations. Philadelphia: Matthew Carey & Sons, 1818.
45. Miller WD. The human mouth as a focus of infection. Dent Cosmos 1891;33: 913–919.
46. Hunter W. Oral Sepsis as a Cause of Septic Gastritis, Toxic Neuritis and Other Septic Conditions. London: Cassell, 1901.
47. Billings F. Mouth infection as a source of systemic disease. JAMA 1914;63: 2024–2025.
48. Mayo CH. Mouth infection as a source of systemic disease. JAMA 1914;63: 2025–2026.
49. Moorehead FB. The prevalence of chronic mouth infections and their management. Dent Cosmos 1916;67:845–847.
50. Moorehead FB. Abstract of discussion of symposium on mouth infections. JAMA 1914;63:2029–2032.
51. Rosenow EC. The relation of dental infection to systemic disease. Dent Cosmos 1917;59:485–491.
52. Gibbons RV. Germs, Dr. Billings, and the theory of focal infection. Clin Infect Dis 1998;27:627–633.
53. Hughes RA. Focal infection revisited. Br J Rheumatol 1994;33:370–377.
54. The Moore pyorrhea remedy fraud. JAMA 1925;85:994–995.
55. More dento-medical quackery. JAMA 1929;92:828.
56. The Rector Company declared a fraud. JAMA 1930;95:612–613.
57. Newman HN. Focal infection. J Dent Res 1996;75:1912–1919.

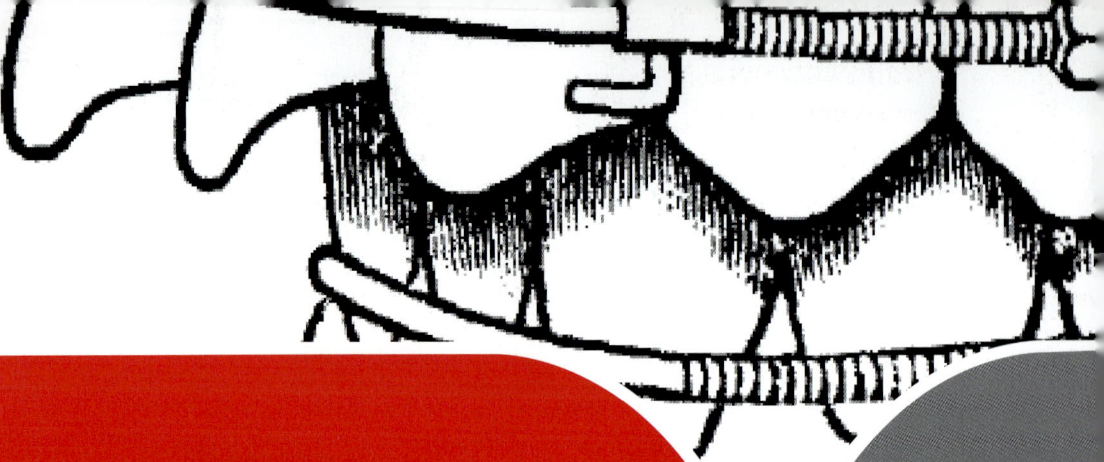

13

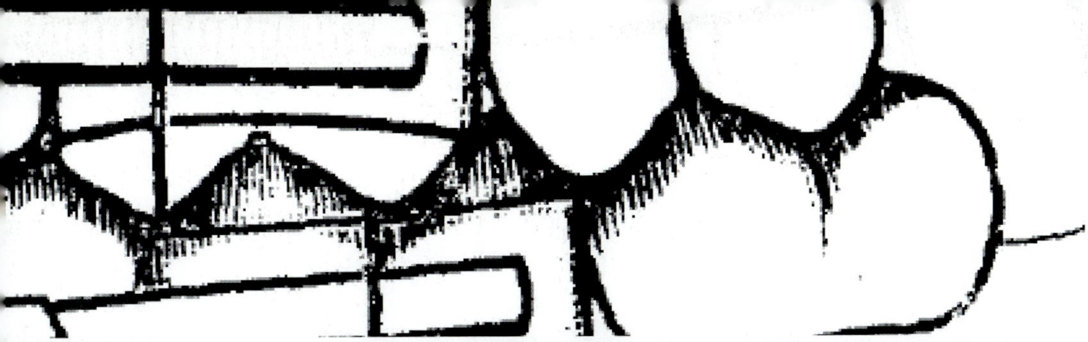

Orthodontics

Prior to the 18th century, there is little mention of the treatment of misaligned teeth in medical or dental publications.[1] Fauchard's book (1728) provides the first direct evidence of the practice of correcting abnormalities in the alignment of teeth. He described the correction of abnormalities in the placement and alignment of teeth in a process he called the "regulation of teeth." Misaligned teeth were forced into correct position by the use of the pelican (forceps) (Fig 13-1) or moved in a gentler and slower manner by applying force with threads anchored to a silver plate (Fig 13-2). In both methods, it was usually necessary to gain space by reducing the width of the teeth by filing tooth structure from their lateral margins. Fauchard also gained space for realignment of teeth by extracting one or more of the permanent premolars. He described 14 cases involving regulation of teeth, most of which were accomplished by luxating and moving the teeth into position with forceps:

> *Some years ago the wife of M. Gusset, Correcteur des Comptes, who lives at rue Bourlabbe, having asked me to examine the teeth of her daughter, then aged twelve years, I found that this young lady had the lesser incisor in the upper jaw very misplaced and inclined towards the palate. Her mother asked me if it were possible to give to this tooth its natural position and to remove by this means the deformity which it caused. I replied that I could do this very easily in eight or ten days by means of threads: provided she would send mademoiselle every day to me: but as different masters of studies came to the house*

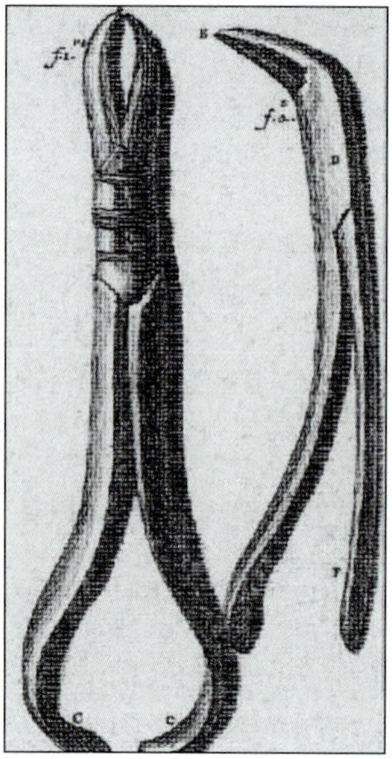

Fig 13-1 Instruments used in filling cavities and small plates used in realigning teeth. (From Fauchard,[2] 1728.)

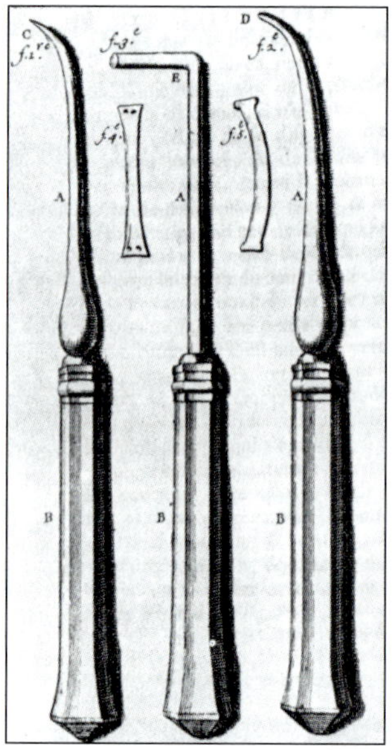

Fig 13-2 Forceps used for extractions and tooth regulation. (From Fauchard,[2] 1728.)

each day to instruct her at certain hours, my proposal was not accepted, because they did not want to interrupt her studies. This obliged me to say that if she wished it I could put this irregular tooth in position in a few minutes. Surprised at the short time I required to execute this operation, she consented without thinking that I should operate at once. I began by separating with a file the misplaced tooth, because it was very crowded by its neighbours, which had diminished the space which the misplaced tooth should occupy. This done, I pulled the tooth forward with my pelican, and placed it in its natural position, as I had proposed, to the astonishment of this lady, her sister, and several others who were present, and told me that they had often seen teeth regulated by the late M. Carmeline and by several others: but that this had never been by a like method in so short of time. As soon as I had placed this tooth in line with the others, I fixed it to the neighbouring teeth by means of common thread which I left for eight days; and during this time I made the young lady rinse her mouth four or five times a day with iron water mixed with half of healing water or woundwort, all-heal. This tooth is so well set that it does not appear that it had ever been out of place.[2]

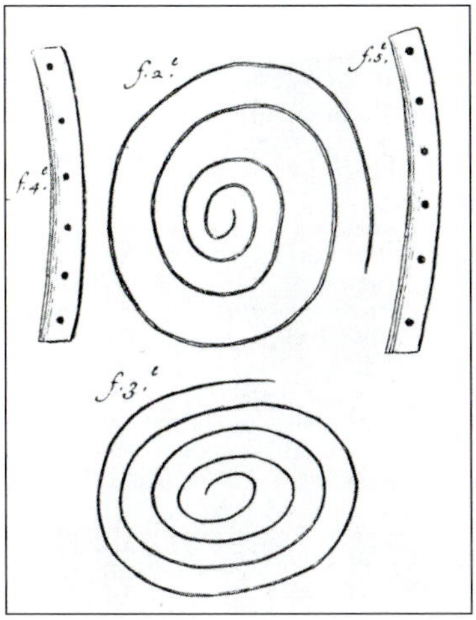

Fig 13-3 Gold plates and wire used in correction of misaligned teeth. (From Fauchard,[2] 1728.)

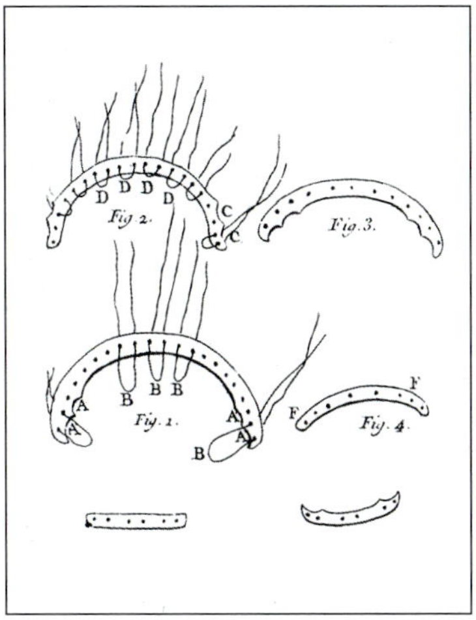

Fig 13-4 Bourdet's sketch of the use of silk ligatures and alignment plates fabricated from hippopotamus ivory or gold. (From Bourdet.[4])

Orthodontics in France

The dental historian Bernard Weinberger gives credit to Fauchard for the first use of an expansion arch, but there is no supporting evidence for this method in Fauchard's 1728 or 1746 edition of *The Surgeon Dentist; Or, Treatise on the Teeth.*[3] Fauchard described small silver bands (Fig 13-3) for moving one or two misaligned teeth, but he did not describe the use of a full-arch band secured on the permanent molars, as illustrated by Bourdet[4] (Fig 13-4).

In all 14 cases described by Fauchard, the patient sought care out of a desire to correct a disfigurement and/or a functional disorder, not from acute discomfort. Thus, by the early 18th century, the cosmetic manipulation of teeth had become a significant component of dental practice in Paris.

In the 100 years following the appearance of Fauchard's treatise, the dental profession blossomed in France, as several dentists published a remarkable series of books describing the rapidly developing craft of dentistry. Competition engendered controversies over the best approach to treatment of abnormalities in tooth alignment.

In 1746, R. Bunon noted that a well-aligned set of primary teeth signaled a well-ordered set of permanent teeth. At the first sign that the permanent teeth were erupting in a crowded condition, Bunon advocated extraction of certain primary teeth to provide space. He emphasized that crowding of teeth was not only disfiguring but a significant risk for development of caries. According to Bunon, it was better to have fewer well-spaced teeth than a full complement of crowded teeth.[5]

The Parisian dentist Etienne Bourdet illustrated various alignment arches (plates), made of gold or hippopotamus ivory, pierced by 20 holes to accommodate silk ligatures for securing the plates to the molars and simultaneously exerting tension on misaligned teeth (canines and incisors)[4] (see Fig 13-4). These plates were positioned on the lingual or labial side of the arch, depending on whether the teeth needed inward or outward force. Bourdet described the use of two alignment arches to correct a case of protruding mandibular canines and incisors. The silk ligatures were replaced or retied every few days to maintain pressure on the misaligned teeth. Bourdet recommended that the dentist make his own plates from hippopotamus ivory because gold plates fabricated by jewelers were never quite precise enough.

Orthodontics in England

With the exception of John Hunter's classic contributions to dental science, the English lagged behind the rapid growth of dentistry in France. However, in the early 19th century, they began to find their authoritative voices. Joseph Fox of London published the first English description of the eruption of the teeth with consideration of the treatment of irregularities in 1803 (Fig 13-5). Fox recognized Hunter's previous work on the natural history and anatomy of the teeth *(The Natural History of the Human Teeth)* as "the best book upon this subject," but regarding the irregularity of the second set of dentition (permanent teeth), Fox noted that Hunter spoke only in generalities: "Neither has he given an exact or precise description of the proper treatment, so as to lead any person to undertake with confidence the right management of the teeth during this period."[6]

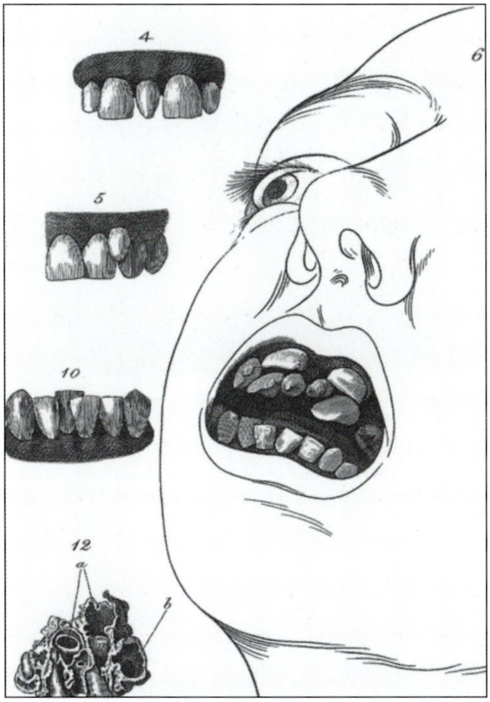

Fig 13-5 A case of irregularity caused by the growth of two supernumerary teeth. (From Fox.[6])

In the introduction to his book entitled *The Natural History and Diseases of the Human Teeth*, Fox spoke of the increasing popularity of preserving a healthy dentition among Londoners:

> *The practice arising from the diseases and other circumstances of the teeth, has of late years become very extensive, and the great comfort experienced when they are preserved in a healthy state, will cause them to be attended to, more universally. The same consideration of their importance, with which the minds of the inhabitants of the metropolis have been impressed, is fast spreading through the country, so that surgeons who from their situation are obliged to undertake every branch of practice, will soon find a new object presenting itself, and calling for their particular attention.*[6]

Fox confirmed Hunter's observation that the size of the anterior jaw remained stable during the eruption of the permanent teeth:

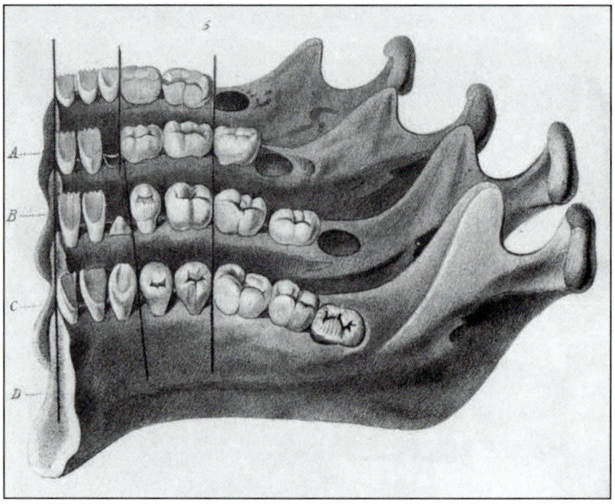

Fig 13-6 Changes in the teeth and mandible from age 6 years (A) to adulthood (D). (Adapted from Fox.[6])

After a child has obtained all the temporary teeth, the jaw in general grows very little, in the part which they occupy [Fig 13-6]. In those children who are an exception to this rule, the temporary teeth become a good deal separated from each other, and these are the cases in which the shedding of the teeth is effected without any assistance of art. When the jaw of a child is compared with that of an adult, very striking difference is observed; that of a child forms nearly the half of a circle, while that of an adult is the half of a long ellipsis. This comparison clearly points out the part in which the jaw receives its greatest increase, to be between the second temporary molaris and the coronoid process; and this lengthened part of the jaw is destined to be the situation of the permanent molare. By the elongation of the jaw a great change in the form of the face is produced; that of a child is round, the cheeks are plump and the chin flat; in an adult the face is more prominent, with a flatness of cheek and a considerable length of chin. The temporary incisores and cuspidati are much smaller than the permanent, while the molares of the temporary set are larger than the bicuspides which succeed them. Hence it is, that the incisores and cuspidati are so frequently irregular, and they never could be otherwise were it not that some space was gained from the molares, in consequence of the bicuspides being much smaller. This circumstance is rendered intelligible, by examining jaws at various ages, and observing in what particulars they differ from each other.[6]

On the practice of extracting teeth to create space for tooth regulation, Fox stated:

> *During the progress of the second dentition, an opportunity presents itself for effecting this desirable object; but everything depends upon a correct knowledge of the time, when a tooth requires to be extracted, and also of the particular tooth; for often more injury is occasioned by the removal of a tooth too early, than if it be left a little too long; because a new tooth, which has too much room long before it is required, will sometimes take a direction more difficult to alter, than a slight irregularity occasioned by an obstruction of short duration. If an improper tooth be extracted irreparable mischief will ensue; as in the case where young permanent teeth have been removed; instead of the obstructing temporary ones, which I have several times known to have been done. Irregularity is often occasioned by the teeth being much too large for the space allotted them, and then it will be necessary to remove one or more of the permanent teeth. When the incisores are perfectly regular, and the bicuspids have appeared before the cuspidati, there is so little space left, that the cuspidati are thrust too forward. It has been the common practice to admit the cuspidate to grow down to a certain length and then to extract them. This operation certainly removes the deformity of projecting teeth, but it destroys the symmetry of the mouth, and takes away two teeth of great importance. The cuspidate are exceedingly strong; they form the support of the front of the mouth, and in the advanced periods of life, to those persons who have the misfortune to lose the incisores, they furnish an excellent means of fixing artificial teeth. On these accounts they should be preserved, and therefore it will be right to extract the first bicuspides on each side.*[7]

Fox demonstrated his method of moving teeth by describing the treatment of intruded permanent maxillary incisors:

> *When the permanent incisores of the upper jaw have cut the gum behind the temporary teeth, and have been suffered to remain until considerably advanced in growth, they always stand so much inwards, that when the mouth is shut, the incisores of the under jaw stand before them, which is always an obstacle to their acquiring regularity, and occasions a great deformity. The time to affect any material alteration in the position of the teeth is before thirteen or fourteen years of age, and as much earlier as possible; for after that time the sockets of the teeth acquire a great degree of strength, and the teeth are so fixed that they cannot be moved without much difficulty. If the irregularity be left to a much later period, it becomes a great deal more difficult to produce any alteration, and frequently all attempts are fruitless. To remove the kind of irregularity abovementioned, two objects must be accomplished; one, to apply a force which shall act constantly upon the irregular tooth, and bring it forward; the other, to remove that obstruction which the under teeth, by coming before the upper, always occasion. The first of these objects may be attained by the application of*

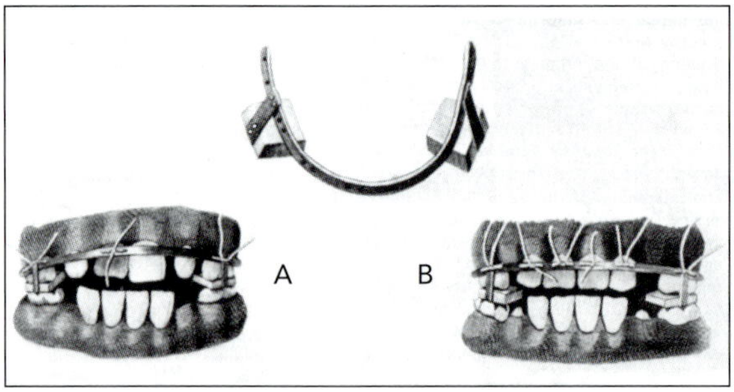

Fig 13-7 Archwire with bite blocks *(center)* to bring a central incisor (A) or all four incisors (B) forward. (From Fox.[6])

an instrument adapted to the arch of the mouth, which, being attached to some strong teeth on each side, will furnish a fixed point in front, to which a ligature previously fastened on the irregular tooth may be applied, and thus, by occasionally renewing it, a constant pressure is preserved, and the tooth may be drawn forward [Fig 13-7]. The second object, that of removing the resistance of the under teeth, must be attained by placing some intervening substance between the teeth of the upper and under jaws, so as to prevent them from completely closing, and be an obstruction to the coming forward of the irregular tooth [see Fig 13-7]. This instrument may be made of gold or silver; it should be so strong as not easily to bend; if about the sixteenth of an inch in breadth, and of a proportionate thickness, it will be sufficiently firm. This bar of gold must be bent to the form of the mouth, and should be long enough to reach to the temporary molares, which are the teeth to which it is to be tied. Holes are to be drilled in it at those places where ligatures are required, which will be on the parts opposed to the teeth designed to be the fixed points, and also at the parts opposite to the place where the irregular tooth or teeth are situated. Then to the bar a small square piece of ivory is to be connected, by means of a little piece of gold, which may be fastened to the ivory and the bar by two rivets. This piece of ivory passes under the grinding surfaces of the upper teeth, is kept there fixed, and prevents the teeth from closing and consequently takes off all obstruction in front. The bar is to be attached by a strong silk ligature to the teeth at the sides, so that if possible, it may remain tight as long as it is required; a ligature is then to be tied around the irregular tooth, and the ends, being brought through the holes in the bar, are to be tied in a firm knot. In two or three days this ligature must be removed and a new one applied; the tooth will soon be perceived to move. A fresh ligature must be used every three or four days, in order to keep up a constant pressure, sufficiently powerful to bring the tooth into a line with the others. The same mode of treatment is to be observed

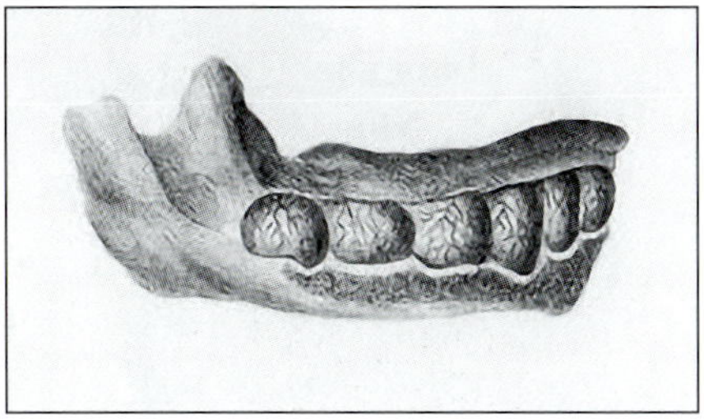

Fig 13-8 Vascular follicular tissue surrounding developing teeth in a child at birth. (Adapted from Fox.[6])

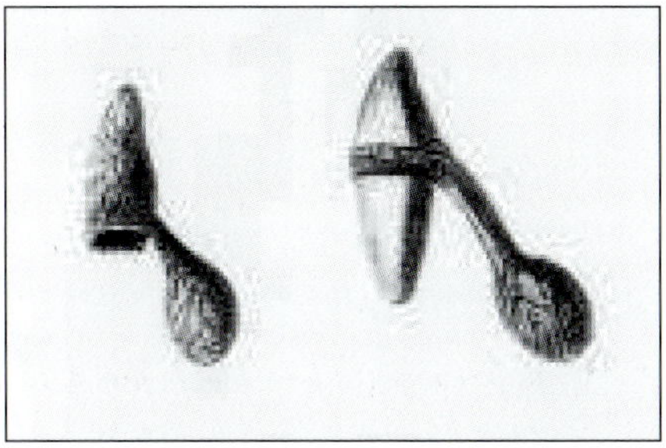

Fig 13-9 Continuity of vascular sacs (follicles) of the primary *(left)* and permanent *(right)* teeth. (Adapted from Fox.[6])

whether there be one, two, or three teeth growing in a similar manner. The teeth are usually brought forwards in about a month or five weeks, and as soon as they are so much advanced as to allow the under teeth to pass on the inside, the piece of ivory may be removed, and the bar only be retained for a few days, until the teeth are perfectly firm, which will prevent the accident of the teeth again receding.[7]

Fox studied the development of teeth by dissecting fetal jaws and by injecting the vascular supply and observed that teeth grew within a highly vascularized follicle or sac (Fig 13-8). He noted that the membranous sac that enveloped each tooth was continuous with the overlying oral mucosa and that the follicular sacs of the permanent teeth were connected to similar sacs of the primary teeth (Fig 13-9). Fox also noted that the manner by which the permanent teeth were formed had not been properly understood until described by Dr Blake. In confirming Blake's observation, Fox stated:

When the rudiments of the temporary teeth are somewhat advanced, a new sac is given off at the upper and posterior part of their membranes. These sacs are at first contained in the same socket, and are so intimately connected with the membranes of the temporary teeth, that they cannot

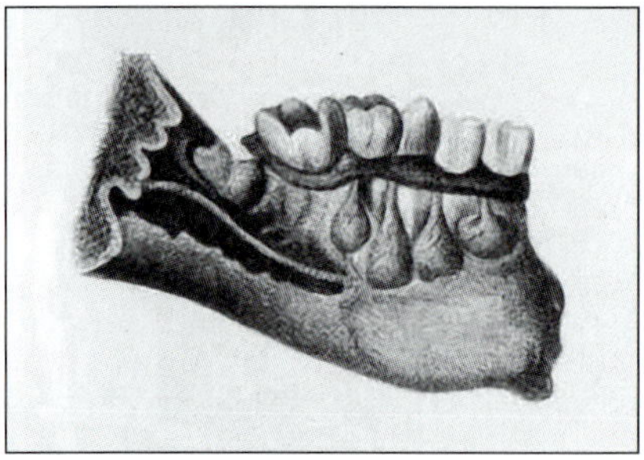

Fig 13-10 Elongated sacs of the permanent teeth are connected to the follicular membranes of the primary teeth. (Adapted from Fox.[6])

> *be separated without tearing one or both. As the sacs of the permanent teeth advance, the sockets of the temporary ones become enlarged, and little niches are formed in the internal plate of the alveolar processes; these increase in proportion with the size of the permanent sacs, and gradually form a distinct socket round each of them. There is however an opening left immediately under the gum, through which the membranes of both sets of teeth continue to be connected. When the temporary teeth have risen in the socket, the membranes are much elongated, and remain attached to the gum at the neck of the tooth, small foramina being left in the jaw for them to pass through; thus they continue to derive their vessels from the gums.*[7]

The continuity of the membranous sacs of the permanent teeth to the overlying mucosa, clearly illustrated by Fox (Fig 13-10), would be taken up by A. Serres in his development of the notion that in eruption the teeth progressed through a fibrous channel he called the *gubernaculum dentis*.

Arch Growth and Eruption

How to gain space in the dental arch to accommodate teeth that were erupting out of alignment became an early subject of controversy. Delabarre noted with regret that there were many dentists of limited talent who regulated teeth based on textbook routines without evaluating the validity of the methods that they were employing. He boasted that his method, labeled as the "natural method," was based on knowledge obtained from dissections at autopsies and not on imagination, as so many others were inclined to accept. Delabarre was critical of dentists who readily extracted teeth to correct malocclusions, even calling Fauchard's and Bourdet's methods of handling

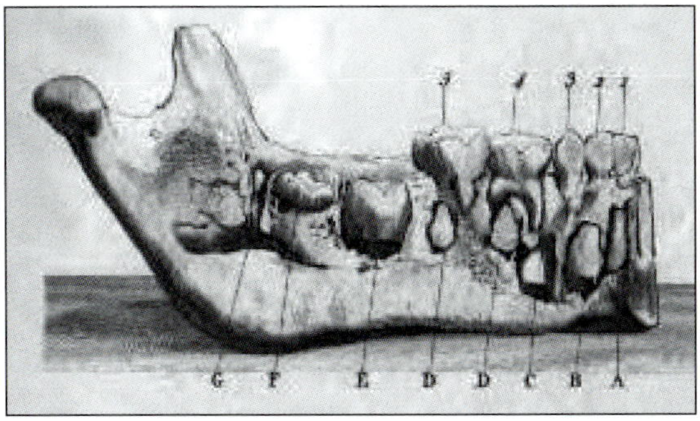

Fig 13-11 Mandible depicting the position of the permanent teeth in the process of eruption. Serres theorized that growth of the anterior segment accompanies the eruption of the canine (C), which is positioned beneath the anterior root of the first primary molar. (Adapted from Serres.[9])

such irregularities deplorable. The major premise of his approach was that there was growth in the maxillary anterior jaw coincident with the eruption of the permanent teeth and that this growth was accompanied by increased spacing between the primary teeth. Delabarre proposed that the mechanical inductive force that led to expansion was created by the erupting primary teeth acting as wedges to transmit pressure on the primary teeth and jaw and thereby cause bone growth.[8] Based on this principle, he advocated the use of interdental wooden wedges to expand the dental arch. Extraction of primary teeth to facilitate eruption and alignment of the permanent teeth was deplorable because it removed the very elements involved in applying the force for expansion. There were cases of overcrowding, however, where it was advisable to file teeth to gain space and to extract a tooth erupted out of alignment, but only when the patient had reached 15 to 16 years of age, the period at which expansion of the arch was no longer possible. When it was deemed necessary to extract a permanent tooth, the second premolar was the tooth of choice.[8]

The notion that the anterior segment of the dental arches grew in size during the transition from primary to permanent dentition was also supported by A. Serres in his book *Essai sur l'anatomie et la physiologie des dents ou nouvelle théorie de la dentition*, published in 1817.[9] As chief of anatomical instruction at Paris hospitals, Serres completed a detailed study of the embryonic development and eruption of teeth in autopsied human fetuses and young children (Fig 13-11). Although the embryonic stages in the development of the dentition had been described earlier by Vesalius, Eustachi, and Hunter, Serres's treatise was the first detailed anatomical study of the location and sequence of the development of all the dental follicles (buds) and the sequence of eruption of the primary and permanent teeth. He stated that in a 2-month-old fetus, he was able to locate the dental buds of the primary incisors and molars. The bud of the primary canine was observed at 2 and a half months and that of the permanent teeth at 3 months. Serres states that he was the first to locate the buds of the permanent premolars, small as pinheads, attached at the base of the primary molars. He noted the presence of a fibrous channel connected to the dentals sacs of the developing permanent teeth that guided their movement through the jaw into the alveoli vacated by primary teeth. He named this structure the *gubernaculum dentis*. In this manner, the permanent teeth erupted within the same arch as the primary teeth.

Serres called attention to the fact that the primary canine did not erupt before the primary molars, as had previously been described by earlier anatomists. He confirmed this sequence in 15 separate autopsies. The physiologic basis of this pattern was found in the earlier calcification and root development of the primary molars compared with that of the canine. This finding demonstrated the futility of attempting to hasten the eruption of the primary canine in children by incising the gums.

Serres stated that the replacement (permanent) teeth, with the exception of the premolars, were larger than their primary counterparts and could only be accommodated by anterior bone growth during the period from 4 to 6 years of age. The space gained by the replacement of the larger primary molars by the smaller permanent premolars afforded additional room for the eruption of the permanent canine. He noted that there were few irregularities in the placement of the primary teeth. The problem of misalignment of the permanent teeth arose mainly from deficient bone growth during the period of transition. The permanent canine, last in the anterior segment to erupt, was most often found to be out of alignment or impacted. Serres viewed the long period of the mixed dentition as necessary for, and proof thereof, bone growth in accompaniment with eruption of the permanent dentition.[9]

Delabarre's and Serres's theories on the growth of the maxillary arches were not without their critics. E. M. Miel raised a serious objection to Delabarre's "natural method" by stating in 1811[1] that the dimension of the primary dental arch at the time when all 10 primary teeth

[1] Miel had presented his thesis in 1811 in volume 7 of the *Memoires de la Societe medicale d'emulation* in Paris.

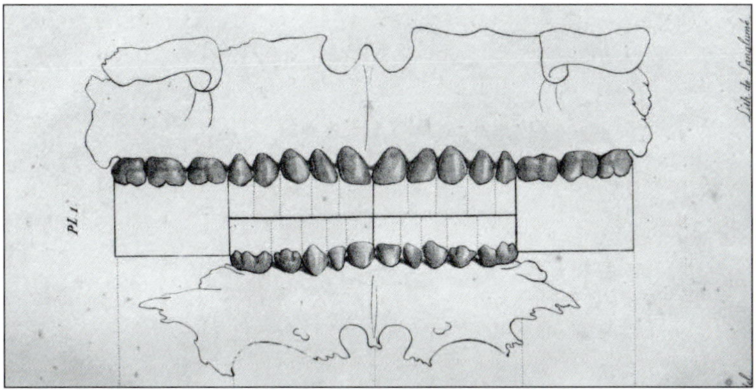

Fig 13-12 Diagram illustrating that the anterior segments of the primary and permanent dentitions are equal in length and that the space occupied by the primary molars is less than that needed for the permanent premolars. (Adapted from Miel.[10])

were fully erupted was constant and that no subsequent growth in this segment was possible.[10] He pointed out that what Delabarre and Serres mistakenly assumed to be new space due to bone growth in the anterior segment (canine to canine) was space gained by the fact that the four permanent premolars were smaller than the four primary molars that they replaced (Fig 13-12). The additional space needed to accommodate the increased size of the permanent incisors over their predecessors was "created" by the smaller size of the permanent premolars over their predecessors. Growth of the dental arches occurred only posterior to the primary molars during the maturation and eruption of the permanent molars. Miel's ideas were fully developed in his book *Researches in the Art of Regulating the Second Dentition*, published in 1826.[10] Unknown to Miel in 1811 was the work of John Hunter, who at an earlier date (1778) had maintained "that part of each jaw which holds the ten fore-teeth is exactly of the same size when it contains those of the first set as when it contains those of the second; and as these last often occupy a much larger space than the first, in such cases the second set are obliged to stand very irregularly." Having learned of Hunter's supporting observation, Miel in 1826 was quick to quote the famed anatomist in supporting an attack on Delabarre's ideas of growth in the anterior part of the dental arches. Miel's concept was later confirmed by E. Magitot.[11]

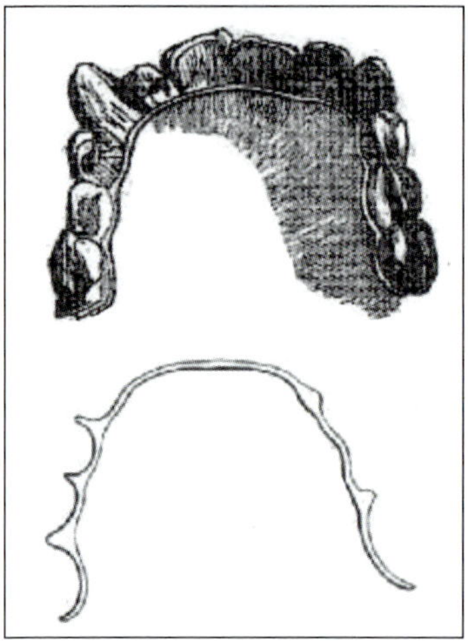

Fig 13-13 Lefoulon's spring archwire used to expand the arch and to realign incisors and canines by means of silk ligatures tied to the gold archwire. (Adapted from Lefoulon.[12])

Regulation of Teeth

P. J. Lefoulon, in his book *Nouveau traite theorique et pratique de l'art du dentiste*, published in 1841, was the first to apply the term *orthodontia* to define the art of regulating teeth.[1] *Orthodontia* was defined as that part of dentistry pertaining to the treatment of congenital and accidental dental deformities in the arrangement of the teeth. Lefoulon deplored the fact that most dentists charged with the care of children (as in boarding schools) were insufficiently prepared to manage problems arising during the transition from primary to secondary dentition. Most had been discouraged by imagined difficulties and had resorted to luxation in repositioning teeth or in unnecessary extraction of teeth. Lefoulon described a technique of applying finger pressure twice a day to expand the dental arch to be carried out by the parents or the children themselves.[12] Delabarre called this a ludicrous idea, not worthy of pointing out its uselessness. On a more practical level, Lefoulon described an original method that he claimed could be used to realign malpositioned teeth as well as to expand the palatal arch using a horseshoe-shaped archwire of elastic gold (Fig 13-13). Being bent slightly outward before insertion, the archwire exerted an outward force on the molars and premolars when in place. It also served as an anterior anchor from which force was applied via silk threads to the teeth needing to be tipped posteriorly. The merits of his appliance were that it was painless, posed no great hindrance to the patient, and was quick-acting. Lefoulon's approach to treatment was

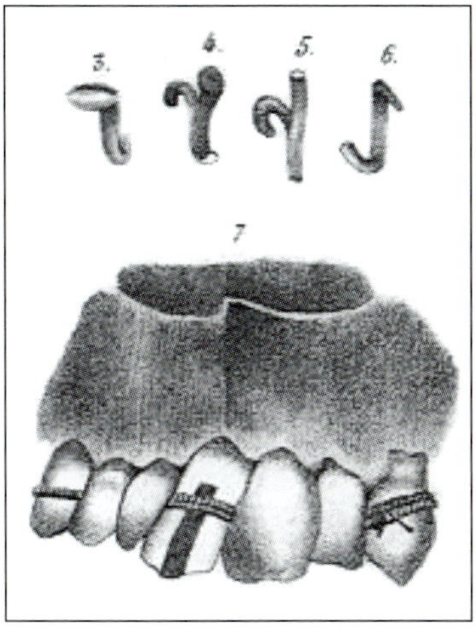

Fig 13-14 *(bottom)* Silk ligature tied to a protruding incisor and passed on the palatal side of the adjacent incisors before being secured to the anchorage teeth. *(top)* Small hooks for securing ligatures. (From Maury.[13])

based on the concept that the shape and size of the dental arch was not invariably fixed but could grow in response to appropriate forces. He called the view held by Hunter, Fox, and Miel—that the size of the anterior dental arches was fixed—erroneous and one that led to abuse of early and needless filing and extraction to gain space.[12]

Among the causes of malpositioned teeth was a neglect to supervise the transition through the mixed dentition—too early extraction of primary teeth or waiting too long before extraction. He was a strong opponent of luxation to forcibly reposition teeth, considering it a brutal and painful technique not to be imposed on children. Similarly, he did not approve of the disfiguring result obtained when filing teeth to gain space. Among Lefoulon's ideas of the causes of disharmonies in the alignment of teeth was the amusing notion that the repetitious enunciation of English words could cause the tongue to exert outward pressure on the maxillary anterior teeth, resulting in eventual flaring.

In 1841, F. Maury of Paris described moving misaligned teeth with silk ligatures secured to the crowns by small hooks to prevent slippage of the ligatures toward the gingiva and tied some distance away to anchorage teeth[13] (Fig 13-14). Shrinkage of the ligatures in the humid atmosphere of the mouth exerted a force on the misaligned teeth. Maury stressed that the force exerted must be slow and constant, without causing pain. This was accomplished by replacing the ligatures every 3 to 4 days over the 2 weeks needed to reposition a tooth into its normal alignment. When patients were unable to bear the presence of ligatures or plates, he recommended luxation and manual repositioning of the offending tooth as practiced by Fauchard. But he cautioned that this was a dangerous method because it was often complicated by ruptured alveolar bone, lacerated gums, and accidental extraction. He stated that the extraction of some permanent teeth to provide room for others, as recommended by several reputable dentists, was repugnant and not to be followed.

In his extensive study of the history of orthodontia, Weinberger concluded that France "must be given credit for making more rapid and direct professional advancement than any of her neighbors.... Between 1728 and 1888 over sixty-six excellent textbooks were prepared treating on dentition and irregularities of the teeth."[1]

Orthodontics in the United States

With the publication of Chapin Harris's textbook *The Principles and Practice of Dental Surgery*, the advancement of orthodontia shifted to the United States. Harris revealed a detailed knowledge of the work of the French and English authorities.[14] He noted that great progress in dental science had been made in France since the publication of Fauchard's work. On the topic of regulating teeth, Harris discussed the contributions of Delabarre, Serres, Miel, Schange, Maury, and Lefoulon. Harris supported Delabarre's concept of the gubernaculum dentis as a guiding force in the eruption of the permanent teeth. In the destruction of the roots of the primary teeth, he agreed with Laforgue and Delabarre that resorption was caused by a "carneous substance" formed on the root apices:

> *The manner of the destruction of the roots of the temporary teeth has been a subject of close and critical enquiry with me for several years, and the more I have examined the subject, the more fully have I become convinced, that it is the result of the action of this fleshy tubercle upon them.*[14]

He stressed the importance of preserving the primary teeth until they underwent their natural replacement:

> *The temporary teeth, however, should, if possible, be retained, until, from the spontaneous destruction of their fangs, they drop out of themselves; nor should their extraction ever be determined on, unless required by some pressing emergency; for their premature loss generally occasions a contraction in the span of the alveolar arch, and a consequent irregularity in the arrangement of the permanent teeth.*[14]

Harris noted that the early appliances developed by Fauchard and Bourdet were awkward and seldom used. He attributed the development of orthodontic treatment to have started with Fox: "His method of treatment has formed the basis of the established practice for more than fifty years."

Harris stated that misaligned teeth may be made to change their position under the influence of pressure:

> *The pressure must be constant; it must be sufficient to cause motion, yet not so great as to set up destructive inflammation; lastly, it must be continued until the teeth can be kept in place by antagonism with the opposing teeth; or in case there is no such antagonism, the regulating appliance must be worn more or less constantly for a year, or even longer. The regulating appliance should be as simple in construction as is possible to accomplish the purpose, so that both time and labor may be saved, and the patient be able to attend to its removal and adjustment when it becomes necessary to cleanse it; this should frequently be done.*[14]

Commenting on the practice of moving teeth by forceps or by extraction and immediate replacement, Harris cautioned that

> *if a tooth is extracted or turned in its socket, the vessels and nerves from which it derives nourishment and vitality are severed; hence, though its connection with the alveolus may be partially reestablished, it will be liable to act as a morbid irritant, and be subject to inflammation from comparatively slight causes.*[14]

On the practice of filing teeth to gain space, as recommended by Bell and Delabarre, Harris stated that:

> *Notwithstanding the deservedly high authority of those two gentlemen, my own experience compels me to disprove the practice. The apertures thus formed by the file, soon close, but not so perfectly as to prevent small particles of extraneous matter from getting in between the teeth, and being retained there until they become putrid...occasioning decay.*[14]

The potential for growth of the anterior jaw, as Hunter and Fox had ruled out, was affirmed by Harris. He believed along with Delabarre that bone growth accompanied the eruption of the permanent dentition. Arguing that Bell's measurements made of the same jaw at different ages had proved that anterior permanent teeth occupied a somewhat larger arch than the primary teeth, Harris stated:

> *The ten anterior permanent teeth occupy a somewhat larger space than that which was taken up by the temporary ones that preceded them, and that, where there is no increase in the size of this portion of the arch, the uniformity of their arrangement would be more or less disturbed. But*

> *there is not always an increase in the anterior part of the jaws; on the contrary, the premature loss of one or more of the temporary teeth, often occasions a contraction, that frequently causes much irregularity in the arrangement of the second set.*[14]

Harris recommended that:

> *The mouth should be frequently examined from the time the shedding of the deciduous teeth commences, until the second set is completed; and when the growth of the permanent teeth so far outstrips the destruction of the roots of the temporary, that they are caused to take an improper direction, the primitive teeth, that have occasioned the obstruction, should be immediately removed.*[14]

Harris recognized Delabarre as having provided the most explicit directions for the management of the transition to the permanent dentition.

Although the earliest editions of Harris's textbook contained few specifics for the regulation of misaligned teeth, confined mostly to discussing Delabarre's and Catalan's use of the inclined plane for correcting crossbites, in later editions he used the term *orthodontia* and illustrated various primitive appliances for employing ligatures, elastics, and gold plates for regulating the alignment of permanent teeth.[15] In recognizing the invention of vulcanized rubber, Harris noted that it had great promise for correcting dental abnormalities:

> *A closely fitting vulcanite plate can be worn with comfort; hence the patient is not tempted to remove it. It has no motion; hence does not wear the teeth or irritate the gums. Its firmness of adaptation makes an excellent fixed point, from which to make pressure or traction in any required direction upon the irregular teeth: the counter pressure, being distributed over all the regular teeth, is not felt.*[15]

Vulcanite denture bases were soon applied in regulating teeth, but not without limitations. Problems encountered with the plate method were described by Dr A. Westcott, a dentist who had been in practice for over 20 years, during which time "the regulating of teeth has constituted a prominent feature."[16] In the case of a young woman whose maxilla was unnaturally small and mandible unusually large, such that she presented "the aspects of a matron of seventy," Westcott set out to expand the maxillary arch using a plate with various fixtures attached to it. Although having made initial progress, he described how

> *just as soon as the teeth and jaw began to move, the fitting of the plates became correspondingly imperfect, both in respect to the clasps, and its adjustment to the roof of the mouth; and during the two, or two and a*

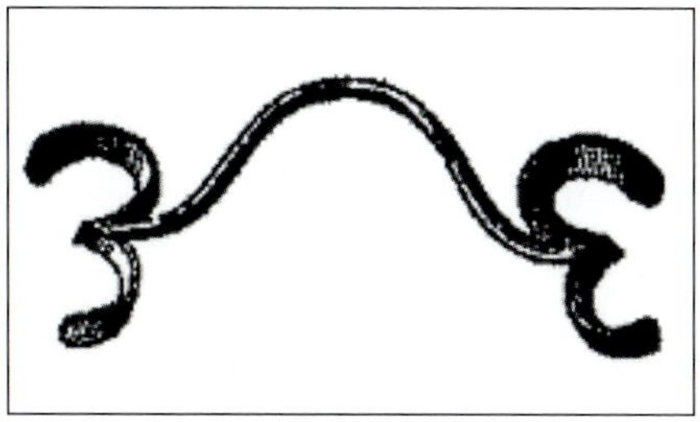

Fig 13-15 Expansion bar described by Westcott.[16]

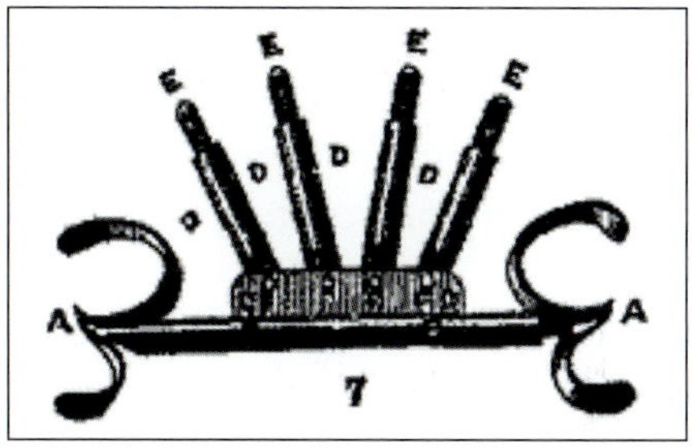

Fig 13-16 Maxillary bar with screws (E) to push incisors forward. (From Westcott.[16])

> *half months referred to, I made no less than six plates, to keep pace with the progress, which was by no means too great.*[16]

Concluding that plates were useless in expanding the maxilla, Westcott created a device consisting of a crossbar attached by double clasps to the premolars (Fig 13-15). The pressure against the teeth was regulated by periodically straightening the crossbar. Once having expanded the arch, he created a second appliance involving a straight crossbar with tubes and screws to push the maxillary incisors forward[2] (Fig 13-16). Westcott concluded from his experience that

> *this cross bar encumbers the mouth less than any other fixture that can be rendered at all available as the basis of levers, springs, or any other appliance for the purpose of moving teeth, and I shall adopt it as the foundation of all other fixtures in my future operations for regulating teeth.*[16]

He underlined the virtues of the appliance as exerting a firm and steady pressure, requiring the least possible alterations, and easily allowing for periodic adjustments to be made, often by the patient.

[2] Angle called this appliance "a monstrosity" in contrast to his simplified and innovative system.

Appliances

In 1881, L. Coffin, a London dentist, introduced the vulcanite expansion plate.[17] The driving force of this appliance was created from bent piano wire arranged to push apart the two halves of a split plate and thereby expand the arch. Other configurations of the bent wires (spring wires) embedded in vulcanite plates were adapted to move individual teeth into alignment. Ingenious adaptations of the spring-wire method were introduced by several dentists. V. H. Jackson constructed a "crib" appliance from piano wire snapped firmly into place over the anchorage teeth. Additional wires were joined to the crib to exert pressure on the teeth that were to be repositioned. Jackson claimed that his devices were inexpensive and quickly constructed. His devices were light, occupied minimal space in the mouth, and could be removed for cleaning.[18]

J. Foster Flagg of Philadelphia, in writing of his experiences in correcting dental irregularities, noted that he had enjoyed a gratifying amount of success while at the same time submitting to a fair share of failures. In making a case for the use of a simple system, Flagg stated that he had repeatedly demonstrated that protruding teeth could be drawn back by "a simple apparatus which does not require five minutes for its construction, no more than ten minutes for its adaptation."[19] Flagg regarded orthodontics as

> *that portion of his practice as decidedly compensating, and that too, at quite moderate charges; and I would wish to be distinctly understood as referring to pecuniary compensation, and by no means to that charming, but slightly theoretic, equivalent, the satisfaction of confirming the benefits of science upon one's fellow creatures!*[19]

Flagg was critical of dentists who caused much injury by the premature extraction of primary teeth, noting that this could be avoided only if dental students were made to study "dento-anatomical preparations which demonstrate the stages of dentition."

Norman Kingsley

One of the first American textbooks devoted to orthodontics was written by Norman W. Kingsley in 1880.[1] He viewed the treatment of irregularities of the teeth as a form of "mechanical surgery." The dentists who hoped to be successful in this enterprise must have a thorough knowledge of mechanics and must be able to command the powers of levers, pulleys, inclined planes, wedges, and screws to form new appliances for each case.[20] Kingsley believed that "it is quite as

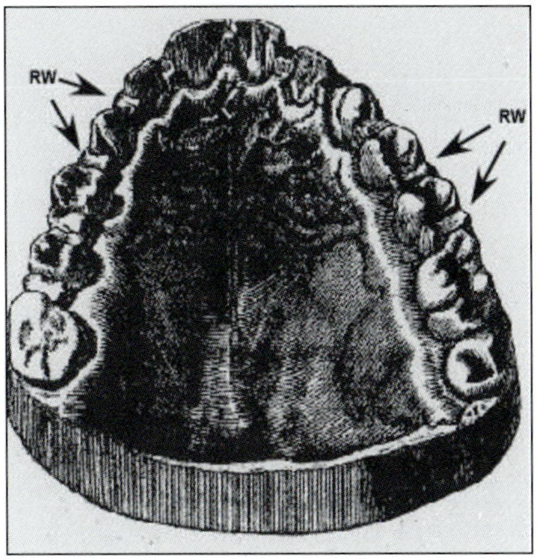

Fig 13-17 Kingsley approach to expanding the maxillary arch by placing interdental rubber wedges (RW). (From Kingsley.[21])

impossible to describe an apparatus, such as would be applicable to every case, as it would be to anticipate the future and describe every invention that the fertile mind of man may make for his comfort or convenience." Each new case demanded a new approach: "No complex case that I have ever seen could be corrected by following the exact steps of any preceding case." He provided numerous examples of how screws, wedges, levers, inclined planes, and elastics could be applied to constructing corrective appliances. Years before his book was published, he had described how treatment of anterior crossbite by expansion of the maxillary arch could be done simply with interdental rubber elastics acting as wedges[21] (Fig 13-17). A vulcanite palatal plate helped to secure the position of the rubber wedges. He claimed that with this method he moved the maxillary teeth into proper alignment within 20 days. For Kingsley, this case "illustrates that the simplest of all mechanical powers wrought all that could have been done by jack-screws, levers, inclined planes, straps, bands, and pulleys combined."

Kingsley was cognizant of the current ideas on bone resorption and that attempts had been made to identify a "physiologic" level of pressure best suited to moving teeth:

> *Different opinions are held as to the kind of pressure most in accordance with physiological action; some maintaining that the pressure must be constant and uninterrupted, while others claim that interrupted pressure will produce the most beneficial result. I doubt if either can be shown to be the best in all cases.*[20]

Here Kingsley took aim at John Farrar (see later section):

> *A recent writer has claimed that there is an exact limit to the distance to which teeth can be moved in a given time without injurious action, and places it at 1/240 to 1/180 of an inch in every twelve hours. It is hardly necessary to show the absurdity of placing physiological or pathological action under a mathematical law, no matter how broad.... It has been maintained by some that teeth cannot be moved with safety faster than bone can be absorbed or reproduced, but an extended experience has shown that in the outward movement of the superior arch and in the movement in either direction of the anterior teeth of the lower jaw, the idea is fallacious.*[20]

For Kingsley, the importance of facial esthetics and the contours of the lips and cheeks were just as important as the occlusal relationship of the teeth in orthodontic treatment. He was of the opinion that it was not possible to apply a single standard for arch form or the number of teeth to all facial types. He maintained that it was wrong to assert

> *that all irregularities in the position of teeth are deformities, and require our interposition. A fine esthetic taste may maintain that there are multitudinous departures from a normal type where neither the utility nor the beauty of these organs, nor the symmetry of surrounding features, is seriously affected by the malposition.... Every human figure differs from every other human figure; face from face—even the two sides of the same face are not mechanically mated. Variation from mathematical precision in nature is universal, and any appearance of absolute regularity always suggests the interference of man.*[20]

Kingsley deplored the fact that "there are seen all over the country prevailing patterns of teeth made in rows, devoid of grace, and inserted indiscriminately in the mouths of the beautiful and the mouths of the ugly." He advocated extractions when indicated to achieve an esthetic result:

> *An erroneous teaching has maintained that the full number of teeth must be retained in the mouth, regardless of their organization, the progress of decay, the limited capacity of the arch, or the external features. An experience of sufficient length to determine results has shown very conclusively that the retention of every tooth in the mouth is not necessary to the efficiency of the masticating apparatus, is not required to maintain the contour of the jaw, and the loss of certain teeth produces no visible external effects.... It is not necessary to the contour, symmetry, or harmony of the features that everyone of the masticating organs should be retained in the mouth. In the treatment of irregularities, the comfort and permanent good of the patient are secured in larger measure by not moving organs that are not themselves offending members.... It is often better to extract a malposed tooth than disturb a whole arch to bring it into line.*[20]

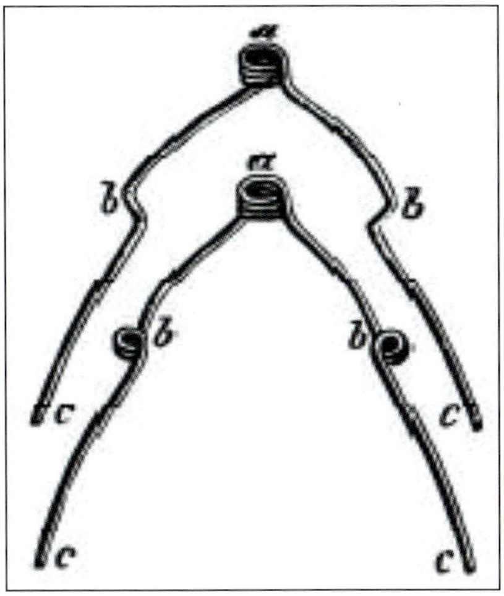

Fig 13-18 Piano wire springs. (From Talbot.[23])

Kingsley achieved international fame for his construction of palatal obturators for the treatment of congenital cleft palate and the related cure of defective speech. He was also honored at the 1853 New York World's Fair and at the 1855 Paris Exposition for his creation of porcelain teeth. Kingsley's artistic abilities were also expressed in sculptures in marble and "flame painting" (wood burning) reproductions of Rembrandt's works.[22]

Eugene Talbot

Eugene Talbot's textbook *Irregularities of the Teeth and Their Treatment*, published in 1888, provided a summary of the many systems then available for correcting misaligned teeth.[23] Talbot explored Patrick's bow-spring wire appliance, Byrne's spring-bands of thin gold, Coffin's split expansion plate, and Farrar's "positive system" for intermittent force application. Talbot's system consisted of piano wire spring devices specifically designed for each case. The elastic force of the wire was increased by coiling the wire several times around a mandrel to form a spring (Fig 13-18). Talbot noted that the wire spring worked on the same principle as the mainspring of an American watch. The springs could be used in connection with vulcanite plates (similar to that used by Coffin in his expansion plate) or to gold or platinum bands fastened to the teeth. The arms of the spring delivered a mild uniform pressure to the teeth that needed realignment.

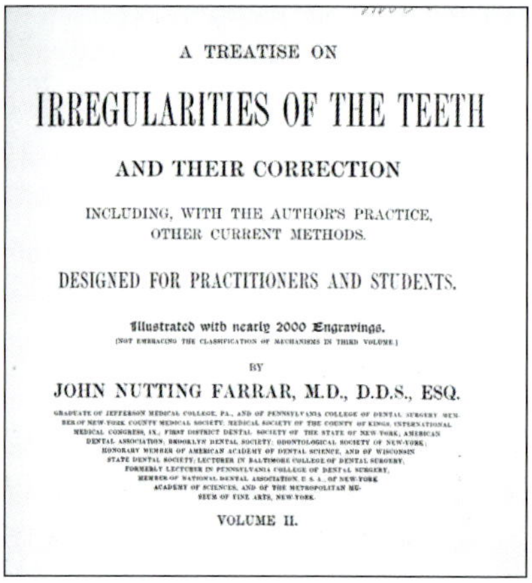
A TREATISE ON

IRREGULARITIES OF THE TEETH

AND THEIR CORRECTION

INCLUDING, WITH THE AUTHOR'S PRACTICE, OTHER CURRENT METHODS.

DESIGNED FOR PRACTITIONERS AND STUDENTS.

Illustrated with nearly 2000 Engravings.
(NOT EMBRACING THE CLASSIFICATION OF MECHANISMS IN THIRD VOLUME.)

BY

JOHN NUTTING FARRAR, M.D., D.D.S., ESQ.

GRADUATE OF JEFFERSON MEDICAL COLLEGE, PA., AND OF PENNSYLVANIA COLLEGE OF DENTAL SURGERY. MEMBER OF NEW-YORK COUNTY MEDICAL SOCIETY, MEDICAL SOCIETY OF THE COUNTY OF KINGS, INTERNATIONAL MEDICAL CONGRESS, IX.; FIRST DISTRICT DENTAL SOCIETY OF THE STATE OF NEW-YORK, AMERICAN DENTAL ASSOCIATION, BROOKLYN DENTAL SOCIETY; ODONTOLOGICAL SOCIETY OF NEW-YORK; HONORARY MEMBER OF AMERICAN ACADEMY OF DENTAL SCIENCE, AND OF WISCONSIN STATE DENTAL SOCIETY; LECTURER IN BALTIMORE COLLEGE OF DENTAL SURGERY, FORMERLY LECTURER IN PENNSYLVANIA COLLEGE OF DENTAL SURGERY, MEMBER OF NATIONAL DENTAL ASSOCIATION, U. S. A., OF NEW-YORK ACADEMY OF SCIENCES, AND OF THE METROPOLITAN MUSEUM OF FINE ARTS, NEW-YORK.

VOLUME II.

Fig 13-19 Title page of Farrar's voluminous textbook of orthodontics published in 1888. The inclusion of nearly 2,000 illustrations is an indication of the complexity of the practice at that time.

Talbot's description of the many different methods then employed for correcting irregularities of teeth illustrates the ingenuity of dentists during this time of rapid growth in the clinical practice of orthodontics. But at the same time, it revealed the haphazard state of the field, soon to be shown by John Farrar, the chief critic and reformer of clinical orthodontics.

John Farrar

In 1888, John Farrar published *A Treatise on the Irregularities of the Teeth and Their Correction*[1,24] (Fig 13-19). Farrar, considered to be the "father of American orthodontics," introduced the scientific approach to orthodontic treatment.[25] Farrar stated that he hoped to create some order and standardization out of the chaos of the rapidly evolving art of orthodontia. In his opening chapter, he stated that prior to 1874 very little had been written upon regulation and that it was of a miscellaneous character:

> *There had not been, so far as I know, any attempt to definitively classify mechanical devices, no nomenclature indicating the position of teeth; no classification of expression for individual teeth, nor of types of the arch; little definite concerning harmony between the facial expression and the arrangement of the teeth; no closely marked differentiation of the principles adopted in manufacturing appliances, nor any differences*

recognized in the character of force; no mathematical demonstrations of the philosophy of action and reaction in the bearings of the apparatus of the teeth; no accurate demonstration of the effect of irregularly developed teeth upon undeveloped ones nor upon their sockets by the process of regulating; no definite explanation as to the action of the alveolar tissues under the influence of the different kinds and degrees of force; nor any clear statement as to the difference between moving teeth by causing absorption and moving them by taking advantage of the flexibility of the alveolar tissue. Above all, the fact that pain may be avoided with certainty by conducting the operations within the domain of the physiological functions of tissues was wholly unknown.[24]

In addressing these deficiencies, Farrar assembled the results of over 20 years of patient care previously described in a series of papers in *Dental Cosmos* from 1871 to 1887.[25]

Farrar stated that one of the cardinal principles of his work was "the observance of the physiological law which governs tissues during movement of the teeth, the object being to prevent pain." He argued, "To ensure exemption from pain, the pressure by which the movement is to be affected should be under the control of the patient, a requirement which implies the use of instruments capable of being operated and adjusted at will." Farrar advised that by following these principles, it was possible to move teeth painlessly. His system involved controllable mechanisms generating intermittent forces whenever practicable.

Farrar noted that "early on, operations for correcting irregularities of the teeth were based chiefly upon forcing them into position without any regard to the injury of the tissues in which they stood." He went on to say that "This philosophy appeared to me in some respects to be unscientific, as I believed that most if not all of these operations should be founded upon the physiological law to which I have alluded."[24]

Over time, Farrar reduced the number of tooth-moving mechanisms to a manageable number. According to him:

The cases of irregularity are so various, each apparently requiring more or less difference in construction of the appliances used to remove it, that an impression is prevalent that it is impossible to establish any system of principles, the knowledge of which would facilitate the efforts of the dentist. At first, it appeared so to the writer; but upon reflection he was surprised to find how simple and few are the mechanisms necessary to accomplish nearly all that is desired, whether turning, drawing, pushing, elevating or depressing the teeth, or holding them in place.[24]

Farrar determined the appropriate rate of force application by experimentation:

> *The idea of taking advantage of the functional laws of the tissues to prevent pain, appeared to me (at the time of its conception) novel, and yet so rational that, when fully appreciated, it would be available in general surgery as well as in dentistry. To determine this rate and test its value, I made a series of experiments which extended over a period of several years. The results were made known to several professional gentlemen in 1873; and in February, 1874, this topic was the subject of my graduation thesis at Jefferson Medical College, and afterward read in the main before the Brooklyn Dental Society.*[24]

Farrar, always fascinated by mechanics, did not confine his talents to dentistry; it is said that he invented elastic car wheels, a water meter, and a typewriter.[26]

Farrar had studied the histologic works of Xavier Sudduth and G. V. Black and knew that, under certain conditions, alveolar bone resorption was a physiologic response carried out under the agency of giant cells. Furthermore, it was well known that physiologic bone resorption was a painless process. Quoting extensively from the publications of Sudduth and Black, Farrar described the biologic events occurring in the alveolus and periodontal membrane during tooth movement to include the resorption of bone along the pressure side combined with formation of new tissue in the tension (stretched) side. He observed that these physiologic processes could be best activated by slow, intermittent application of force. The art of regulating teeth resided in the ability of the operator to design appliances for application of appropriate forces: "lightly if continuous, or periodically if greater, the latter allows the tissues to act, and then grants them a period of rest." By keeping the forces to a physiologic level and by applying force intermittently, pain could be avoided.

Through clinical experimentation, Farrar concluded that teeth could be moved 1/120th of an inch per day without causing pain. These findings were obtained by employing a band and screw appliance activated daily with a key. Farrar concluded that in a "patient of fourteen to twenty-five years of age, forty to sixty days was sufficient time to move a tooth, painlessly, through solid alveolar tissue one-fourth of an inch by absorption."

In describing his system, Farrar explained that the mechanical appliances for regulating teeth could be classified according to the different principles of mechanics on which their construction was based:

> *Known as the probable and the positive; so called because one is certain and definite in action, while the other is not. These two plans not only act upon different mechanical principles, but also, as suggested in previous chapters, are thought to be capable of exercising peculiar characteristic influences upon the functions of the tissues involved. The plan of*

construction by probable mechanics implies the use of elastic materials, such as springs and rubber, in such a way that a continued force is maintained upon the teeth to be moved; the management of which force is not only usually beyond the control of the patient, but is also difficult even for the dentist to so manage as to harmonize sufficiently with physiological functions, to insure the highest success with the least pain in the majority of cases. The positive plan consists in constructing the apparatus in such a way that the force acts intermittently at will, to any desired degree, and is not only manageable by the dentist, but also by the patient, who, as before said, is really the best judge of the greatest degree of force that can be applied without causing pain. This intermittent principle of action may be approximately reached by the use of the old and well-known wooden wedges, pegs set in a plate, metallic fingers projecting from the plate, so that they may reach out to bear upon the teeth by being occasionally bent, or by the inclined plane, but generally can be better and more accurately applied by the use of the screw.... It has been said that all regulating apparatus constructed purely upon the screw principle, belong to the positive plan of mechanism, and are capable of an intermittent motion of any degree at will; while devices constructed so as to act purely upon the principle of elasticity, and which are not capable of causing an intermittent force that can be made to act at will, but are continuous in their action, belong to the probable plan.[24]

Based on his experiments, Farrar concluded that:

1. In regulating teeth, the force should not exceed the bounds of physiological functions. 2. That the plan of moving teeth by elastic materials, though practical if kept under perfect control, is so difficult to manage that it often leads to pain and inflammation, and is sometimes dangerous to the future usefulness of the teeth, while a properly constructed apparatus, intelligently operated by means of screws, insures beneficial results, without pain or nervous exhaustion. 3. That if teeth are moved by absorption through the alveolar process about 1/240th of an inch every morning, and the same distance in the evening, no pain or nervous exhaustion follows. 4. That while these tissues will allow an advance of a single tooth at this rate (1/240th of an inch) twice in twenty-four hours, without exceeding physiologic functions, if a much greater pressure be made, the changes will become pathological.[24]

For Farrar:

The absorption and formation of new tissue, when kept within certain limits, is painless, and if pain is the result of over-stepping the domain of healthy action, it is evident that the painless method is more scientific because it is more humane. Again, if pain is the result of perverted physiological action, whether caused by continued force or by too great a degree of intermittent force, it logically follows that, notwithstanding the circumstances of cases may justify it at certain periods in some very difficult operations, or even where the saving of time or money is a matter of consideration, it cannot be denied that to the extent that pain is unnecessary it is wrong to cause it, and that to the degree that pain is caused it is a violation of the law of harmony.... If intermittent force of a definite degree, alternated with proper intervals of rest, will more generally attain the highest success with the least pain and least annoyance to the patient, then the interests of humanity suggest that, as a general rule in adult cases, teeth should be regulated by this plan whenever circumstances will permit. I say "whenever circumstances will permit."[24]

He noted that the use of intermittent force was gaining acceptance:

Although some dentists (in public) profess to be guided by eclecticism, and assert that in their practice they select from all plans the one best suited to the case in hand, yet in private continue to use old and crude methods, the profession generally is making honest endeavors to investigate the matter, and is practicing (more and more) the plan of using intermittent force whenever possible. Many of those who at first strongly opposed it, now appear to accept most of its cardinal principles; and others, although failing to admit openly that there is a limit to the degree of pressure proper to each case, indirectly imply its acceptance through different words meaning practically the same thing, and directly by adopting the plan of construction and method of operating the kind of apparatus recommended.[24]

In an often combative style, he criticized fellow colleagues for having claimed priority of discovery for certain technical innovations and of having used the patent process to gain financial rewards, an exercise he was not averse to conducting himself (Fig 13-20). He urged his colleagues to publish descriptions of their mechanical inventions so as to date them and thereby prevent others from fraudulently obtaining patents to which they were not entitled. He stated that "the recording of dates is not for the purpose of preventing people from obtaining patents for things that they originated, but to prevent the restraining by patents of the use of the inventions of others, who have, through a love of the science and the welfare of the dental profession, given them free to all."[24]

Farrar emphasized that:

It has for some time been evident that the day will come when the elements that are necessary to construct apparatus will be so systematized and simplified that the latter will be kept in stock (in parts, not made up) at dental depots, in readiness for the profession at large, so that they may be ordered by catalogued numbers to suit the needs of any case.[24]

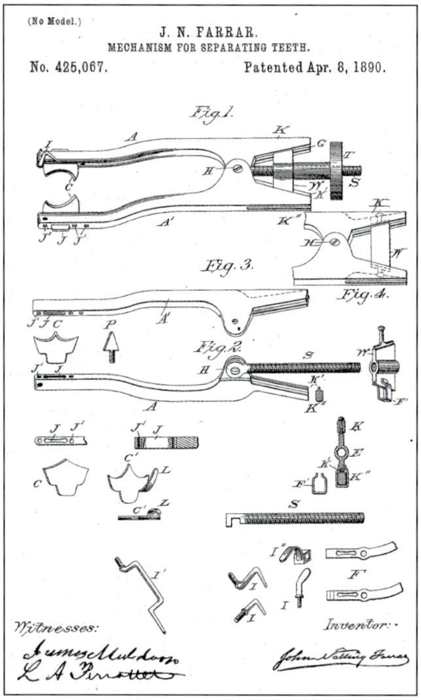

Fig 13-20 Illustration of various clamping devices patented by Farrar in 1890.

Farrar hoped to execute that dream by manufacturing and marketing his many devices to the profession. S. H. Guilford, in his textbook of orthodontics, stated that Farrar's appliances "were beautifully constructed and for a time had a ready sale, but their elaborateness and complexity caused them to be superseded by others of simpler form and different construction."[18] Dr R. Ottolengui, in writing Farrar's obituary, stated the following:

> *Unfortunately for his system, with the exception of a few basic principles first announced by him, it is likely that Dr. Farrar's system will die with him. His appliances though tremendously ingenious required great skill in their construction, and something more than genius for their application, because in the main each case was treated by Dr. Farrar with an appliance devised by himself to meet its individual peculiarities.*[26]

It was not until 1887 that "ready-to-wear" orthodontic appliances became a reality when Dr Edward Angle introduced his system.

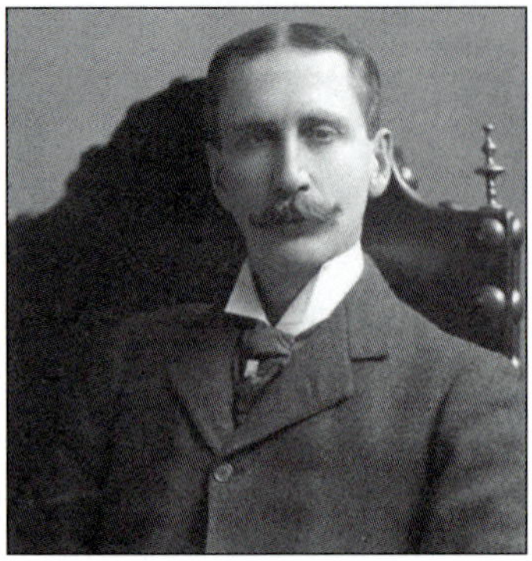

Fig 13-21 Edward H. Angle.

Edward Angle

The individual who did more to systematize and bring order to the often-chaotic state of affairs in orthodontic practice was Dr Edward H. Angle (Fig 13-21). Assessing the state of orthodontic care at the close of the 19th century, he wrote:

> *Two plans are now followed in the designing and construction of regulating appliances. The first is based upon the belief that each case so radically differs from all other cases that an appliance must be invented and constructed from raw material to meet its special requirements. The second plan recognizes the division of malocclusion into a few clearly defined classes, with requirements of treatment clearly indicated by each class, and having fixed standard forms of ready-made regulating appliances acting upon definite principles, which amply provide for all requirements of all cases belonging to each class. The first plan is the one that has been most universally employed, and has come down to us from the earliest history of orthodontia; indeed the greater part of the literature of the science consists of descriptions of appliances which have been invented to accomplish tooth movements in special cases until some thousands are recorded, one author alone boasting of many hundred.*[3] *Although much may be accomplished in skillful hands following this plan, it should require no argument to prove that for many reasons it is most defective and unscientific.*[27]

The first plan, according to Angle, was empiric, requiring the invention of a new apparatus for each specific case. It was a tedious and

[3] Angle is probably referring to Farrar, a chief competitor for leadership in the new field of orthodontics.

costly system that often resulted in failure. In contrast, the second plan (Angle's plan) "recognizes the practicability of fixed, standard forms of devices for performing the different tooth movements necessary in all the various classes of malocclusion having been arrived at as a result of careful experimentation and close observation." He went on:

> *Instead of handmade productions by the dentist, which, with his limited experience and meager facilities must always fall far short of the ideal in delicacy of proportion, temper, accuracy of fit and interchangeability of parts and in finish, they are made upon the elaborate machinery, like fine watches or high-class dental or surgical instruments, by the most skilled workmen who have become experts, not only through natural ability but from close study and long experience, ensuring the most perfect product at the minimum of expense.*[27;4]

After many years of dealing with a vast array of appliances, Angle concluded that "force was exerted upon misaligned teeth in one of three ways, namely by pushing, pulling, or twisting." Based on these three applications of force, it occurred to Angle that "it might be possible to construct a few instruments of simple form and standard pattern which would meet the requirements of all cases."[27] He then devised three instruments, one for each type of force application, "each of form to admit of almost universal application, and all to be of standard pattern; delicate yet efficient, with interchangeable parts, to be attached to the teeth used as anchorage as well as to the teeth to be moved, by means of plain bands made from ribbons of band material."[27] Angle adapted the jack screw for pushing, the traction screw for pulling, and the lever for exerting rotary force. These were assembled along with auxiliary items (wire, small tubes, and band material) in kits made commercially available (Fig 13-22). Angle stated that these three devices were quickly recognized for their simplicity, efficiency, and range of ready adaptability and soon superseded the limitless number of old, made-to-suit-the-case forms of appliances. The new kits were being extensively used by dentists not only in the United States but also in other countries. In designing his appliances, Angle followed the principles of simplicity, delicacy, inconspicuousness, stability of attachments, and the use of nickel silver (German silver).[27]

Guilford, in discussing the fabrication of regulating appliances for sale to the profession, stated that the first effort in this endeavor was

[4] Here Angle, with a bit of sarcasm, quotes Farrar's prediction that simplified appliances would someday be commercially manufactured and readily available to the profession.

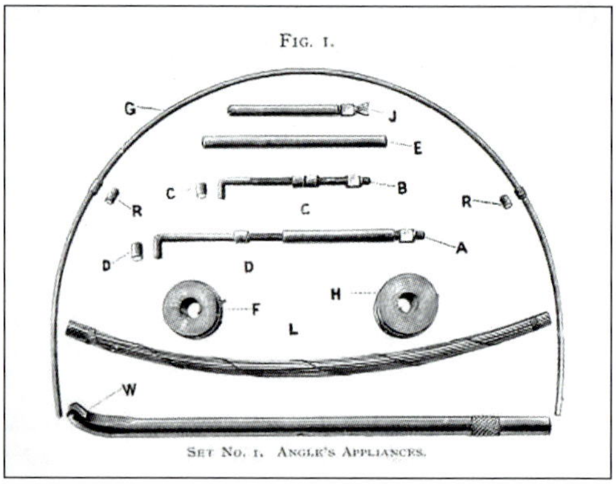

Fig 13-22 Angle's set no. 1, consisting of retaining wire (G), 10 sections of anchor pipes (R), traction screws (A and B), a jack screw (J), and band material (F and H). (From Angle, 1897.)

by Farrar in 1876[18] (see page 353). Dr Angle's systems were placed on the market in 1887, and they "met with such favor that with modifications and additions they have increased in popularity and are today more generally used than any other ready-to-wear appliances."[18]

Early on, Angle had recognized the significance of the occlusal relationship of the first molars to malocclusion.[28] This concept formed the keystone to his classification of malocclusions and the basis for appliance design and treatment. The first molars were to a large extent "the molders of the dental apparatus and the locators of all the other teeth. They are also the true points, and the only true points, from which to begin the study and diagnosis of all cases of malocclusion."[28] On the basis of the occlusion of the first molars, Angle devised a classification of the most common forms of malocclusion:

> *The first molars are in normal relationships when the mesio-buccal cusp of the upper occludes between and buccally to the mesio- and disto-buccal cusps of the lower, as shown in the normal occlusion [Fig 13-23]. It is only with this arrangement of the molars that it is possible for each subsequent tooth upon its eruption to assume its correct mesio-distal relation. However, the teeth anterior to the normally locked molars may, and often do, assume malpositions on their eruption.*[28]

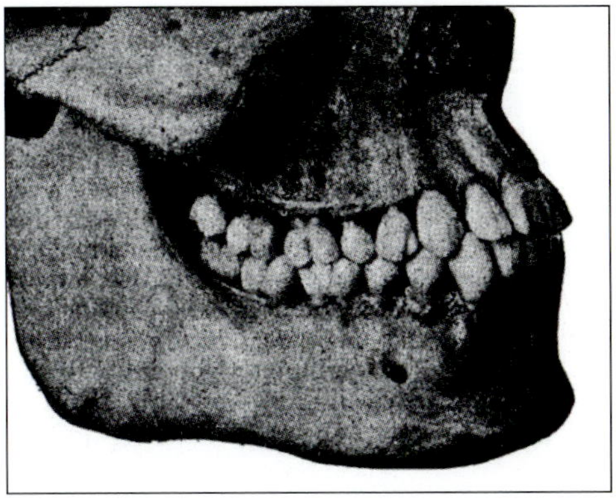

Fig 13-23 Correct occlusal relationship of the maxillary and mandibular first molars in Class I cases. (From Angle.[28])

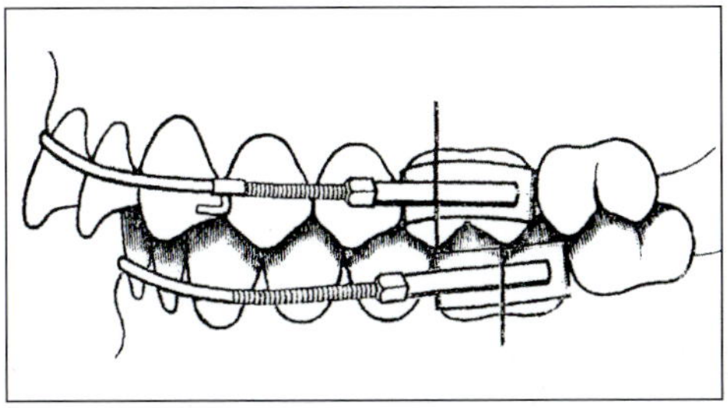

Fig 13-24 First molars in a Class II relationship. (From Angle.[28])

These types of malocclusions he classified as Class I malocclusions. Furthermore:

> *If the lower first molars in eruption should lock with their antagonists distally to normal, the entire misarrangement of all the other teeth must result. All of the remaining lower teeth will be forced to take positions of distal occlusion to those of the upper and there will be complete malarrangement and malocclusion of each occlusal plane both anterior and posterior to the first molars.*[28]

These conditions he called Class II malocclusions (Fig 13-24). But if "the lower first molars in erupting take their positions mesially to normal, each lower tooth subsequently erupting is forced to take a position mesial to normal in its relation to the upper teeth." These conditions he called Class III malocclusions (Fig 13-25).

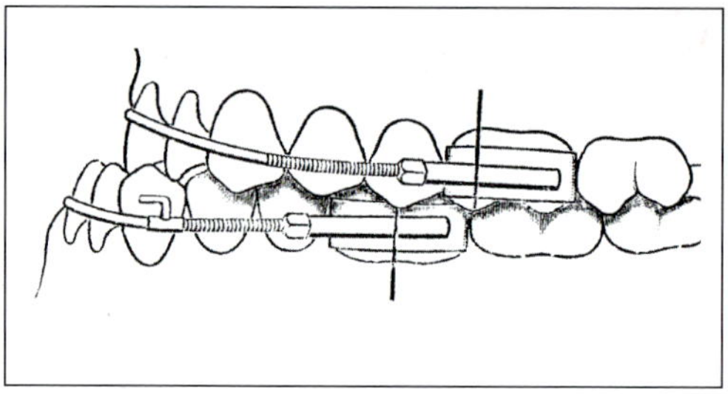

Fig 13-25 First molars in a Class III relationship. (From Angle.[28])

Impressed with the work of Dr Frederick Noyes in the area of histology, Angle was struck with the discovery that bone grew as a result of mechanical stimulation.[29] He had come to the conclusion that malocclusion was due to a lack or a perversion of bone growth. A corollary of this realization was the belief that, with the proper appliance, bone could be remodeled and teeth moved bodily in the jaw:

> *Instead of tipping the crowns of the teeth into the line of occlusion and leaving the roots at abnormal angles of inclination, to be adjusted by nature during the period of retention, the teeth should be moved bodily, as a result of force so gentile and so evenly distributed as to stimulate normal cellular activity and growth of bone. In other words, the work of the orthodontist should be the intelligent assisting of nature in her process of developing bone, thus making it possible for her to normally build the denture in its entirety.*[30]

These ideas led to his invention of the "working retainer" as the means of stimulating bone growth.[29] This appliance used very gentle pressure rather than pronounced force to stimulate bone modeling, a method supported, according to Angle, by the work of Dr Albin Oppenheim of Vienna, whose experiments in moving teeth in monkeys revealed the activity of bone remodeling in response to pressure.

Tooth Movement and Extraction

James David McCoy, in his book *Applied Orthodontia* (1922), stated:

> *It is a lamentable fact that teeth are constantly being moved by those who have but a vague knowledge of the processes involved within the tissues, their ideas and aims being wholly mechanical and empirical in nature. If it were not for the fact that the structures involved are capable of standing considerable abuse, more damaging results would be brought to light than are demonstrable at the present time.*[31]

It behooved those who intended to practice orthodontia to gain a thorough knowledge of the biology of bone and bone cells. According to McCoy, "Those unwilling to do this have no moral right to attempt orthodontic operations." He noted that up until the experiments of Oppenheim, which explained tissue changes occurring incident to tooth movement, none were based on anatomical or histologic research but rather relied on theoretical considerations and ingenious deductions.[31] The net result of Oppenheim's research was to demonstrate that physiologic tooth movement was achieved by constant application of light forces. Strong forces caused injury to the circulation and the periosteum and retarded the intended tooth movement.

Calvin Case

The bodily movement of teeth was first reported by Dr Calvin Case in 1893, but it took 20 years for his ideas to be fully accepted.[32] Case reviewed the application of his "contouring apparatus" as a method for correcting facial deformities in conjunction with the bodily movement of teeth before the European Orthodontia Society in 1914. In the discussion that followed Dr Case's presentation, it was noted by Dr A. Rubbrecht of Brussels that the contouring apparatus was useful only for the bodily movement of the six front teeth and that the new Angle appliance could be applied to the movement of all the teeth. Dr E. A. Bogue of New York City commended Dr Case for enunciating the principle that "a tooth must be moved bodily and kept upright." But Bogue was critical in that Dr Case had been too prone to advocate extractions and had not related his failures.[32]

Edward Angle

In contrast to Kingsley's acceptance that extractions were often permissible, Angle believed that the loss of teeth by extraction was responsible for many cases of malocclusion and disharmony of the face:

> *The interdependence of the teeth is so great at all times that the loss of one or more at any period of their history must have a marked influence upon the remaining teeth. Each tooth is such an important part of occlusion that its laws should be seriously considered before deciding upon its removal. Occasionally we hear of someone advocating the sacrifice of the first permanent molar as a prevention of or cure for malocclusion. The author has yet to see a single case where the loss of this tooth has not been followed by malocclusion.*[27]

For Angle, the loss of no other tooth was followed by so many evil effects as when the permanent first molar was removed. He also condemned the extraction of lateral incisors and canines:

> *The evil effects arising from extraction of the upper lateral incisors in order to provide space in the crowded arch for the canines are so apparent that arguments against the practice seem out of place in a modern textbook. The abnormal appearance given the face in the region of the nose consequent upon the diminished size of the upper jaw, together with the carnivorous appearance of the mouth by the resulted prominence of the canines is as repulsive as it is inexcusable. Still greater deformities are caused by the inexcusable practice of sacrificing the permanent canine. Indeed the enormous prevalence of the practice of extraction of teeth by dentists of this and other countries is a reflection upon the degree of their comprehension of the science of dentistry. Radical reform in this respect or to be instituted. The trivial excuses often given by men of high standing in dentistry for extraction of teeth are amazing.*[27]

Guilford emphasized that "premature loss of anyone of the deciduous set may be but the paving of the way for an irregularity in the permanent set," while "the diminishing of the size of a crown by extensive caries will tend toward the same by lessening the size of the arch." Therefore, he argued that "No deciduous tooth should be prematurely lost if at all possible" and that "in any loss of tooth substance through caries the part affected should be restored to its original outlines by filling; only in this way can we preserve the size of the arches."[18]

On the all-important question of extraction in orthodontia, Guilford noted the following:

> *The results of the practice are so far-reaching that we must be careful not to err in deciding whether to resort to it or not in cases that come to us for treatment. It would be unfair and possibly misleading to say that any particular line of practice is only good or wholly bad, or that it should always be practiced or never. The resort to extraction in the treatment of cases of irregularity was at one time quite common but careful observation of the results has caused it to fall more and more into disfavor. Experience has taught that it is very seldom necessary*

and that while it does simplify the procedure it does so usually at the expense of other valuable desiderata.[18]

Orthodontic technique had reached such a high point at the turn of the 20th century that Guilford could claim that "scarcely any deformity of the mouth and teeth is beyond mechanical remedy."[18]

Orthodontics As a Specialty

Angle felt sure that orthodontia had made its greatest progress since the introduction of his fixed, standard forms of ready-made regulating appliances. With the availability of the new commercially manufactured appliances, dentists were no longer faced by a confusing array of appliances but could devote their time to mastering standard devices that were readily available. The introduction of his system would also have benefits in the dental curriculum:

There was simply no system or order, and the difficulties and discouragements in teaching orthodontia at that time can at this date hardly be comprehended....A few of the writers and teachers, it is true, are still linking the present with the past in commending to dental students the acquirement of skill in the construction of regulating appliances, which can only be very crude at best. The custom is archaic and illogical, and the long, tedious hours which students are usually compelled to devote to their making, should by a more advanced standard of teaching be directed to purposes more in keeping with the requirements of true orthodontia. The successful, up-to-date orthodontist classes himself on a different plane from that of a mechanic.[33]

Angle, based on his understanding of the complexity of orthodontia and the failure of the dental school curriculum to adequately prepare graduates to provide orthodontic care, made strong arguments for teaching orthodontics as a specialty divorced from the rest of dentistry. Commenting on the teaching of orthodontia to the alumni association of Tufts College in 1902, Angle stated the following:

In a very large percentage of schools in this country it is of the most superficial character, being made secondary, both in teaching and appointments, to all else in the school, and that students on leaving college usually possess about as accurate a knowledge of orthodontia as of astrology, for the teaching is usually without system and has been truly said to begin nowhere and end nowhere...a smattering knowledge of orthodontia is of the least use. I believe such knowledge, besides being of practically no benefit, is more often positively harmful.[33]

The end result of the dental school experience was that few dentists understood orthodontia or could intelligently practice it. The remedy was to establish separate schools of orthodontia where a minimum of a year-long exposure to all phases of the subject would be offered to graduates of dental and/or medical schools. The Angle School of Orthodontia was opened in 1900 in St Louis and later moved to Pasadena, California, in 1922.[34]

In considering the advances that had been made in the field of orthodontics during the early 20th century, Frederick B. Noyes suggested that key advances were the development of techniques for "using the support of the bone on the apical third of the root as a means of tipping the crowns distally" and for bodily movement of teeth. Furthermore, Noyes stated that the development of appliances for moving all of the teeth together to correct malocclusions was the greatest advance in orthodontic thought, "accounting more than any other one thing for the possible reduction in the necessary time of treatment."[35]

Recounting his experience in orthodontics, Noyes underlined the fact that there were different fundamental philosophies underlying the practice of dentistry and orthodontia. Noyes said that after about 10 years of practicing orthodontics as part of his dental practice, he came across Angle's school of orthodontia:

> *I knew at the end of the first week that I had not the most fundamental conceptions of orthodontia; that I was thinking of alignment and of occlusion in the sense of teeth hitting together, and of the moving of teeth without any reference to whether that was where they belonged in the denture or not. I had little conception of the denture as a unit and less knowledge of the forces involved in its development. I quit practicing orthodontia. I went home and did not undertake another orthodontic treatment until I gave up the practice of dentistry.*[35]

Causes of Misalignment

Many dental misalignments were acquired following birth due to a wide variety of causes. Long retention of primary teeth or early loss of primary teeth were known to alter the normal eruption pathway and/or sequencing and space for replacement teeth. Delayed eruption of permanent teeth, the presence of supernumerary teeth, and the injudicious extraction of primary and permanent teeth were common causes of misaligned teeth. Developmental abnormalities in contiguous parts of the face and nasal apparatus were associated with abnormalities of the jaws and teeth. Mouth breathing caused by adenoidal growths led to formation of a high palatal arch and anterior crowding.

Thumb and lip sucking, when allowed to continue over a long time, caused elevation of the hard palate and flaring of the maxillary incisors. Beyond these rather obvious etiologies, there was a great deal of confusion over the inheritance of dental disharmonies.

During the latter half of the 19th century, when scientific research had yet to make its impact on dentistry, there was a great deal of pseudoscientific speculation on the causes of dental disharmonies. Farrar expressed that race was a factor:

> *It was widely held that abnormalities in the size of the teeth and jaws were caused by intermingling of the races. The union of different races, types, nationalities, physical characteristics as to size, etc., cannot but be detrimental to general harmony of structure in the offspring. That such unions do not bring about an orderly blending of the forms and qualities of the parents, but rather an apparently hap-hazard and often in harmonious combination of them, is too frequently noticed to need much argument.*[24]

He further noted that in "all nations that have lived within themselves for a great length of time, and that seldom intermarry with people of other nations, are generally harmonious in their anatomical structures, thus teaching the advantage of marriage within the same type." For example, he argued:

> *The teeth and jaws of Italians are seldom irregular; the same may also be said of the Chinese. Wherever there is the crossing of types, so common in the United States, a nation made up of all nationalities, irregularity of teeth naturally follows. In parts of New England, prior to 1850, when there was but little mixing of other nationalities with the Puritan stock, the relations of the jaws were in better proportion with the other parts of the physique, and the teeth were more regular, than was the case in and about the cosmopolitan city of New York.*[24]

Similarly, Guilford wrote in 1905:

> *The Teutons, Anglo-Saxons and Scandinavians have large frames and large teeth while the Latin races have smaller bodies and similar teeth. In the United States, where mal-arrangement of the teeth seems to be unusually common we have constant intermarriage of members of the European races.*[18]

Eugene Talbot, in his book entitled *Osseous Deformities of the Head, Face, Jaws and Teeth*, revealed his extreme ideas on the origin and causes of such pathologies. He devoted chapters to deformities of the jaw as seen in criminals; prostitution and sexual degeneracy; moral insanity, pauperism, and inebriety; intellectual degeneracy; neurotics; idiocy; consanguinity of parents; and intemperance.[23] By the end of the first decade of the 20th century, the talk of racial mixing as a cause of dental malocclusions seemed to fade away as more scientific conceptions came forward.

Summary

In the space of about 40 years, orthodontia progressed from a confusing assortment of mechanical inventions for regulating teeth into a system for bodily movement of large numbers of teeth in concert with improvement of facial esthetics. Progress in the science of bone physiology explained the tissue changes activated by the application of orthodontic force and revealed the potential for tension-induced bone growth in the jaws. Orthodontics became recognized as a special branch of dentistry taught at the postdoctoral level. The attempt to place the cause of dental irregularities on the mixing of the races or on the declining moral values of city dwellers was proven false as the science of human development progressed from pure speculation to factual explanations arrived at by scientific research.

References

1. Weinberger BW. Orthodontic bibliotheca. Dent Cosmos 1921;63:1126–1140.
2. Lindsay L. The Surgeon Dentist; Or, Treatise on the Teeth by Pierre Fauchard (as translated from the French). Pound Ridge, NY: Milford House, 1969.
3. Weinberger BW. The history of orthodontia. Int J Orthodontia 1916;2:103–117.
4. Bourdet E. Recherche et observations sur toutes les parties de l'art du dentiste. Paris: J. T. Herissant, 1757.
5. Bunon R. Experiences et demonstrations faites a l'hopital de la salpetriere et a S. Come en preferences de l'academie royale de chirurgie. Paris: Briasson, 1746.
6. Fox J. The Natural History and Diseases of the Human Teeth. London: T. Plummer, 1803.
7. Fox J. The History and Treatment of the Diseases of the Teeth, the Gums, and the Alveolar Processes, with the Operations Which They Respectively Require. London: Thomas Cox, 1806.
8. Delabarre CF. Traite de la partie mecanique de l'art du chirurgien-dentiste. Ouvrage orne de 42 planches. Paris: Croullebois, Gabon et Mequignon-Marvis, 1820.
9. Serres A. Essai sur l'anatomie et la physiologie des dents. Paris: Mequinon-Marvis, 1817.
10. Miel EM. Recherches sur l'art de diriger la seconde dentition. Paris: Firmin Didot, 1826.
11. Magitot E. Traite des anomalies du systeme dentaire ches l'homme et les mammiferes. Paris: L'Academie de Medecine, 1877.
12. Lefoulon J. Nouveau traite theorique et pratique de l'art du dentiste. Paris: Fortin, Masson et Cie, 1841.

13. Maury F. Traite complet de l'art du dentiste d'apres l'etat actuel des connaissances. Paris: Rouvier, 1841.
14. Harris CA. The Principles and Practice of Dental Surgery. Philadelphia: Lindsay and Blakiston, 1845.
15. Harris C. The Principles and Practice of Dentistry. Philadelphia: P. Blakiston, Son, and Co, 1882.
16. Westcott A. A case of irregularity. Dent Cosmos 1860;1:60–68.
17. Coffin WH. A generalized treatment of irregularities. Dent Cosmos 1882;24:463–471.
18. Guilford SH. Orthodontia or Malposition of the Human Teeth: Its Prevention and Remedy, ed 4. Philadelphia: T. C. Davis & Sons, 1905.
19. Flagg JF. Orthodontia. Dent Cosmos 1866;7:14–15,64–66,468–469.
20. Kingsley NW. A Treatise on Oral Deformaties As a Branch of Mechanical Dentistry. New York: D. Appleton, 1880.
21. Kingsley NW. Treatment of irregularities. Dent Cosmos 1872;14:62–65.
22. Ottolengui R. Norman William Kingsley, M.D.S., D.D.S. Dent Items Interest 1913;35:308–313.
23. Talbot ES. Irregularities of the Teeth and Their Treatment. Philadelphia: P. Blakiston, Son, & Co, 1888.
24. Farrar JN. A Treatise on the Irregularities of the Teeth and Their Correction. New York: The De Vinne, 1888.
25. Asbell MB. A brief history of orthodontics. Am J Orthod Dentofacial Orthop 1990;98:176–183.
26. Ottolengui R. Dr. John Nutting Farrar, D.D.S., M.D. Dent Items Interest 1913;35:547–550.
27. Angle EH. Treatment of Malocclusion of the Teeth. Philadelphia: S. S. White, 1907.
28. Angle EH. The importance of the first molars in their relation to orthodontia. Dent Cosmos 1903;45:173–178.
29. Angle EH. Bone-growing. Dent Cosmos 1910;52:261–267.
30. Angle EH. Evolution of orthodontia—Recent developments. Dent Cosmos 1912;54:853–866.
31. McCoy JD. Applied Orthodontia. Philadelphia: Lea & Febiger, 1922.
32. Case CS. The bodily movement of teeth in orthodontia. Dent Cosmos 1916;58:877–893.
33. Angle EH. Orthodontia as a specialty. Dent Cosmos 1902;64:905–910.
34. Hoffmann-Axthelm W. History of Dentistry. Chicago: Quintessence, 1981.
35. Noyes FB. Undergraduate teaching of orthodontia. Dent Cosmos 1930;72:514–524.

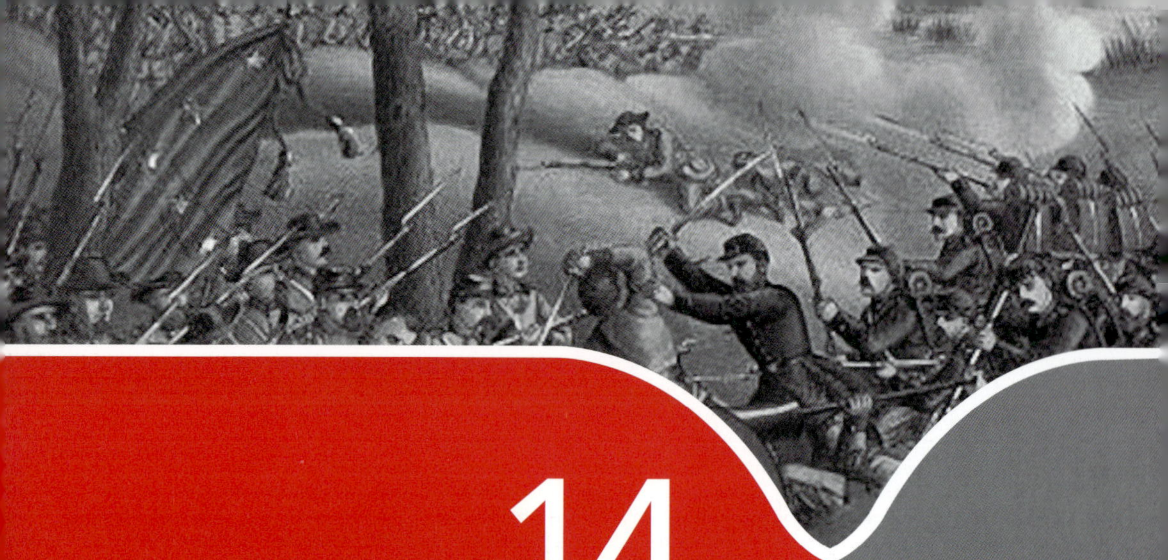

14

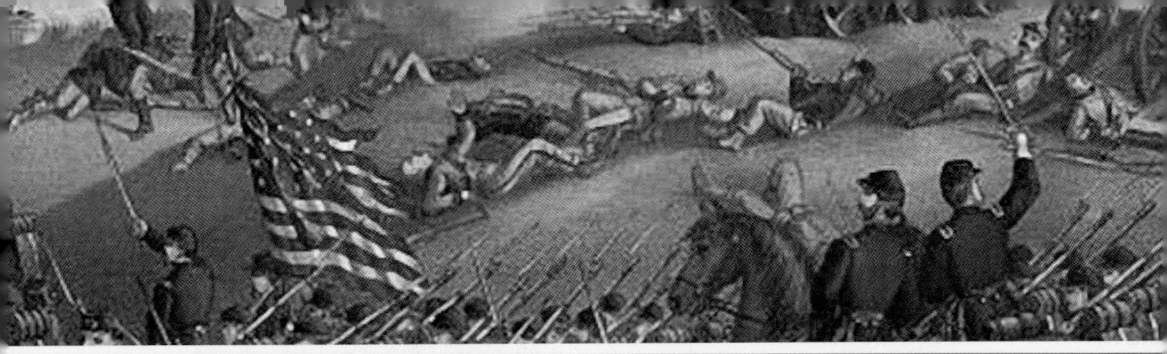

Oral Surgery and Oral Radiology

Surgery of the oronasal region can be traced to da Vinci's anatomical descriptions of the mouth and nasal sinuses in 1489 and in the more detailed treatise of Nathanial Highmore in 1651.[1] Early recognition of the association of chronic sinusitis with dental infections led to the development of surgical approaches to establish drainage, irrigation, and medication of the maxillary sinuses. William Cowper is given credit for curing a maxillary sinus infection by gaining access through the alveolar socket. During the 16th to 18th centuries, German and French surgeons described several surgical methods for dealing with diseases of the oronasal region, including the correction of cleft lip and palate.[1] It was not until 1778 that a comprehensive description of the scope of oronasal surgery was attempted with the publication of Anselme Jourdain's *Traite des maladies et des operations reellement chirurgicales de la bouche, et des parties qui y correspondent*.[1] Jourdain noted that no complete description of the treatment and management of the surgical diseases of the mouth existed. According to him, there were many isolated, fragmented, and "chaotic" contributions to this part of surgery, yet no one had yet assembled a comprehensive description of the field. Jourdain maintained that effective surgical treatment of diseases of the mouth required special, and often unique,

[1] A Treatise on the Diseases and Surgical Operations of the Mouth and All Contiguous Parts.

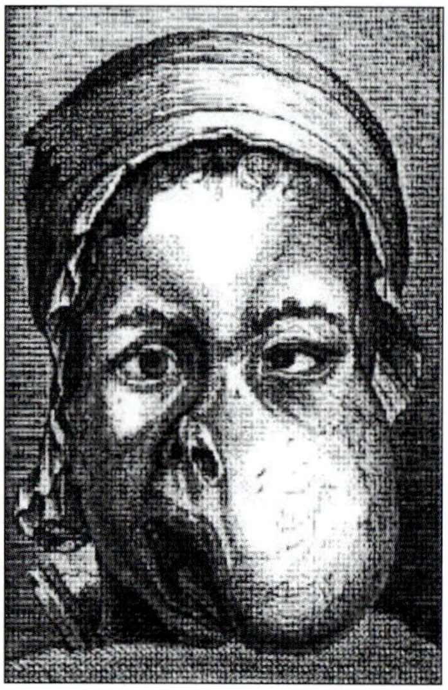

Fig 14-1 Case of a solid tumor of the maxillary sinus of a young child. Jourdain, supported in consultation by the chief surgeons of the Hotel Dieu, La Charite, and Les Invalides (the three major hospitals in Paris), decided that the lesion was inoperable. (From Jourdain.[2])

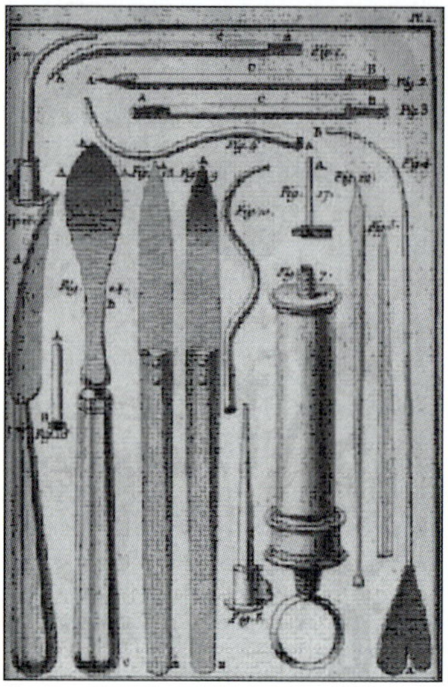

Fig 14-2 Instruments for perforating the maxillary sinus from the alveolar route and probing the sinuses, cannulas and syringes for introducing medications and lavage of the sinuses, and lancets and scalpels for extirpation.

techniques. General surgeons, otherwise of established merit, often failed when attempting treatment of oral lesions using routine methods.[2] Although Jourdain praised Fauchard for his description of the mechanical art of dentistry, he found him and his contemporaries deficient in knowledge of oral surgery.

In his treatise, Jourdain provided an extensive discussion of the various diseases affecting the maxillary sinuses (Fig 14-1), the interrelationship with carious molars, and the various routes of access to the sinuses for introducing medications and establishing drainage of purulent exudates. Like many of the pioneers of surgery, Jourdain developed special instruments (Fig 14-2). He cautioned against overaggressive surgery, favoring conservative medical regimens whenever possible. Like several contemporary surgeons, Jourdain advised against unnecessary shedding of blood in cases that were unlikely to benefit from surgery. Although he included case reports to support his treatment modalities, Jourdain failed to provide the anatomical and technical illustrations that would have greatly aided his readers and improved his treatise.

Contending that the mouth was the window to the body, Jourdain maintained that oral diseases were often early indications of more

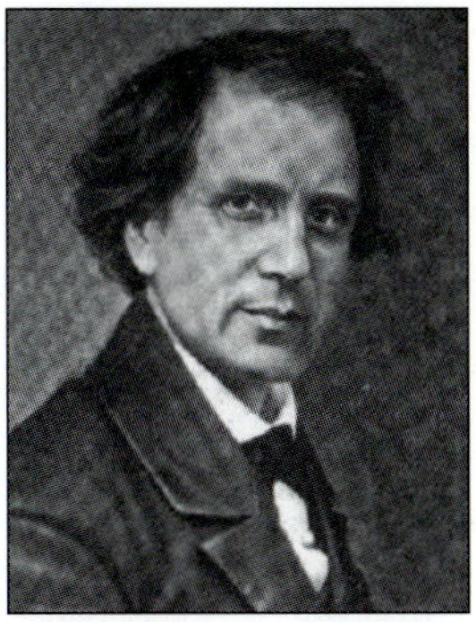

Fig 14-3 Simon Hullihen.

serious systemic diseases, such as syphilis, scurvy, and malignant fevers. He stated that failure to recognize and deal with certain types of oral diseases until they involved the eyes, ears, or nose or impaired the ability to masticate and swallow food often resulted in death of the patient.

In the United States, in the period following the Civil War, oral surgery was practiced as a special branch of surgery by a small number of physicians who also practiced or had developed knowledge of dentistry. These men formed an unofficial network, engaging one another at dental or medical association meetings, sharing their common interests in dealing with congenital diseases or traumatic injuries to the teeth, jaws, and facial region. From this group, there arose several leaders who were to define the domain of the oral surgeon and in the process effect changes in dental education. Two of the earliest were Simon Hullihen and James E. Garretson.[3,4]

Simon Hullihen

Simon Hullihen (Fig 14-3), born in 1810, was attracted to medicine early in life, reading every medical book he could get his hands on, until he attended and graduated from Washington Medical College in 1832.[5] He established his practice of medicine and dentistry in Wheeling, West Virginia, where he soon became noted for his skill in plastic and oral surgery. Hullihen's notebooks, listing the scope of his practice during the last 10 years of his life, reveal that he performed 100 operations for cleft lip, 50 for cleft palate, 150 for cancer, 200 for diseases of the antrum, and 85 for plastic reconstruction of lips, noses, and mandibles. In addition, he performed hundreds of general surgeries and cataract operations.[5] Hullihen published case reports in the earliest editions of the *American Journal of Dental Science* and lectured at the Baltimore College of Dental Surgery. Prior to entering medicine, Hullihen worked as a silversmith, perfecting mechanical skills that later helped him design and fabricate special dental appliances used for wound stabilization and facial reconstruction.[6]

Hullihen became renowned for his skill in operating on cleft lip and cleft palate patients at a time when inhalation anesthesia had yet to be discovered. He introduced "adhesive straps" to assist in closure of the alveolar arch by exerting constant forward tension on the jaw bones.[5] He advocated operating on cleft lip cases at an early age:

> *I am therefore, decidedly in favor of early operations on infants, for the cure of harelip [cleft lip]. I have operated on thirteen cases before dentition had commenced; three infants of this number were only four weeks old; and I have yet to witness the first untoward event, or the slightest unfavorable indication resulting to an infant from the operation.*[7]

Hullihen is also known to have invented several instruments and was held in acclaim for his description of the surgical correction of a severe facial deformity caused by a burn. Treatment of this case involved resection of the mandible, immobilization with a specially fabricated silver plate, reestablishment of the lower lip, and elevation of a skin flap from the shoulder to correct skin defects created during the release of the wound contractions.[5] In 1843, Hullihen received the honorary degree of DDS from the Baltimore College of Dental Surgery.

In addition to his skill as an oral surgeon, Hullihen gained recognition for his community service. With the help of Bishop Richard Whelan and the Sisters of Saint Joseph, Hullihen founded a patient-care facility that later evolved into the Wheeling Hospital of Wheeling, West Virginia.[6]

James E. Garretson

James E. Garretson (Fig 14-4) is generally hailed as the founder of the specialty of oral surgery. At 22 years old, he entered a dental apprenticeship in Wilmington, Delaware, and later completed dental school at the Philadelphia College of Dental Surgery in 1856. After establishing his dental practice in Philadelphia, Garretson attended

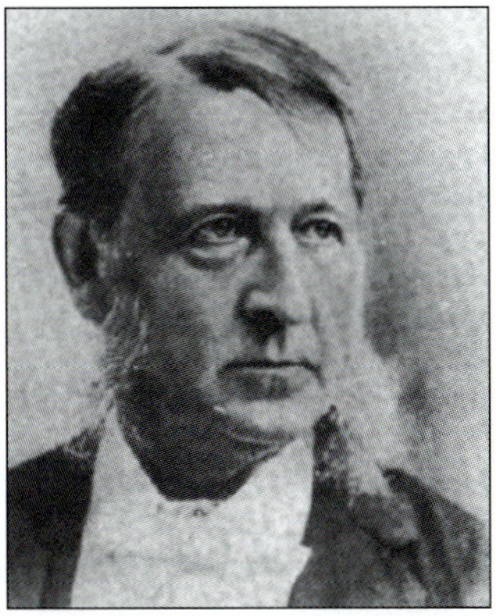

Fig 14-4 James E. Garretson.

the University of Pennsylvania, earning his MD degree in 1859.[8] Combining the mechanical dexterity of a dentist with his medical education, Garretson perfected surgery of the orofacial region.

In 1870, Garretson was appointed lecturer in the newly established lectureship on oral and associated surgery at University of Pennsylvania.[9] His clinical lectures, open to both medical and dental students, were held every Wednesday, forming the basis of nearly 100 publications in *Dental Cosmos*. In 1869, Garretson published *A Treatise on the Diseases and Surgery of the Mouth, Jaws, and Associated Parts*, a monumental textbook that defined the territory and scope of the specialty of oral surgery. It was later expanded and better illustrated under the new title *A System of Oral Surgery*. The editors of *Dental Cosmos* declared: "Dr. Garretson's new work furnishes the missing link needed to unite dentistry with medicine and surgery, supplying a deficiency on either side, and creating, if we mistake not, a new specialty,—that of Oral Surgery—in which, at a time not remote, the dentistry of today will be merged and lost."[10] The 1,364-page fifth edition was praised by the *New York Independent Practitioner*: "So much new matter has been introduced as to make it obligatory upon every dentist, who desires to keep abreast of the advance of thought, to add the latest edition of the standard work to his library."[11] The *Dental Practitioner* stated that "could the dental profession have but one of the textbooks now in existence, Garretson's 'System of Oral Surgery' would be, *par excellence*, the book."[2] The editors of *Dental Cosmos* hailed the new edition with a glowing review:

[2] Quoted in volume 4 of the Philadelphia medical quarterly *International Clinics* in 1894.

> *This is in fact the only book in print entitled to be denominated a system of oral surgery. This much may fairly be said, without detracting from the merits of the various dental text-books which had preceded it; for, however complete they may have been in the particular sphere which they designed to fill, none have aimed to furnish, associated with ordinary instruction in dental manipulations, compact and comprehensive teaching of the physiology and pathology of contiguous parts with the therapeutic and surgical indications for treatment. We cannot omit calling attention to the happy faculty by which the author leads his reader, from a consideration of the elementary facts involved, to a full appreciation of the subject treated upon; so that the student can find here rudimentary lessons, and the practitioner, seeking information about complex operations, can fortify himself by precedents. A capital illustration of this faculty is afforded in the author's consideration of tumors. We know of no chapter in medicine in which a complex subject is treated more philosophically; none more successful in rendering an obscure class of abnormities thoroughly comprehensible. This book, therefore, fills a hitherto unoccupied place in the literature of the profession, and bridges the chasm which has separated dentistry from medicine; for, while it aims to present whatever is directly and practically important in the more ordinary manipulations of the office, even to an extent which to some may seem unnecessary and tedious, it leads the inquirer to a comprehension of pathological and therapeutical truths,—the rationale of conditions and of treatment as the author understands them."*[10]

The reception across the Atlantic was quite different. The *Journal of the British Dental Association* in 1891 faulted Garretson for including material

> *not commonly included under the heading of oral surgery... skin diseases, keloid of neck, gumma of forehead, ringworm, ligature of occipital artery, fractures and trephining of skull, neuralgia of lumbar muscles due to uterine trouble, the diagnosis of aortic aneurism and diseases of lungs, matters which, however interesting, can scarcely be regarded as coming within the scope of the title.*[11]

Passages were quoted to illustrate vagueness, inaccuracies, and scientific errors, after which was written the following:

> *After reading our quotations, no one can be surprised that we should endorse the opinion which we expressed about a previous edition as applying equally to the present one. The general anatomy, pathology and surgery are so incomplete as to in no wise take the place of the current text-books upon those subjects, while the dental anatomy, as far as it is attempted at all, is generally inaccurate and often ridiculous. At times during its perusal we were forcibly reminded of De Quincey's excitement over a German life of Shakespeare, when he read a passage*

> *and then rushed to the window, flung it open, and called loudly for the police.*[11]

Garretson, professor of anatomy and surgery of the Philadelphia Dental College and oral surgeon of the hospital of the University of Pennsylvania, was soon acclaimed to be America's foremost authority in this "new" special branch of dentistry and medicine. He gave the discipline the name "oral surgery" and made it an important component of the dental curriculum.[4] In his short biography of Garretson, dental historian R. C. Koch wrote:

> *The whole complexion of his operations, whether viewed as to their technique or as to the character of the results, differed essentially from the work done by any of his predecessors and the majority of his contemporaries. His work was distinctly conservative in character, always keeping in view the importance of the cosmetic feature of his results, and as a consequence his operations were designed and done with a distinct purpose to avoid to the utmost extent permanent mutilation.*[9]

Oral Surgery As a Specialty

Educated both as a dentist and as a physician, Garretson held the position that oral surgery was a medical specialty and that it encompassed dental surgery (ie, all mechanical and operative procedures as described in his textbook). This radical view created a great deal of controversy in both medical and dental educational circles. Most physicians viewed "oral surgeries" as just part of general surgery, not a special branch of dentistry, and much of what was described in Garretson's textbook could be found in textbooks of general surgery.[12,13] Operations on tumors and traumatic injuries to the jaws and mouth were normally performed by general surgeons. Bernard and Huette's extensive textbook of surgery, illustrated with numerous colored plates, described several operations on oral tissues, including repair of cleft lip and palate, and resection of tumors of the tongue, jaws, and maxillary sinuses (Fig 14-5). Among the surgeries described in Henry H. Smith's *The Principles and Practice of Surgery* are the following instructions for excisions of the mandible. Smith's terse directions summon the swift, solid incisions of the surgeon as he races against the clock:

> *Make a horizontal incision along the inferior border of the bone, extending from the symphysis to the angle of the jaw; make a vertical*

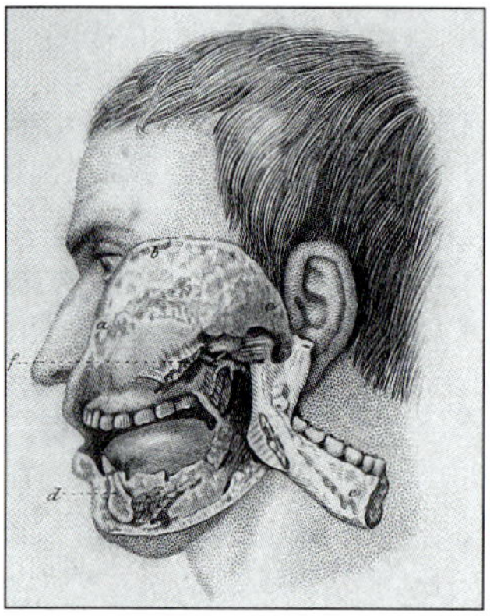

Fig 14-5 Resection of the mandible illustrated in Bernard and Huette's *Illustrated Manual of Operative Surgery and Surgical Anatomy.*[13]

> *section at each extremity of this incision; the internal, dividing the lower lip through the median line; the external, carried from the zygomatic arch behind the ramus of the jaw. This makes a quadrilateral flap, which is to be dissected and turned up. Saw through the jaw at the median line, and keeping close to the bone, detach with the bistoury all the soft parts adhering to its posterior surface as far as the angle of the jaw. Carry a probe pointed bistoury beneath the zygomatic arch and behind the coronoid process, and with it divide the tendon of the temporal muscle while depressing the bone to disengage the process and luxate the condyle. Pull the bone strongly outwards, as far as possible from the vessels, in order to avoid especially the internal maxillary artery, and complete the operation by dividing the pterygoid muscles and the articular ligaments. The whole, or only a part, of the horizontal portion of the lower jaw may be removed, according to the exigencies of the case.*[12]

In a time when there were no antibiotics and no general anesthetics, it is remarkable that patients survived such procedures. According to Smith, the operation had been performed more than forty times by American surgeons prior to 1860, and in 160 cases of resection of the mandible reported by the French surgeon Velpeau,[3] only forty resulted in death: "a success which is very great when compared with the serious character of the operation."[12]

Garretson proposed to consolidate such operations into a new specialty of oral surgery. In addressing the Association of the Colleges of Dentistry in 1866, Garretson, representing the Philadelphia Dental College, proclaimed that the "scientific attainments and sphere of duties" of dentists were too limited: "Graduates of dental colleges manifest to the world their inability to treat any disease outside of those associated with a few simple semi-vital organs, and which dis-

[3] Alfre-Armand Velpeau (1795–1867), chief of clinical surgery at the University of Paris.

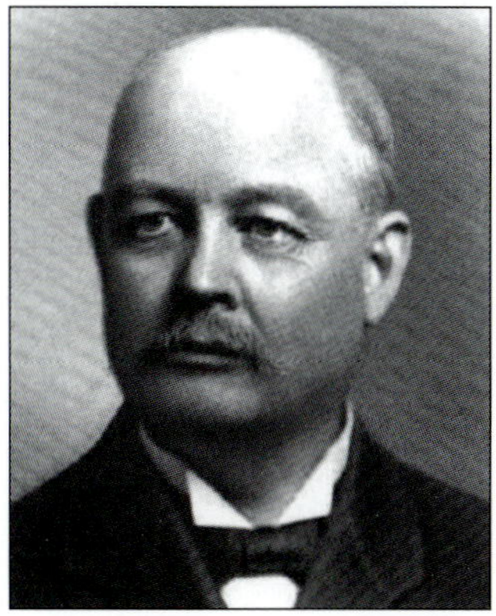

Fig 14-6 Eugene S. Talbot.

eases require for treatment much more the skill of a mechanician than that which the world recognizes as a doctor." In his enthusiasm to improve dentistry by elevating it to a specialty of medicine, Garretson recommended abolishing the DDS degree and, by expansion of dental curriculum, including medical training and qualifying new dental graduates for the MD degree and the title of oral surgeon. For Garretson, the term *dentist* was limiting and no longer reflective of the evolving and rapid growth of the profession. Koch noted that Garretson's textbook made "all departments of dental science and art a part of oral surgery and substitutes the title or designation of 'oral surgeon' and 'oral surgery' for 'dentist' or 'dental surgeon.'"[8] Garretson noted that the Philadelphia Dental College had evolved to correct this deficiency by instituting a new curriculum to include aspects of general surgery, with dissections and appropriate "demonstrative courses."[14] Its graduates were "surgeons by education, equal to any demand that emergencies may at any time make upon them, whether at the railway train, on the battlefield, or called hastily from the privacy of the office."

Pressure to increase the medical content of the dental school curriculum continued well into the 20th century. Many of the most successful dentists and oral surgeons of this period held the MD degree in addition to the DDS degree. Many deans of dental schools and department heads were both physicians as well as dentists. Dr Eugene S. Talbot[4] (Fig 14-6) had been a longtime advocate of greater

[4] Dr Eugene S. Talbot was a graduate of Pennsylvania College of Dental Surgery (1872) and the Rush Medical College (1880). A strong believer that dentistry should be a specialty of medicine, Talbot was instrumental in establishing chairs of dental and oral surgery in five medical colleges in Chicago and in creating the Section on Stomatology in the American Medical Association.[13]

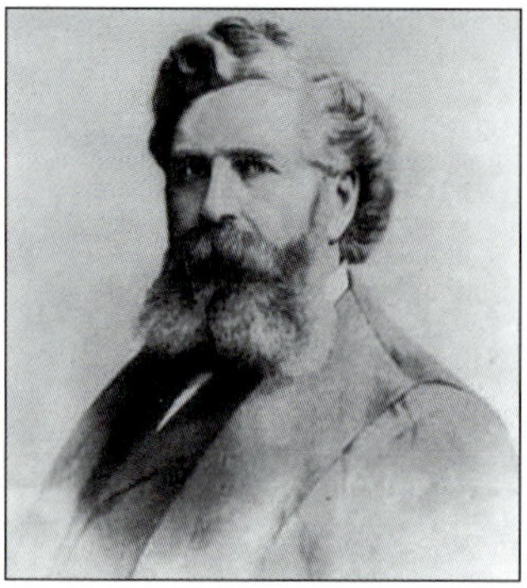

Fig 14-7 Truman W. Brophy.

exposure to medicine in the dental curriculum, even to the point that would qualify the dental student for the MD degree[15]:

> *All dental schools should be actual departments of universities, preferably state universities. The first year should be devoted to the fundamental branches of medicine, and due credit should be given for the same toward a future medical course. The student may now enter the dental school for two years and graduate with the degree of D.D.S. If he is desirous of continuing his studies in medicine and to become a stomatologist, he may now enter the medical school and finish his studies in this department, obtaining the M.D. degree.*[16]

Dr Truman W. Brophy,[5] (Fig 14-7) was a leading oral surgeon of the late 19th century, best known for the "Brophy operation" for correction of cleft palate and for his strong support of joint medical and dental education.[15] Brophy, founder and dean of the Chicago College of Dental Surgery, one of the largest dental schools in the United States, blamed excessive extraction of teeth on the failure to educate physicians in dental pathology:

> *The ruthless extraction of teeth is little less than criminal. An X-ray picture made by one who will attempt to make a diagnosis, though not educated in dental pathology, oftentimes seems to be a guide to the extraction specialist who declares that the patient has infected teeth and consequently removes them without further investigation. The X-ray specialist has been a most important factor in the community and has rendered a valuable service. Some are eminently qualified to make a diagnosis. But when one attempts to make a diagnosis, marking charts indicating morbid conditions which he often does not understand, and*

[5] Truman W. Brophy, a classmate of Talbot's (Pennsylvania College of Dental Surgery in 1872 and the Rush Medical College in 1880), joined him in advocating greater integration of medicine and dentistry.[13]

> *advises the patient to have certain teeth extracted, he is going too far and doing that which should be left only to the thoroughly educated man in this field of pathology.*[17]

In 1915, Brophy requested P. Blakiston's Son & Company to write to the leading medical colleges of this country and ask the following questions: "Have you a professor of oral surgery?" If so, "How many lecture hours per year, and how many clinical hours in oral surgery are given?" The results showed that

> *out of sixty-four replies, six were in the affirmative as to having a chair of oral surgery. It may easily be seen that persons suffering from dental diseases and getting opinions from medical men as to what should be done with their teeth, will continue to suffer and continue to sustain irreparable losses so long as the medical colleges fail to give their students instruction upon these subjects... The medical student should be taught the origin and development of the teeth, their minute anatomy and physiology, the many morbid conditions to which they are subject, the influence of certain diseases of the teeth upon the general health, their part in forming the initial lesions of trigeminal neuralgia; how to make a correct diagnosis of dental pulpitis.*[17]

Drs Talbot and Brophy were part of a small group of dentists/physicians who in 1881 led a successful effort to form a new special section on dentistry within the American Medical Association (AMA), later renaming it the Section of Stomatology.[18] The main objective of the Section of Stomatology was to introduce physicians to the ever-increasing clinical and basic dental science, particularly in view of the apparent association of dental diseases with systemic disorders.[19] The initial enthusiasm declined over time as attendance at the stomatology section meetings waned during annual AMA conventions: "Time and time again have excellent programs been prepared and presented to an audience so small as almost to discourage the essayist and embarrass the members."[19]

Part of the attendance problem resided in a failure to recruit dentists (with just a DDS degree) into the membership of this section. Dental school graduates who did not hold the additional MD degree were welcomed into the AMA and the Section of Stomatology but were enrolled as "associate members"; despite assurances that no discrimination was intended, many dentists saw the distinction as demeaning.[19]

The stomatology movement in the United States highlighted a significant problem: "Medicine leaves the oral cavity to dentistry, and dentistry, largely a technical procedure concerned with the preservation and restoration of tooth structure, does not adequately supplement medical science."[20] The no man's land between the two professions gained greater importance due to the upsurge of publicity given to the focal infection theory. Although the medical school curriculum continued to slight dental diseases, the dental school curriculum did eventually include greater exposure to medical and basic science; as a result, the DDS degree gained in stature (see chapter 17).

Dr Kurt Thoma, in reviewing the history of oral surgery, made the claim that oral surgery had become a "well established branch of dentistry...In spite of this fact, certain medical groups, perhaps because of economic conditions affecting their own field, are eyeing with envy the grass on the other side of the fence and, from a strictly legal point of view, trespass into a field and profession that are definitely not theirs."[4] Thoma felt confident that dentists as "rugged individualists" would protect oral surgery as a dental specialty. Oral surgery became an established part of dental education, with separate departments and clinics within most dental schools. Efforts to define the oral surgeon as strictly a "medically educated dentist or one who held both degrees" gradually lost importance.[9] By the turn of the century, dental school graduates who intended to specialize in oral surgery completed an additional year in a graduate program and 1 to 2 years of hospital internship.[4]

War and Oral Surgery

History teaches us that the development of surgery was closely related to treating wounded soldiers. Ambroise Paré perfected his techniques alongside the French armies of the 16th century. In the American Civil War, dentists and physicians were called upon to minister to great numbers of casualties, often involving disfiguring and critical head wounds. American oral surgery began rapid development after this period and would soon be called upon to progress to a new level in the battlefield hospitals of World War I.

The surgeon general of the United States reported that from the beginning of the Civil War to October 1864, there were 4,167 cases of gunshot wounds to the face, 107 proving fatal (mostly due to secondary hemorrhage).[21] The oral surgeon John H. McQuillen[6] recounts his experience in treating John McGouisk, aged 42 years, of the 83d Regiment of Pennsylvania Volunteers, who suffered a life-threatening facial wound by an exploding shell on June 2, 1864, at the Battle of Cold Harbor, Virginia (Fig 14-8).[7] Shell fragments had broken away parts of his maxilla and mandible, torn parts of the lower lip, and destroyed numerous teeth (Fig 14-9a). Hemorrhaging

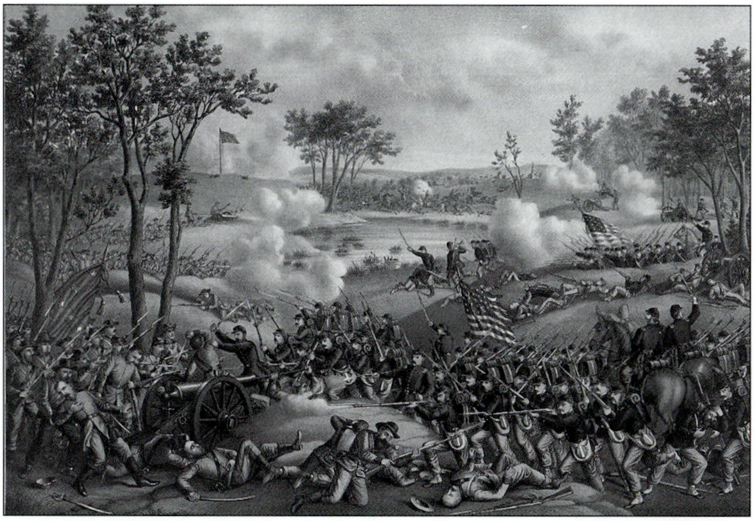

Fig 14-8 *Battle of Cold Harbor* by Kurz and Allison. (Courtesy of the United States Library of Congress.)

profusely, McGouisk was expected to die at a field hospital. But he survived. Six weeks later, he was transported back to Philadelphia, where he was placed under the care of Dr John McQuillen. Although some wound healing had occurred, McGouisk was in critical condition:

> *A portion of the lower lip had been lost, and what was left had fallen in and become adherent to the jaw. The incisors, canines, bicuspids, and their alveolar processes in the upper and lower maxillae had been carried away by the fragment of shell, leaving also a compound fracture of the lower jaw. The under surface of the tongue, from the tip, had become adherent to the lower jaw, while the fractured ends of the maxilla were drawn towards each other by the contraction of the mylohyoid muscle. The pressure of the lower molar teeth on the sides of the tongue produced constant irritation of that organ, which was very much swollen, so much so as to interfere with respiration. It was with great difficulty that the patient could swallow, being restricted to*

---

[6] John Hugh McQuillen studied dentistry as an apprentice to Elisha Townsend of Philadelphia. While in practice, he attended Jefferson Medical College, earning the MD degree in 1852. He received an honorary DDS degree from the Philadelphia College of Dental Surgery in 1853. McQuillen is best remembered as an organizer, prominently involved with the foundation of the American Dental Association, the Association of Colleges of Dentistry, and the Pennsylvania Dental Association. McQuillen also served as editor of *Dental Cosmos*.[8]

[7] Grant said of the battle in his memoirs, "I have always regretted that the last assault at Cold Harbor was ever made.…No advantage whatever was gained to compensate for the heavy loss we sustained."

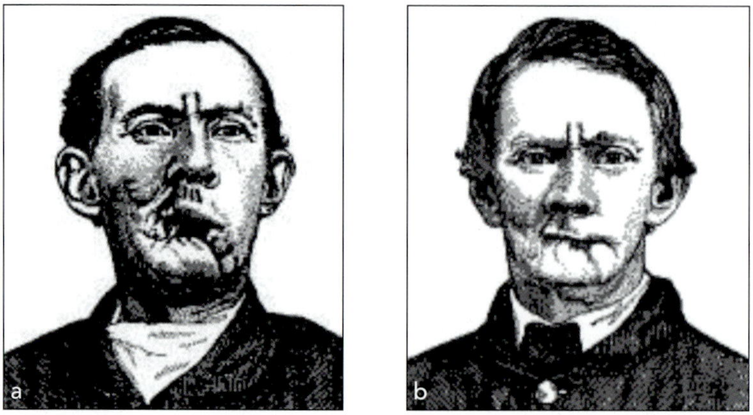

Fig 14-9 *(a)* John McGouisk as he presented upon arrival in Philadelphia. *(b)* McGouisk after surgical repairs by Dr McQuillen.

> *soft food. He could not articulate a word, and was compelled to make known his wants by writing on a slate.*[22]

McQuillen proceeded to remove the pressure of muscular contraction "by propping apart the fractured ends of the lower jaw," thereby allowing the tongue to slowly return to its normal size. Soon respiration and deglutition were markedly improved. A submandibular abscess was corrected when teeth that were no longer useful or infected were extracted. After performing plastic surgery to correct the V-shaped fissure of the upper lip, McQuillen performed an operation to restore the patient's speech and to correct the condition of the lower lip:

> *An incision an inch and a half in length and an inch in depth was made on the posterior side of the lower jaw, severing the unnatural relation existing between it and the tongue; this liberated that organ, and he was able to protrude the end of the tongue from the mouth. What remained of the lower lip was then carefully dissected up from the lower jaw... The edges of the lip on each side were attached to the adjacent soft parts by means of metallic sutures. For two days the indications were quite favorable for perfect union, which would have left an opening of somewhat limited size to the oral cavity in comparison with the mouth originally. At the expiration of this time, however, some of the sutures sloughed out, and a portion of the lip was drawn back into its abnormal position. Although not entirely successful, important results were gained by the operation: the flow of saliva and mucus from the mouth was arrested, examining the mouth; I discovered a portion of necrosed bone of considerable size, the presence of which was a constant irritation to the soft parts, and maintained*

a fistulous opening in the mouth and another under the chin.... The fistulous opening in the mouth was enlarged with a bistoury, and the necrosed portion easily removed with a pair of forceps. I found that it was a portion of the base of the lower jaw, and in three or four days he was enabled to speak freely and do entirely without the slate, which had heretofore been indispensable in communicating his thoughts and making known his wants. His appearance was markedly improved [Fig 14-9b].... The patient is now living in Lancaster, Pa., in the enjoyment of excellent health.[22]

Trench warfare and Dr Varaztad H. Kazanjian

Trench warfare in World War I led to a high incidence of facial trauma, creating a great need for oral surgeons and dentists with experience in reconstructive prosthodontics. Exposure of the head and neck above the trench line meant death or certain disfigurement from enemy fire. Dr Francis Wilson,[23] chief of the Dental Service of the American Ambulance Hospital at Juilly, France, described the enormous number of cases of fracture of the jaws:

In September, 1915, I had 52 cases of fracture of the maxillae enter the hospital in one afternoon; of these I saw only 2 completely cured—all the others were sent to hospitals away from the war zone some ten days later. Among these 52 cases were some of the worst that have ever come under my observation. In fact, it would be difficult to imagine how many of these could have been worse. One poor fellow had the entire face below the eyes blown off, nothing remaining of the inferior maxilla. Among the simpler cases a great many multiple fractures, particularly of the lower jaw, some fractured in five, six, seven, or eight places. My work was to wire these together so the man could eat soft food besides being more comfortable. The mouths were washed out with a mild antiseptic or normal salt solution as many as six or eight times a day. When the inflammation subsided sufficiently, we took impressions, extracted useless roots and made cast splints which were cemented to place. I might mention that very often portions of the inferior maxilla would be found missing ranging in size from slight splits to even half or all of the jaw.[23]

Before the United States joined the conflict, numerous physicians and dentists from the States had volunteered to aid the French and British armies. As early as June 1915, Harvard University assembled a team of 32 physicians and 3 dentists as the First Harvard Surgical Unit. Dr Varaztad H. Kazanjian (Fig 14-10), a demonstrator of prosthetic dentistry at the Harvard Dental School, led the dental team. Assigned to the British General Hospital No. 22 at Dammes-Chamiere in upper Normandy, Kazanjian began to deal as best as he could with a never-ending stream of wounded. Following the initial

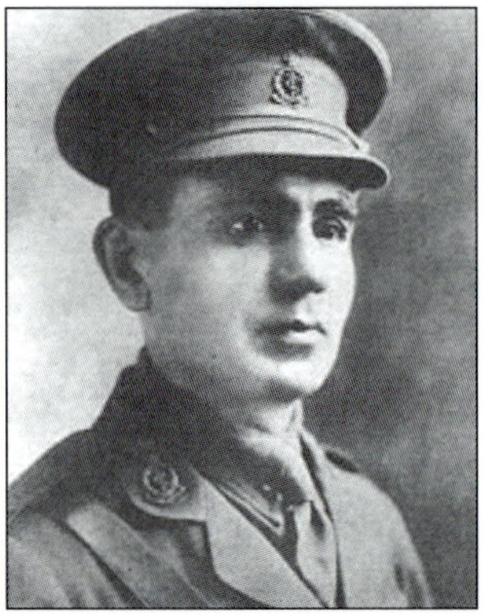

Fig 14-10 Major Varaztad H. Kazanjian.

phase of treatment, each case of craniofacial wound required the design and fabrication of a new device to stabilize segments of the fractured jaws. During 4 years of service at the field hospital, Kazanjian treated over 3,000 cases of jaw fracture.[24] Scores of wounded soldiers owed their physical and mental recovery to his surgical skill and imaginative improvisation. Earning a reputation as "the miracle man of the Western Front," Kazanjian was made a Companion of the Order of St Michael and St George by King George of England.[24]

Shortly after his return to the United States in 1919, Kazanjian presented a paper before the New Jersey Dental Society recounting some of the lessons learned in managing war injuries to the face and jaws. Kazanjian explained that:

> *The treatment of wounds of the face and jaws may be divided into two distinct periods. The first or early period, which covers the three to four weeks following the receipt of the wound, is the most critical for the patient. This is the period of initial exhaustion, of loss of blood, of pronounced sepsis, and of great pain and mental depression. This is also the time at which alarming complications, as broncho-pneumonia, secondary hemorrhage, and general infections are most likely to occur. After this critical first period, the patient passes through the second period, and the convalescent period is in sight. At this time, depending upon the severity of the case, the treatment of the patient is confined chiefly to the further repair of the bony tissue by means of splints, to the construction of prosthetic appliances, to minor operations, and to plastic operations for the reduction of the facial deformity.*[25]

In describing his new method of splinting for mandibular fractures, Kazanjian stressed the importance of early fixation, pointing out that

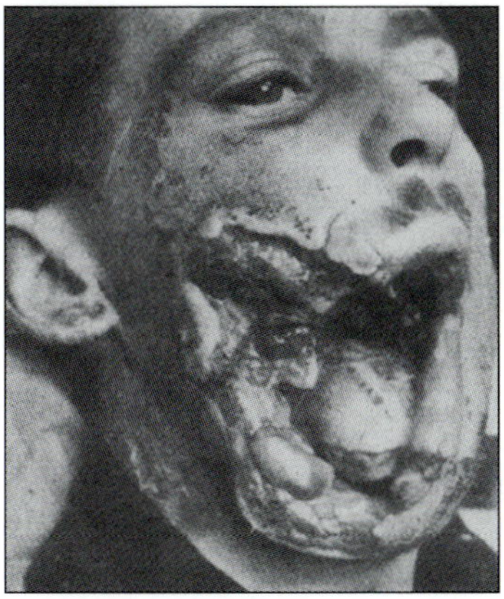

Fig 14-11 Soldier wounded in 1917 and treated by Kazanjian. (From Kazanjian.[25])

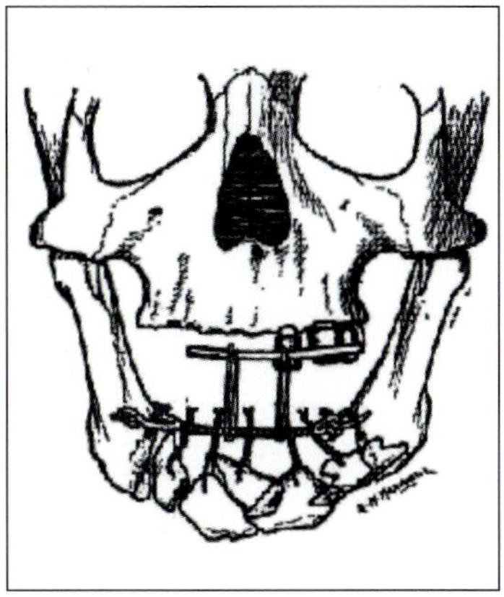

Fig 14-12 Alignment and stabilization of mandibular fragments in the patient shown in Fig 14-11. (From Kazanjian.[25])

the "mobility of the bony parts which exists immediately after injury facilitates the technique of fixation."[25] Furthermore, he recounted that he had:

> *noticed that on account of the unsightly appearance of the external wound there is a strong temptation to give attention to the wound, to the neglect of the setting of the bones. The wound should undoubtedly receive proper care, but the fundamental treatment must begin with the bony structure [Figs 14-11 and 14-12]. If the patient has a fractured arm we do not wait several weeks or months before applying our splints or bandages. This rule holds equally true with fractured jaws.*[26]

Kazanjian noted that an initial lack of cooperation between general surgeons and dentists was soon resolved:

> *During the earlier part of the war the failure of the general surgeon and the dental surgeon to agree on the part which each should play in the treatment prevented the appreciation of the value of immediate fixation of the bony tissues, and many cases of gunshot wounds of the face and jaws became grossly deformed as they passed to and fro, now under the care of the surgeon, now under the care of the dentist, while each in his own way attempted to carry out a scheme of treatment. The better results were obtained only after genuine co-operation of the dental and general surgeon, and after one scheme of treatment made possible the application of splints immediately, while at the same time the general condition of the patient received proper attention.*[26]

It was also learned that placing the teeth and jaws into correct occlusion at the time of fixation provided a "true guide for the reduction of the fracture."

As noted in chapter 11, the introduction of inhalation anesthesia during the latter half of the 19th century facilitated the successful growth of oral and general surgery. The application of the discovery of x-rays greatly assisted oral surgeons in the advancement of their art.

Dental Radiology

One of the most important advances in physics from the point of view of medicine and dentistry was the discovery of x-rays by Wilhelm Roentgen (Fig 14-13) in October of 1895. While investigating the conduction of electricity through evacuated glass tubes (Crookes tubes), Roentgen observed that a fluorescent plate was illuminated by radiations emanating from the activated tube.[27] Unexpectedly, the rays had the power of penetrating through matter. Because the new rays had properties not shared by the known forms of radiation, Roentgen called them *x-rays*.[28] Dr George Manes, a student of Roentgen, recalled the excitement and joy caused by this discovery:

> *I was sitting with my friends in a coffee-house when one of our group came in, pulled out the Frankfurter Zeitung from his pocket and read aloud the following report: "The physicist of the University of Wurzburg, Wilhelm Konrad Roentgen, has discovered a new kind of ray which penetrates all materials with the exception of bones, metals and similar matter. It also affects a photographic plate. Still uncertain about the true nature of these rays, he has named them 'X-Rays.' A photograph of the hand of the famous anatomist, Professor Koelliker, taken with the X-Ray, shows the skeleton very distinctly." We gave a cheer, and walked in high spirits to the Physics Institute to hear a lecture by Roentgen. When he came in, we stamped the floor enthusiastically for minutes, the customary form of applause in German universities.*[29]

The most startling of Roentgen's findings was that x-rays could penetrate flesh to reveal an image of the underlying bones. He had demonstrated this property by exposing his wife's hand to the penetrating x-rays.[28] Newspaper accounts of the discovery were illustrated with Roentgen's x-ray "photograph" of the bony skeleton of the hand of his colleague, the famous anatomist Albert von Kölliker[29] (Fig 14-14). News of the discovery of the mysterious x-rays, also referred to as *Roentgen rays*, spread rapidly and soon led to applications in the medical field.

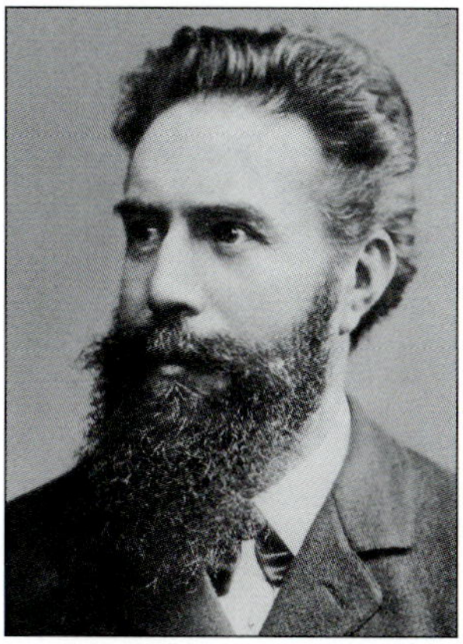

Fig 14-13 Wilhelm Roentgen.

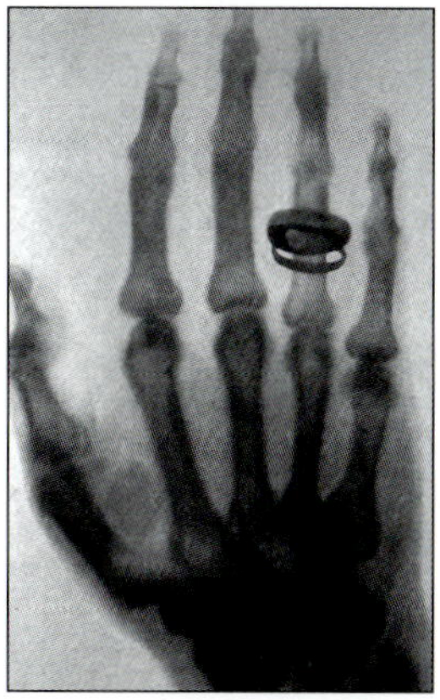

Fig 14-14 Radiograph of Kölliker's hand taken in Roentgen's laboratory.

It was relatively easy to assemble the needed equipment to produce x-rays, because Crookes tubes, electrical generators, and photographic plates were relatively available at scientific supply houses. An instrument-maker advertised in the magazine *Nature* that all the components needed to build a machine for Roentgen photography were available by postal order. Within a few years of Roentgen's discovery, numerous scientists, physicians, and self-promoters entered the free-for-all to exploit the new methodology. It has been reported that in 1896 alone, 49 books and pamphlets and over 1,000 papers on Roentgen rays were published.[27] In that same year, 32 different models of Roentgen tubes became available, and the patent offices in America and Europe were flooded with new patent applications.

In January 1896, a German dentist, Dr Otto Walkhoff, published an image of his teeth made during a 25-minute exposure to x-rays. To make this radiograph, Walkhoff held a photographic glass plate wrapped in rubber dam material between his teeth and tongue as he laid on the floor in the path of the x-rays.[30] In February 1896, the Physical Society of Frankfurt published 14 cranial radiographs made by professor Wilhelm Koenig of Frankfurt. He had perfected a new tube designed to reduce exposure time by over 50%. Walkhoff opened the first dental radiology laboratory in 1896.[30] In France, the first hospital radiology laboratory was opened in 1897.[28]

As soon as the news of the discovery of x-rays reached New York, Thomas Edison went to work at his Menlo Park, New Jersey, laboratory to develop materials that would fluoresce when exposed to x-rays. This led to the invention of the fluoroscope and its presentation

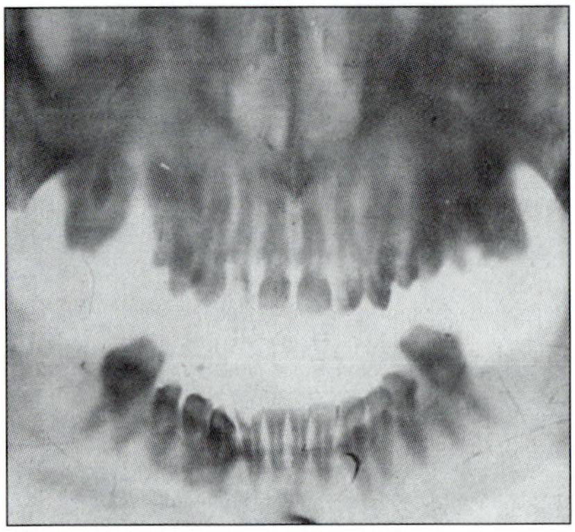

Fig 14-15 Dental radiograph made by William Morton.

to the public at the National Electrical Exposition in New York City in 1896.[30]

At a meeting of the New York Odontological Society held in April 1896, Dr William James Morton, son of dentist William Morton of ether anesthesia ignominy, addressed members of the society on x-rays and their application in dentistry.[31] In opening his talk, Dr Morton noted that he was of the opinion that the x-ray possessed an unusual interest for the dental profession; in fact, he suggested that "it may prove of equal, if not greater, interest to the dental than to the general surgeon." Morton told his audience that he was not going to take up their time by any "abstruse idea" of the science of x-rays but that he proposed to demonstrate, on the spot, how to take a dental radiograph and to show them the potential use of x-rays in dentistry using lantern slides[32] (Fig 14-15).

Morton demonstrated his equipment for generating x-rays and the two methods for capturing the radiographic image (ie, photographic plates and fluorescent plates). Fluorescent plates or screens were developed and manufactured in Thomas Edison's New Jersey laboratories. Morton demonstrated how the fluorescent screen provided an instant image as it became excited by the x-rays emitted from the Crookes tube. Next, he demonstrated a series of dental radiographs made on photographic films, noting that the photographic negatives were superior to prints for providing definition. He illustrated how the radiograph revealed the outlines of the roots of teeth, the extent of metal fillings, the pulp chamber, unerupted teeth, and bony erosions of the jaw. Morton marveled at the power of the new science: "Again and again, I have looked through the human body and seen not only the vertebrae, the ribs, the hip-joint, but also located larger and denser organs like the liver; nay, more, I have watched the heart in its beatings."[32]

In a previous visit to the New York Odontological Society (February 18, 1896) where he was to speak on cataphoresis in dentistry, Morton could not help but digress to speak of his enthusiasm over the new Roentgen rays. In describing his first "shadowgraph," he said:

> *I placed my hand beneath one of my Crookes tubes, and exposed it about thirty minutes, and then developed the plate; and I assure you that for many years—not since I was a medical student—have I felt such a crawly sensation as when I saw my own bones, bereft of their flesh, on that plate. My hair felt as if it were rising. I had not previously seen my own skeleton, and I did not want to see it.*[33]

In concluding his lecture on x-rays in dentistry, Morton said the following:

> *To what perfection, gentlemen, may not the science and art of dentistry reach if some of the new things which press upon your attention are fully realized. Already painless dentistry is within your grasp by aid of electricity and simple anesthetics, and now the X-ray more than rivals your exploring mirror, your probe, your most delicate sense of touch, and your keenest powers of hypothetical diagnosis.*[32]

It is remarkable that this was taking place less than 1 year following Roentgen's discovery. In 1896, in collaboration with E. W. Hammer, an electrical engineer, Morton published *The X Ray or Photography of the Invisible*, which explained the physical principles and electrical engineering of x-ray generation.[34] The book was illustrated with numerous examples of the use of this new diagnostic method in medicine and surgery (see Fig 14-15).

Edmund Kells

American dentists lost no time in introducing x-ray technology in diagnosis of dental problems. First among these pioneers was Dr Edmund Kells (Fig 14-16), a graduate of the New York College of Dentistry in 1878.[28] Kells, the son of a New Orleans dentist, grew up immersed in his father's dental laboratory and in the newly growing fields of electricity and mechanics. While attending dental school in New York City, Kells often visited Thomas Edison's laboratory in nearby Menlo Park, New Jersey, where he immersed himself in the newest advances in electricity.[28] Kells's innate creativity and ingenuity led to a lifetime of discovery and invention. He was reported to have had over 30 patents granted to him for such inventions as the fire

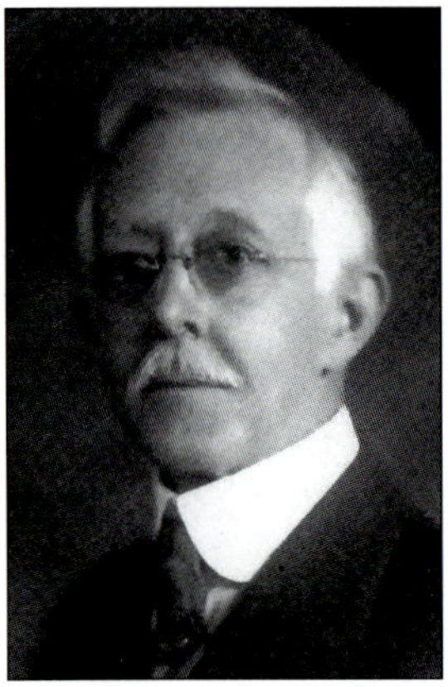

Fig 14-16 Edmund Kells.

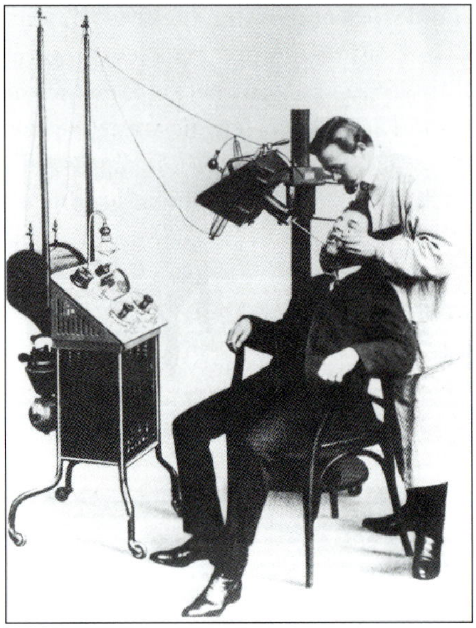

Fig 14-17 Early dental radiographic equipment depicting the dentist exposed to stray radiation.

extinguisher, the automobile jack, and the braking and starter mechanisms for elevators.[35] In the dental office, he was the first to use compressed air to dry teeth and to control dryness of the operative site with a saliva ejector. His dental operatory was the first to be equipped with electricity and with an electric dental drill at a time when most dentists used foot-powered dental drills and operated by gas lamp or daylight only.[36] He was ahead of his time in employing women as dental assistants, an innovation that brought upon him a great deal of criticism from his professional colleagues.

Shortly after reading of Roentgen's discovery, Kells placed orders for building his own dental x-ray machine. He cut dental films from larger sheets of x-ray film, fabricated intraoral film-holders, and, with his dental assistant as subject, began to experiment with the new method. In less than 8 months following Roentgen's discovery, Kells was on his way to Asheville, North Carolina, to demonstrate dental x-rays before the Southern Dental Association.[37] Kells explained to conventioneers that it was essential to place the photographic plate as closely as possible to the teeth, demonstrating that his film-holders were held in place by biting down upon them. Although he had his equipment set up and ready to take radiographs on a volunteer, lack of electricity during daylight hours prevented the demonstration. Kells did, however, provide examples of the potential diagnostic use of x-rays using "skiagraphs"[8] made previously. Skiagraphs were invaluable in "locating broken roots and ascertaining to a certain extent their shape...partly erupted or encysted third molars...and examination of the roots of replanted or implanted teeth."[38] A second attempt to make skiagraphs at the evening session, when electricity was available, was again foiled by a demonstration of fluoroscopy.[37] Conventioneers lined up to see their bones imaged on the fluoroscope in such numbers that there was no room for Kells's demonstration; even the evening's charity ball was poorly attended.[39]

When Kells began experimenting with dental radiographs at age 40 years, he was unaware of the danger that x-radiation posed. It was then common practice to hold films in position for the patient with one's own hands and to remain within the path of the x-rays during several minutes of exposure (Fig 14-17). Kells was able to reduce exposures to 30 seconds to a minute (for molars) and with the intraoral "bite-film" stand aside during the exposure. Nevertheless, he exposed himself to indirect radiation while making radiographs and during many experiments. In 1903, Kells opened a New Orleans x-ray laboratory in the same building that housed his dental offices. It is assumed that he was directly involved in making radiographs for medical diagnostic purposes, most likely exposing himself to additional and longer periods of exposure to x-rays. By the time he reached 50 years of age, he had developed cancer in his right hand. Despite dozens of surgeries to amputate parts of his fingers, the cancer spread, requiring the amputation of his left arm. He underwent periodic experimental treatment under ultraviolet irradiation to stop the cancer but to no avail. After several years of suffering, Kells reached the breaking point. With a gun pointed to his head, he committed suicide in his dental office.[28, 39]

Other Americans significant to dental radiology

Dr William H. Rollins, another American pioneer in dental radiology who by July 1896 had developed an intraoral fluoroscope, was one of the first dentists to warn of the danger of radiation exposure.[40] Rollins, a graduate of the Harvard University Dental School at age 21 years and later a graduate of the Medical School as well, had conducted experiments that showed that prolonged exposure to x-rays could kill guinea pigs. As a member of the x-ray department at the Boston

[8] Kells preferred to use the term *skiagraph*, from the Greek for shadow or ghost, rather than *radiograph* or *Roentgengraph*.

City Hospital, he invented the Rollins box, a lead-lined box to house the Crookes tube, thereby restricting the passage of the x-rays to a small aperture. This precaution reduced the exposure for both the patient and the radiologist from stray radiation. Rollins also protected his patients from excessive exposure with lead-lined aprons.

But at the turn of the twentieth century, the excitement over radiology was so strong that for many innovators it swept away any thoughts of caution until it proved too late. Exposure of the hands to prolonged or repeated x-radiation produced erythema, swelling, and pain. Over time, the skin cracked and ulcerated and areas of carcinoma developed. Fingers had to be amputated but usually too late to prevent the spread of cancer to other parts of the body. Rebecca Herzig has discussed how the culture of late-nineteenth-century natural science acted to valorize voluntary sacrifice in the cause of the scientific progress of medicine.[41]

Entrepreneurs saw a chance to profit from this new medical advance by setting themselves up as radiographers. There being no special educational requirements and no legal obstacles to establishing x-ray laboratories, such enterprises rapidly materialized in the major cities. Dr F. Collar of Alameda, California, described this development:

> *One of the leading dental supply salesmen of Los Angeles foresaw the commercial possibilities of the X-ray game, as he terms it, and procured the necessary financial backing to equip an x-ray laboratory. On account of his intimate acquaintance and friendship with a large percentage of the dentists, he immediately had a large following as soon as he sent out his announcements and price lists. His technical knowledge of the x-ray, he acquired from selling x-ray machines. His knowledge of pathology, histology, methods of sterilization, diseases and anatomy, he learned while walking the streets and visiting dental offices. He is no longer a hard working dental salesman but after a few years of operating his laboratory, he is the owner of an orange grove and remarked recently, that if they hold off dental legislation governing x-ray laboratories for another year, he will not care what they do, for he can retire.*[42]

Dr James McCoy stated that commercial radiographers, "dental picture galleries," had increased and monopolized the field of oral radiography in Los Angeles to such an extent that "capable, educated dentists do not feel like entering in competition with them."[42]

Collar believed that radiology had proven to be of such importance in diagnosis that no modern dental practice could afford to be without it. He emphasized that only dentists, educated in pathology, histology, and clinically experienced, could make efficient use of radiographs as diagnostic aids. The nondentist radiographer had no place in making diagnostic determinations or in consulting with the patient.[42]

Dr Howard Raper introduced dental radiology into the dental school clinic at Indiana University in 1909 and became the first professor of dental roentgenology to write a textbook on dental radiography.[43] By 1920, dental radiologic examinations took on special importance in the evaluation of the oral and systemic health of a patient. Prominent oral surgeon and histopathologist Kurt Thoma stated the following:

> *The physician often has occasion to inquire into the condition of his patient's mouth, especially when in search of a focus or foci of the disease concerning which the patient is consulting him. The mouth should not be overlooked by the diagnostician when making a thorough physical examination. Some physicians are contented with "The dentist is visited regularly," and "There is absolutely nothing wrong with the teeth," but the thorough diagnostician will not be satisfied except with a report based upon a careful examination and roentgenographic diagnosis made by a dentist or specialist in whose judgment he can trust.*[44]

Summary

During the end of the 19th century and the start of the 20th century, oral surgery and radiology became integral components of dental practice, essential in the further development of other branches of dentistry, especially endodontics, periodontology, and pediatric dentistry. The specialty of oral surgery developed in America at a time when there was confusion as to its rightful place within medicine or dentistry. Hullihen, Garretson, Brophy, and Talbot, leaders in the development of the specialty of oral surgery in 19th-century America, held MD degrees in addition to the DDS degree. Garretson criticized the education provided by dental schools as too limiting with too much emphasis on mechanical procedures. Brophy and Talbot hoped to make oral surgery a discipline within medicine and concurrently expand the dental curriculum to include more exposure to general pathology and basic medical science. They were also critical of medical schools for their failure to teach dental pathology. The focal infection theory lent urgency to these movements. Brophy gathered meager support for his proposal to eliminate the DDS degree by making dentistry a specialty of medicine. As members of the AMA, Brophy and Talbot formed a Stomatological Section within that organization with the dual objective of exposing physicians to dental pathology and recruiting dentists into the AMA. Because dentists were accepted only as associate members, their enthusiasm for membership waned, and the Stomatological Section died a slow death because of low interest on the part of physicians and the failure to recruit dentists. While stomatology as a specialty of medicine flourished in Europe, it failed to develop in America. The bridge between physicians and dentists was strained, and the specialty of oral surgery ultimately remained within the dental profession.

For centuries, wars have been training grounds for surgeons, and World War I proved to be no exception. In treating severe facial wounds, oral surgeons acquitted themselves well in the field hospitals of France during this war. Working in close cooperation with general surgeons and physicians, they achieved recognition for their unique talents. As the specialty matured during the first half of the 20th century, an increasing number of oral surgeons held dual degrees, serving to bridge the gap between the two professions.

Dental radiology developed rapidly following Roentgen's discovery of x-rays. Whether it was due to a pure humanitarian spirit or a propensity to gain clinical stature, dentists were quick to take up radiology without much consideration of its harmful effects. The use of radiology in diagnosis proved immensely useful in dentistry, and its use grew, especially during the focal infection scare.

References

1. Harle F. The history of maxillary sinus surgery—From Leonardo da Vinci until today. Bull Hist Dent 1992;40:79–84.
2. Jourdain M. Traite des maladies et des operations reellement chirurgicales de la bouche, et des parties qui y correspondent. Paris: Valleyre l'anie, 1778.
3. Lufkin AW. A History of Dentistry. Philadelphia: Lea & Febiger, 1948.
4. Thoma KH. The history of oral surgery: The oldest specialty of dentistry. Oral Surg Oral Med Oral Pathol 1957;10:1–10.
5. Goldwyn RM. Simon P. Hullihen: Pioneer oral and plastic surgeon. Plast Reconstr Surg 1973;52:250–257.
6. Thorpe BL. Simon P. Hullihen, M. D., D. D. S., pioneer and expert in oral surgery and founder of the Wheeling Hospital. Dent Rev 1903;17:250–260.
7. Hullihen SP. Hare-lip and its treatment. Am J Dent Sci (1st Ser) 1844;4:244–254.
8. Koch CRE. History of Dental Surgery, vol 2. Chicago: The National Art, 1909.
9. Koch CRE, Brophy TW. Oral surgery. In: Koch CRE (ed). History of Dental Surgery, vol 1. Chicago: The National Art, 1909;387–395.
10. The future of dentistry. Dent Cosmos 1872;14:608–611.
11. Reviews and notices of books: A system of oral surgery, by James E. Garretson. J Br Dent Assoc 1891;12:217–218.
12. Smith HH. The Principles and Practice of Surgery. Philadelphia: J. B. Lippincott, 1863.
13. Bernard C, Huette C. Illustrated Manual of Operative Surgery and Surgical Anatomy. New York: Bailliere Brothers, 1864.

14. Garretson JE. Surgical education. Dent Cosmos 1866;8:186–188.
15. Sperry FM. A Group of Distinguished Physicians and Surgeons of Chicago. Chicago: J. H. Beers, 1904.
16. Talbot ES. The problem of dental education. Dent Cosmos 1915;57:424–428.
17. Brophy TW. A retrospective survey of early dental practice, with reflections on the modern trend of dentistry. Dent Cosmos 1921;63:323–333.
18. Brown GV. The section on stomatology as a factor in the evolution of dental and medical science. J Am Med Assoc 1914;63:2106–2110.
19. Fisher WC. The section on stomatology: Its needs, its duties and its opportunities. II. The field of stomatology. J Am Med Assoc 1914;63:2104–2106.
20. Johnson LR. Stomatology: A problem in education. J Am Med Assoc 1929;92:1500–1503.
21. Marshall JS. Fracture and distasis of the superior maxillae and upper bones of the face, treated by the aid of the interdental splint and cranial support; with three cases in illustration. Dent Cosmos 1891;33:175–187.
22. McQuillen JH. A case of oral surgery. Dent Cosmos 1875;17:397–401.
23. Brown GV. The Surgery of Oral Diseases and Malformations. Philadelphia: Lea & Febiger, 1918.
24. Hapgood RL. History of the Harvard Dental School. Boston: Harvard University, 1930.
25. Kazanjian VH. Splints combined with sutures through the bone for the immobilization of extensive fractures of the lower jaw. Proc R Soc Med Sect Odont 1918;11:67–86.
26. Kazanjian VH. Treatment of maxillary fractures. Br Med J 1916;1(2877):266–267.
27. Sarton G. The discovery of x-rays. Isis 1937;26:349–369.
28. Jacobsohn PH. Making darkness visible: The discovery of x-ray and its introduction to dentistry. J Am Dent Assoc 1995;126:1359–1366.
29. Manes GI. The discovery of x-ray. Isis 1956;47:236–238.
30. Langland OE, Langlais RP. Early pioneers of oral and maxillofacial radiology. Oral Maxillofac Radiol 1995;80:496–511.
31. Morton WJ, Hammer EW. The X-ray: Or, Photography of the Invisible and Its Value in Surgery. New York: American Technical Book Co, 1896.
32. Morton WJ. The x-ray and its application in dentistry. Dent Cosmos 1896;38:478–486.
33. Morton WJ. Cataphoric medication of the mouth. Dent Cosmos 1896;38:400–402.
34. Morton WJ. The X-Ray; Or Photography of the Invisible. New York: American Technical Book, 1896.
35. Kracher CM. C. Edmund Kells (1856–1928). J Hist Dent 2000;48:65–69.
36. Kells CE. The application of electricity in dental practice. Dent Cosmos 1891;33:358–361.
37. Southern Dental Association. Dent Cosmos 1896;38:1007–1013.
38. Kells CE. Roentgen rays. Dent Cosmos 1899;41:1014–1029.
39. Wynbrandt J. The Excruciating History of Dentistry. New York: St. Martin's, 1998.
40. Linton O. Francis H. Williams and William H. Rollins. J Am Coll Radiol 2006;3:478–479.
41. Herzig R. In the name of science: Suffering, sacrifice, and the formation of American roentgenology. Am Q 2001;53:563–589.
42. Collar FJ. Professional radiography vs commercial radiography. Int J Orthod Oral Surg Radiogr 1922;8:445–451.
43. Raper HR. Elementary and Dental Radiography. New York: Consolidated Dental Manufacturing, 1913.
44. Thoma KH. Oral Roentgenology. Boston: Ritter, 1917.

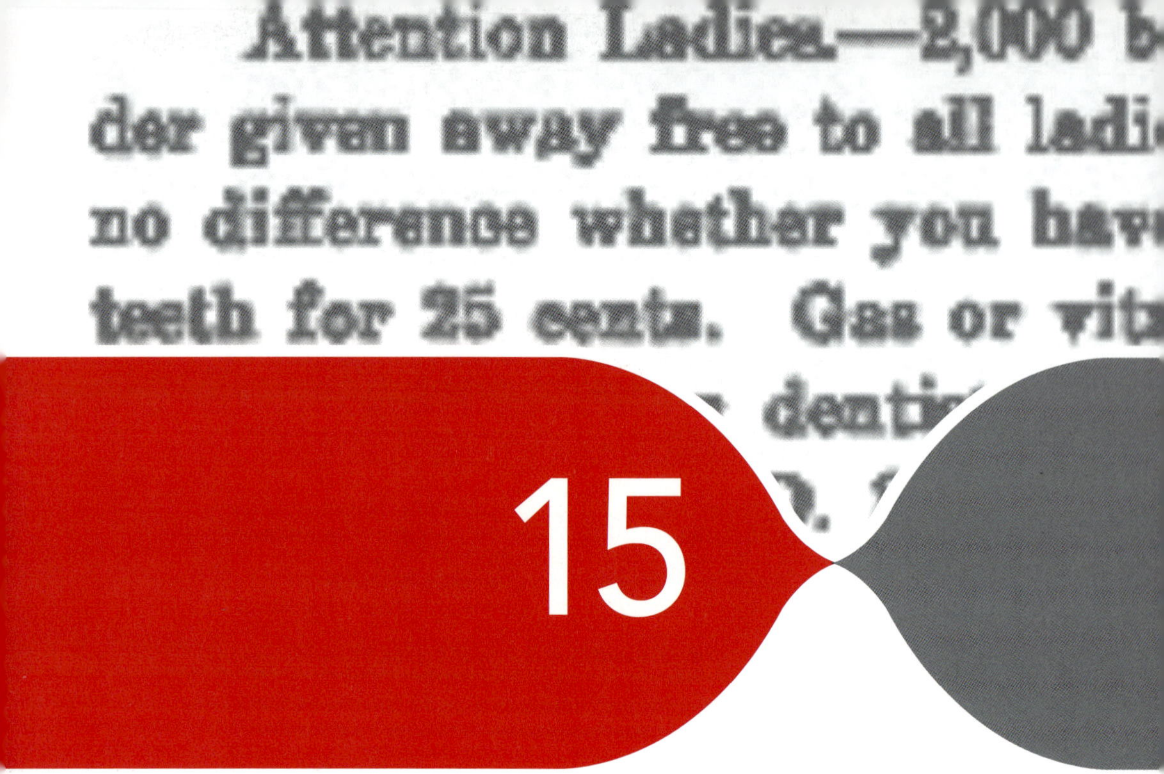
Attention Ladies.—2,000
der given away free to all
no difference whether you
teeth for 25 cents. Gas or

15

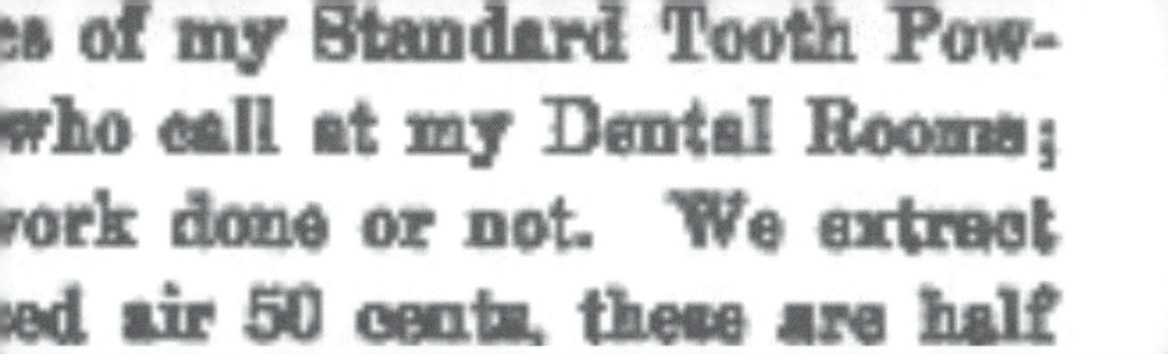

Defining the Ethics of Practice

The process of professionalization of American dentistry began in 1839–1840 with the formation of the first dental societies and the first dental college (see chapter 7). As in every human advance, the professionalization of dentistry received impetus from the determination of a few men of vision. In addressing the third annual meeting of the American Society of Dental Surgeons in 1842, Dr Eleazar Parmly, in an effort to improve dentistry's image, appealed to the membership to exhibit moral leadership in exposing fraudulent practice. He spoke of the large number of men who had taken up dentistry without the "skill, ingenuity and judgment" necessary to fulfill the needs of their patients. He continued:

> *This kind of charlatanism has been and is now practiced to such an extent, that I will venture to say that there is more injury done than benefit conferred by operations on the teeth.... Such fraudulent proceedings exhibit a want of moral principle, and have done much to destroy that confidence in the profession.*[1]

As a leading practitioner of operative dentistry, the most fundamental branch of dentistry, Parmly, along with his colleagues in New York City, Philadelphia, and Boston, led an organized movement to elevate and purge dentistry of its low-grade imposters. Professionalization, started by the elite in New York and Philadelphia, continued during the rest of the 19th century until the Gies Report of 1920 accelerated reforms in the dental educational system, setting dentistry on a course that soon gave it equality with medicine.

The sociologist Paul Starr defines a *profession* as "an occupation that regulates itself through systematic, required training and collegial discipline; that has a base in technical, specialized knowledge; and that has a service rather than profit orientation, enshrined in its code of ethics."[2] During the latter half of the 19th century, the dental profession formulated its own code of ethics, largely following precedents set by the medical profession. For much of the 19th century, the marketplace and the business of practice forced dentistry to compromise between altruism and the entrepreneurial spirit. Dentistry, in not wanting to be viewed solely as a trade, aspired to take its place as a member of the learned professions. But despite advancements in dental education, dental regulation, and dental science, all acting to legitimize the profession, a rising commercialism associated with quackery, dishonest advertising, and the rush to patent every new product pulled the profession downward from its aspired position.

When the topic of ethics was taken up at dental society meetings, the discussion usually centered on the desirability of gentlemanly interaction between professional men, with less attention paid to protecting the rights of patients. C. P. Fitch, writing in *Dental Cosmos* in 1861 under the heading "Professional Ethics," suggested that rules of ethical conduct must apply to the "entire sphere of professional (dental) employments," yet he focused almost entirely on the duty of a dentist to exhibit restraint in passing judgment on the clinical work of other dentists:

> *The practice of an indiscriminate condemnation of all operations found in the mouths of persons whose great misfortune seems to have been in falling into other dentist's hands, is, to speak in the mildest terms, highly censurable; and the person habitually guilty of this charge should be shunned as the plague or pestilence.*[3]

Fitch was comfortable with pointing out the defective "state of the teeth and their artificial appliances" but not in demeaning the dentist who had performed the work. His position was that "a manly and full statement of facts should always be made to those seeking professional advice, abating all reflections calling in question the integrity and ability of a predecessor," furthermore stating that "we should never claim too much for our own performances, especially when it may directly or indirectly compromise the character and standing of a professional compeer."[3] Dr James McCabe, in his address before the

First Annual Meeting of the Virginia Society of Southern Dentists, remarked that "he who is willing to trifle with the reputation of another member of the same profession, or lessen him in the estimation of the public, is either an ignorant quack himself, or grossly deficient in the practice of common honesty."[4]

For Dr C. J. Essig, the "chivalry of professional life" was complicated by the "want of concordance in diagnosis and in treatment" and led to questions of professional ethics that were not easily reconciled.[5] Essig described the difficulties posed by lack of agreement in diagnosis and treatment outcome that often led to condemnation of the work performed by a professional colleague. Was it a breach of professional ethics to indicate to a patient that certain dental work had been ill advised or poorly carried out? Was there a certain "esprit de corps" that protected a dentist from criticizing the work of a fellow practitioner? If such criticism were activated by commercial competition, the public would see it as dishonest and would lose trust in dentistry as an honorable profession.

Code of Ethics

At the Sixth Annual Session of the American Dental Association (ADA), after many hours of deliberation, a committee of three men were given the task of drawing up a code of ethics that was presented to the assembly for approval.[6] It followed closely the Code of Ethics of the American Medical Association (AMA), adopted in 1847.[7] The first clause of the dental code pertained to the duties of the dentist to his patients. The code called on a dentist to rely on "his own sense of right" in the faithful performance of his services. He was encouraged to educate his patients to "appreciate the benefits of dental care" and never to "encourage false hopes by promising success" (the emphasis on *promising*). Temperance in mind and body were seen as the essential matrix wherein good judgment and skill would develop. Each member was expected to acquire the character of a gentleman, show respect for fellow members and patients, and avoid all language and conduct dishonoring the profession.

The code was explicit in condemning all forms of advertising as being detrimental to the good image of the profession. It was the duty of every member to expose quackery and to act to gain the respect and confidence of the public. Acceptance of the scientific spirit and the acquisition of new knowledge were seen as the hallmarks of professional men.

Parts of the code were clearly formulated to protect the business of practice by setting a uniform level of fees, avoiding open criticism of fellow clinicians, and discouraging the use of methods to establish superiority over local practitioners.

The code elicited much discussion, and, despite some opposition, it was accepted at the annual session. It was then referred back to all state and local dental societies for their adoption. Although the more conservative men were generally favorable toward such a code of ethics, there were critics who rebelled against the idea that they were to be subjugated to "arbitrary" rules of conduct. Other men believed that there was no need to spell out in detail what constituted good professional conduct or to ban behaviors defined as detrimental to the profession. They held the notion that all one had to do was be gentlemanly, wrongly presupposing that all men entering the system were innately cognizant as to what constituted the state of gentlemanliness. Dr McQuillen, a member of the Committee on Dental Ethics, stated that he had "read the code, but could claim no credit for its preparation; on general principles was opposed to its adoption, as unnecessary for gentlemen, and its enforcement impracticable upon those who were not."[6]

The Odontographic Society of Pennsylvania unanimously rejected the proposed code:

> *The members of this Society do not recognize in the constitution of the Association [ADA] the right of that body to dictate terms to local societies, either with respect to theory, practice, or ethics, or to deny the right of representation to societies which may decline to adopt what has been agreed upon in such directions by that organization.*[8]

In 1868, the Northern Iowa Dental Association adopted an ethics code "setting forth the relative duties of dentists and patients, dentists and physicians, and the responsibility of dentists, the discountenancing of empiricism, and the duty of maintaining professional character."[9] The Association also adopted a uniform fee schedule.

In a discussion of ethics at the Illinois State Dental Society, Dr M. S. Dean observed that a code of ethics was essential in dentistry, "there being no other pursuit in which those who practiced it were to the same extent the sole judge of their own operations, and no legal standard being required." Yet others stated that if the code interfered with the practice of their business, they would leave the society.[10]

The adoption of a code of ethics was no guarantee that members would follow its recommendations or behave in a more gentlemanly manner toward colleagues. Competition was rampant at the lowest level in advertising cheap and painless dentistry and at the highest level in demagoguery at society meetings and in publishing self-promoting elitist papers in the literature. Competitive struggles escalated as the ranks of the profession were swelled with graduates of the new dental colleges, as well as by the continued entrance of illegal imposters and swindlers.

Toward the end of the 19th century, it was increasingly recognized that despite the adoption of a code of ethics by the American Dental Association, unprofessional conduct remained unchecked. At a convention of New England dentists held in 1890, it was stated by Dr G. W. Hoffman that all were in general agreement that they should abide by the code, "yet, pitiful as it may seem, we all know that nine out of ten dentists break that code deliberately, frequently, and cheerfully, and the dental societies are unable to prevent it."[11]

The code was a product of the professional elite, formulated in part to establish an image of high social responsibility and designed to exclude practitioners who were less educated, poorly trained, and operating by rules of trade. But the average dental practitioner, who may have wanted to abide by the professional code, when faced by the unfair competition of the advertising dentist and by evidence that the elite who professed to be exemplars of ethical dentistry were often guilty of transgressions, lost any reason to practice by the code. In the words of one dentist who believed in the need for a code:

> *It is a hard thing, I know it by practical experience, to sit still hour after hour and day after day, not seeing a patient, and at the same time seeing your advertising competitor thronged. I know what it is to see an advertisement in the paper, and to know that you cannot say anything to the public in answer to it; first, because the rule of the society forbids it, and secondly, because if you do answer it the public will say you are jealous.*[12]

Dr Ottolengui, a leading member of the Dental Society of the State of New York, was surprised to find the names of several highly honored "gentlemen" of the profession (including one who had been president of the society) among the dentists listed in the business directory of the city of New York. Their names were in large type, "same as the other advertising men." Another example of the double standard was in the annual social directory of New York City, wherein a "dental list" contained the names of 36 practitioners, among whom 6 were faculty of dental colleges and 6 had a national reputation, all 36 listed "because they have paid five dollars each for the recommendation."[13] Although these were milder forms of advertising, not meeting the level of unprofessional conduct, they made it easier for a defense of advertising dentists.

One of the most grating aspects of the ban on advertising was the use of various methods to abide by the letter of code while subverting its spirit. Those men who drummed up their practice by using academic titles or by publishing newspaper articles describing their unusual success were castigated at dental society meetings to no avail. The Sunday society pages were another venue where the spirit of the code was evaded:

> *In the society columns of the Sunday paper you will occasionally see a notice reading something like this: "Dr. So-and-so, whose dental parlors are a dream of luxury, whose equipments are second to none, whose clientele is made up of the first families in the city, has gone to take a much needed rest," etc. And then again we have the fraternity man who plays his lodge for all it's worth. A close second to him is the bright young dentist who joins the leading church, and who attends all the means of grace with a pocketful of his cards.*[14]

Could a new and better code provide the answer? Dr J. F. Burket argued that because "the good must still be protected and the bad restrained," the profession needed a new code. But what was most needed was improvement in the matriculation of men with "nobility of character" into the dental colleges.[12] The standards of professional conduct would rise when more attention was paid to recruiting men who were better educated and of higher morals. Dr B. Holly Smith, in discussing the role of the colleges, suggested that they could provide instruction in ethics, "teaching by precept and example a gentlemanly life and behavior," but it was too much to expect the colleges to exact morality of its graduates.

For Dr R. Ottolengui, the code was "enacted by men whom we all respect, but who adopted them in a spirit of imitation. Being anxious to be considered medical men, they aped that profession in the formation of societies and in the adoption of written rules of conduct."[15] The medical code had its origins in the Hippocratic Oath and, in more recent history, Dr Thomas Percival's extensive instructions to English physicians.[16;1] Percival's dictums spelled out the gentlemanliness of medical practice. Ottolengui opined that the medical code, based in part on Percival's rules of medical etiquette set down at the beginning of the 19th century (1803), was not applicable to the dental profession in the 1890s. Dentistry's code of ethics was "utterly useless" because it "does not describe specifically all that which should

[1] Thomas Percival, a physician of Manchester, England, published a "Code of Medical Ethics" in 1804. It contained rules for the conduct of physicians, surgeons, and apothecaries in their interactions within the newly established hospitals.

be against the spirit of the rules...and it permits sins in one direction, which are as bad, or worse, that those designated for punishment.... No amount of written law will convert a blackguard into a gentleman, nor make a charlatan a professional man."[15] Ottolengui said that although he had little respect for the code, he obeyed it "because I am at heart ethical...having been reared in the South, where codes of ethics and codes of honor are obeyed in the spirit and not in the letter."[15]

Dr G. S. Dean viewed dismissal of the code as "a plea for professional anarchy." For Dean, man was "both an instinctive and an intelligent being, needing in matters generally, both instinctive guidance and intelligent direction, the guidance of both the heart and the head."[17] Based on his view of the current debate, Dean found the burning issues to be: *(1)* advertising; *(2)* secrets and patents in the matter of medicaments, processes, and appliances; and *(3)* fraternal assistance and its opposite, "professional jealousy." In such areas, professional men needed to be guided by written rules. Regarding advertising, it was permissible to advertise the profession or the science of dentistry so long as one did not use this method as a subterfuge for self-aggrandizement. Personal advertising that was "derogatory to the dignity of the profession" was prohibited.

Advertising

The Code of Ethics of the AMA was strongly opposed to advertising:

> *Solicitation of patients by circulars or advertisements, or by personal communications or interviews, not warranted by personal relations, is unprofessional. It is equally unprofessional to procure patients by indirection through solicitors or agents of any kind, (as) or by indirect advertisement, or by furnishing or inspiring newspaper or magazine comments concerning cases in which the physician has been or is concerned. All other like self-laudations defy the traditions and lower the tone of any profession and so are intolerable.... It is unprofessional to promise radical cures; to boast of cures and secret methods of treatment or remedies; to exhibit certificates of skill or of success in the treatment of diseases; or to employ any methods to gain the attention of the public for the purpose of obtaining patients.*[18]

The American public was exposed to an increasing number of medical and dental advertisements as the newspaper business flourished from 200 newspapers in 1800 to 4,000 in 1860.[19] Dentists were early in recognizing that the print media was a sure way of attracting new patients. The reading public was repeatedly informed of new and

> **Plain Dealer, Oct. 31, 1894.**
> **Attention Ladies.—2,000 boxes of my Standard Tooth Powder given away free to all ladies who call at my Dental Rooms; no difference whether you have work done or not. We extract teeth for 25 cents. Gas or vitalized air 50 cents, these are half the price of other dentists. 13 Euclid Ave., open nights. E. W. Thompson, D. D. S. Press, Jan. 2, 1893, shows a picture of a steel bridge and under it the word "work".**

Fig 15-1 Dental advertisement appearing in the *Plain Dealer* on October 31, 1894. (From Ambler.[20])

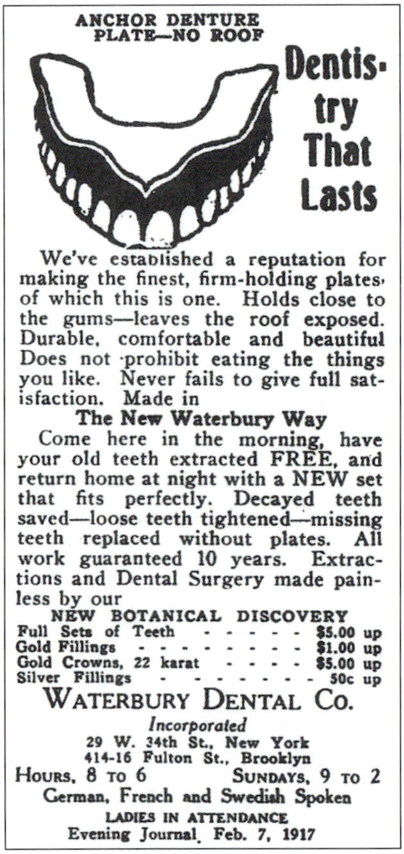

Fig 15-2 Example of a typical dental advertisement in a New York City newspaper, 1917.

improved techniques, painless dentistry, the finest establishments, all work guaranteed, high-class dentistry at half price, teeth filled at night in parlors lighted by electricity, etc.[20] Dental advertisements (Figs 15-1 and 15-2) were so commonly untruthful and misleading

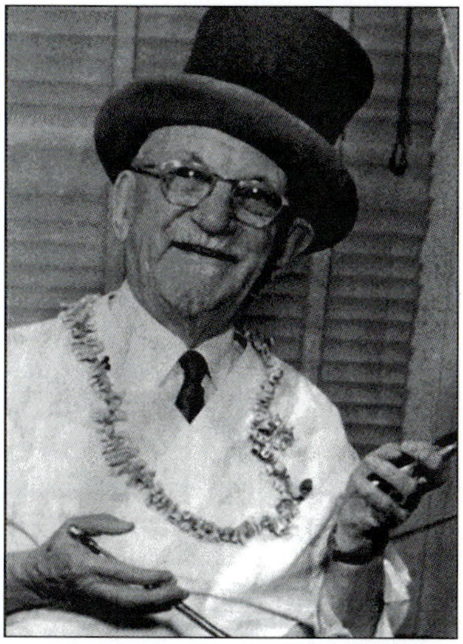

Fig 15-3 Parker wearing his necklace of extracted teeth.

that they were equated with quack dentistry and sure to attract a "less desirable class of people."[18]

The Illinois State Dental Society, in a proposed revision of its Code of Ethics, noted that the most restrictive part of its code dealt with advertising. They reaffirmed that it was unprofessional to "advertise by hand bills, posters, circulars, cards, signs, or newspapers or other publications, calling attention to special methods of practice or claiming excellence over other practitioners."[21] They recognized a man's legal right to advertise, but any man employing such means could no longer remain a member of the dental society. It was even predicted that advertising restrictions would become more exacting as the profession developed to a higher level.

Despite all the talk at dental society meetings and the adoption of codes of conduct, the practice of advertising continued unabated. Among the most notorious of the advertising dentists was Edgar "Painless" Parker (Fig 15-3). A graduate of the Pennsylvania Dental College and a New York City street dentist, Parker would make a mockery of the code of ethics by his flamboyant advertising and outrageous hucksterism (Figs 15-4 and 15-5). He boasted of having extracted 357 teeth in one day and wore them on a necklace as an affront to the elite of the profession and as a symbol of his prowess to the gullible public (see Fig 15-3). Parker proclaimed that "I like being a dentist and a salesman at the same time." Adopting the

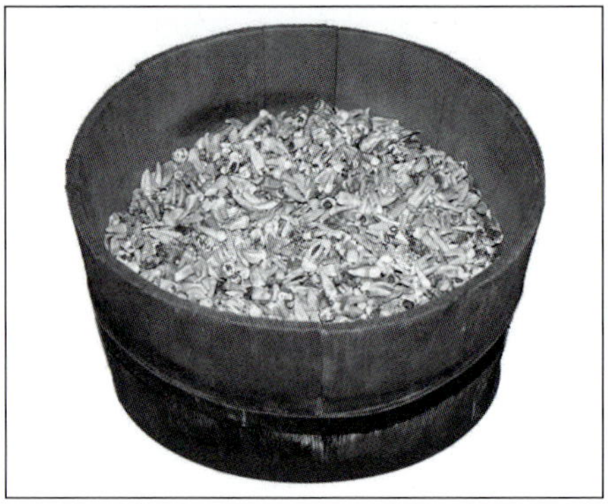

Fig 15-4 Parker's bucket of extracted teeth.

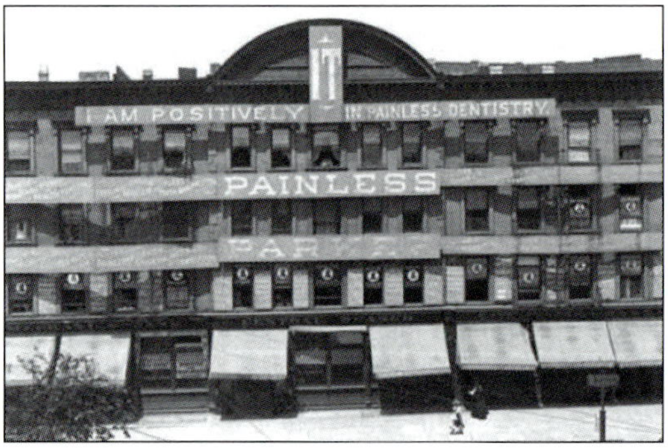

Fig 15-5 Parker's Dental Emporium on Flatbush Avenue in Brooklyn, New York, 1895.

methods of P. T. Barnum, he carried out his early trade from a horse-drawn dental office with girl attendants and bugle players. Through newspaper advertisements and other publicity stunts, he enlarged his practice and was soon employing other dentists and occupying large office facilities. When accused of malpractice by the California State Board of Dental Examiners for his advertising claim to provide painless dentistry, he simply went to court and changed his legal name to Painless Parker.

Dr Norman Kingsley characterized the state of dentistry in 1900 as follows:

> *In the first half of this century, nearly all dentists were regarded as quacks by the medical fraternity. They were empirics, but not charlatans. There were quacks as there always are in any vocation. But, relatively, there was not nearly so much quackery as exists today. Fifty years ago in this city there was very little quackery. The profession contained*

many honored names,—gentlemen of culture and social standing. In the fashionable functions of that day were to be found the names of dentists distinguished alike for their skill and good breeding. The quacks were peripatetic, itinerating from one place to another, but even they were not guilty of the crimes in the name of dentistry that are so frequently found to-day. The profession as a whole did not accomplish as much good as it does now, and on the other hand the quacks did far less harm. As I look over the field at the close of a half-century's observation, I see three grades of dentistry. Dentistry as a profession, dentistry as a trade, and dentistry as a side show to a circus.[22]

Dr H. J. Oldstein of Scranton, Pennsylvania, posing as a patient, visited an advertising dental parlor. Here is his story:

I once went into one of these offices in order to convince myself of their mode of practice. When my turn came to be waited on, I was called into a cage where the contractor examines patients' mouths. After being asked numerous questions, in order, I suppose, to find out how large my bank account was, I was on the verge of getting a bloody mouth mirror placed in my mouth for the examination. I of course refused to be treated thus, and the contractor called to the man in the next cage to hand him a mouth mirror. After two minutes of probing and examination, I was told that I was in need of four gold caps and eight fillings, some gold and some silver, involving an expenditure of thirty dollars. I could have all this done the same day provided I paid in advance, as the day was bargain day; some other day it would cost more. To me it was really a great bargain indeed—considering that my mouth was in no need of any dental care at all! Such is their mode of practice, and thus they fleece the innocent public.[23]

With Parker's dental parlor and many more like it in mind, Kingsley described how such operations degraded the dental profession and the health of the community:

Dentistry as a system of organized and legalized quackery reaches its fullest attainment in the "dental emporiums" of the avenues and streets in which ethics play no part, and the chief and only object is to make money by all the devices known to trade; the main factors being advertising and underselling your neighbor.... All professional ethics have been thrown to the winds, and even the ethics of trade, "honesty is the best policy," are not regarded.[22]

He held little hope that quackery could be cured by legislation:

There are certain diseases and vices which all the legislation in the world up to the present has failed to abate. They continue to flourish in spite of all the sumptuary or prohibitory laws on the statute books. Quackery is a vice, and figuratively a disease. It has not been stamped

> *out by legislation. It is not even abated. It is on the increase, and, most discouraging of all, the community does not look upon it as disreputable or unethical.*[22]

To the men who labored to establish dentistry as a learned, ethical profession, the growth of "dental emporiums" and their unscrupulous hawking of dental services was ruinous of their good names. Kingsley furthermore stated:

> *The mortifying fact stares us in the face that, in the estimation of a large portion of the community, these people are dentists just as much as we are. You and I may know that we are of a different order and so do our personal friends, but to the people at large we are dentists, and so are they. To see one's vocation, which is in itself humanitarian in character, which within its sphere is second to none in the personal benefits it confers, whose methods call for the exercise of more than the average of intelligence and skill, to see such an honorable calling dragged through the mire of charlatanism, makes everyone with any esprit de corps blush with shame and mortification at the name of dentist.*[22]

Kingsley placed his hopes for the future of the dental profession on the "courage and enthusiasm" of the thousands of graduates of dental schools, hoping that they would recognize and resist the fraud through continued promulgation of prohibitory laws.

Dr Maxfield of Holyoke, Massachusetts, expressed his fears as follows:

> *The tendency of the age is toward commercialism. We hear very little of late years of the ideal in dentistry, but it is, "How much are we going to get?" for this or that. It is said that a corporation is being formed in New Jersey, with $2,000,000 capital, to establish dental parlors throughout the country. Are we as a profession coming to this?*

The legislative acts of various states had given police powers to boards of dental examiners to counter the rise of "dental companies" by ruling that dentists must practice under their own personal license. Dr W. D. Winslow of Kansas City had his dental license revoked for practicing under the employ of the Eastern Dental Parlors rather than under his own name.[24;2] The growth of Painless Parker's empire was blocked when he was prevented from opening dental parlors in Denver, Colorado. The Colorado Supreme Court, in overturning a

[2] The Dental Act of Kansas stated that the "board may revoke such license (dental) if issued to the individuals who have by false or fraudulent representations obtained or sought to obtain money or other things of value or have practiced under names other than their own, or for any other dishonorable conduct."

lower court, ruled that the statute governing dental practice applied to a dental company as well as to a personal being. Parker, having no license to practice in Colorado, could not do so under the guise of a dental corporation.[25]

But during the early part of the 20th century, advertising was no longer viewed as a form of exploitation of the public but rather as a legitimate means of educating the masses, even a necessity for building a successful medical and dental practice.[26] Advertising now became acceptable as the new science of marketing. The old notion that advertisers were fakes no longer applied; in the fast-changing world, self-promotion was becoming acceptable.

Patents

Throughout the latter half of the 19th century, the dental profession agonized over the question of patents: Was it ethical to restrict the free dissemination of new knowledge or new technology through restrictive patents? Was it not the essence of professionalism to share in the free exchange of knowledge for the public good? Was the patent system, emblematic of the trade and commercial spirit, a blemish on the altruistic character of the professional man? Dr W. W. H. Thackston, president of the Southern Dental Association, referred to a patentee as a "ravenous beast of prey" acting according to the "soulless and selfish laws of trade."[27]

Because of the inordinate and "illiberal" attempts to patent many aspects of dental care, such as "cutting off a tooth," "the removal of tooth-pulps," "the fitting of a band or ferrule to the end of a tooth," the dentists of northern New Jersey deemed it necessary to frame a bill appealing to Congress to place limits on this practice.

The trade aspect of dentistry was highlighted in 1890 by the U. S. Census Department's classification of dentists as manufacturers. The Philadelphia County Dental Society instructed its members to reject requests to complete "manufacturer's blanks," taking the position that "dentistry is a liberal profession, and a branch of the healing art, and in no sense a manufacturing business."[28]

Dr H. C. Meriam, instructor of operative dentistry in the new dental school at Harvard University and former president of the Massachusetts Dental Society, writing in *Dental Cosmos* in 1889, stated:

> *The doctor's position has always depended on his fidelity as a teacher. Your nostrum-vender, or maker of proprietary articles or medicines, who will not teach the making or their formulas, is one who disgraces*

this position and has no right to the title. So, also, if a discoverer or inventor in a liberal profession patents the requirements of his profession, making them his exclusive property, and, in the language of the Patent Office, secures "the exclusive right to make, vend, and use" them, he violates the pledges of his diploma, and has lost his claim to belong to a liberal profession.[27]

Meriam was in good company, as his position was supported by Dr H. Bowditch, the dean of Harvard Medical School. Dr Bowditch, writing in reply to Dr Meriam, stated:

I have received your letter of Feb. 6 asking my opinion on the probable effects upon the dental profession of its members becoming pecuniarily interested in patent processes and materials used in the practice of their art. As a reason for addressing me on this subject you say that "Dentistry claims to be a specialty in medicine." It seems to me that were this claim generally made and allowed there would be no occasion for discussing the above question, for it would then never occur to a dentist to patent a process for filling a tooth, any more than to a surgeon to patent a method of operating on hernia. It is precisely because so many dentists look upon their business as a trade rather than as a profession that trade methods find so easy application in dentistry. With this tradesman's view it is difficult to find fault. No moral reason can be given why a dentist, if he desires to do so, should not reap the reward of his skill and ingenuity in the same way that is permitted to an engineer or a mechanic. It is only when viewed from the standpoint of a member of a liberal profession that such conduct appears objectionable, for the chief distinction between professional men and traders is that the former are animated by an esprit de corps, and work largely for the good of the community, while the latter have, as a rule, no such motive, and work chiefly for their own individual benefit. It is evident, therefore, that there can be no greater obstacle to the recognition of dentistry as a liberal profession than the interest of the practitioner in secret materials and patent methods. Hence it is clearly the duty of those who desire to see dentistry assume a position as a specialty of medicine to discourage such practices in every possible way. There need be no quarrel with those who see fit to patent their inventions or to hold patent rights, but it should be distinctly understood that in so doing they are working on lines inconsistent with professional standards. When the lines are thus clearly drawn, the strength of the claim which dentistry may make to be regarded as a liberal profession will be apparent.[27]

Meriam's position was also in agreement with that of medical school professor Oliver Wendel Holmes, who wrote that dentistry's "work is so largely mechanical that it necessarily tempts inventors to seek fortunes through improvements in dental instruments. The more exactly they exclude owners of money-making contrivances who patent their inventions; the better will be their claim to be considered a liberal profession."[27]

But not everyone held that view at Harvard's dental school, a school tied by its umbilical cord to the older and prestigious medical school. W. E. Boardman, DMD, president of the Massachusetts Dental Society and member of the dental faculty, argued that if one upheld copyrights for dental books one could not logically prohibit professional men from holding patents: "Consistency would seem to demand that all should accord to the inventor that degree of consideration which is now and has been hitherto demanded for the author."[29] Patent laws, stated Boardman, had produced "quickening of industries, the creation of wealth, the cheapening of all the necessaries of life, the bringing of luxuries within the reach of the poor, and the diffusion of knowledge." Boardman's praise of patent policy was evidence that some in the elite of the dental profession were capable of making accommodation with the commercial elements in dentistry.

Some men recognized positive aspects in the patent system and argued for the right of a professional man to obtain letters of patent for their personal sacrifices and investments of time and money in developing new technologies or instruments that would benefit the public.[17] J. D. White, in an 1865 editorial in *Dental Cosmos*, advised the dental profession that so long as the laws of the land granted every citizen (including dentists) the right to protect their inventions with patents, it was in the best interests of the profession to accept this fact and avoid bitter conflicts and litigation:

> *Let everyone who invents, or thinks he has improved, any mechanical thing, or material, or appliance, have the right which the laws of his country guarantee to him; but he who thinks differently let him set himself aside from association with him, as a true professional man, and let the patentee in turn be satisfied with whatever emolument may accrue to him by the sale of his wares or improvements to whomsoever may choose to purchase them, and use them in his practice.*[30]

In his textbook *Ethics and Jurisprudence for Dentists* (1915), Edmund Noyes stated:

> *The medical code of ethics expressly declares that it is unprofessional for any practitioner of medicine to hold a patent on any surgical instruments or appliances, or upon any medicine or pharmaceutical preparation. It is believed that no similar clause is to be found in any code of dental ethics hitherto adopted by any dental society.*[18]

He noted that the dental profession had little opposition to patents on dental instruments so long as the purchase price included compensation to the inventor, but when the owner of the patent expected to collect a fee for every use of the invention (process fee) as in the case of vulcanite dentures, the profession was greatly embittered. Patents that controlled the process of dentistry (ie, covering things made for individual patients) were condemned because they raised the cost of dentistry and were not in the best interest of the public.

After a half-century of attempted regulation of the dental profession through adherence to a code of ethics, there had been only modest progress. The general malaise was best expressed in this 1898 quotation from H. E. Harlan:

> *Utility is the ultimate appeal on all questions of ethics. The value of material things is determined by their usefulness—a law, a code, a constitution, are men-made things; and when they are insufficient "to make the punishment fit the crime," when they do not meet the exigencies of the case their sacredness falls from them, they are extraneous and, like old clothes that are worn and soiled, they are to be cast aside. The wheels of progress are moving forward in even and definite lines, and the ultimate is the all of life, and our profession owes to itself and posterity the fostering of the spirit of fairness, breadth of thought, liberality of sentiment and freedom of action. If all of the members of the profession were imbued with the spirit of fairness, if we were all unselfish and just, if we could even coerce our fellows into these conditions, there might be some hope for the code of ethics; but as long as our colleges and the profession admit the class of men they do, to the ranks of the profession, as long as the smart and sharp people are allowed to take precedence over strength, character, worth and quality in other men, as long as the hypocrite, the shoddy and snobbish pretender can find a field to operate in, just so long will the delectable mountains of a code-regulated profession be always a dream of the future, a lost golden thread and the ever-eluding mirage of professional fairness.*[14]

Dental Education

From 1900 to 1925, the dental educational system underwent profound changes, raising the educational level of entering students, enriching the scientific content of the dental curriculum, and generally fostering a greater sense of pride among dental school graduates. Many of these changes preceded the Gies Report on Dental Education (discussed in chapter 17). The Gies Report brought the public's attention to needed changes in dental education, legitimizing and ensuring that the reform already started would continue to expand among all dental schools of the United States and Canada.

Yet issues of commercialism and professional ethics remained problematic and would continue to evolve, along with changes in dental practice brought about by progress in dental science and a new postwar social environment. Dr Edmund Pelligrino, professor of medicine and director of medical humanities at Georgetown University, speaking before the New York Academy of Medicine in 1989 on the dilemma of professional ethics, stated:

> *Today, our profession faces the unenviable choice between two opposing moral orders, one based in the primacy of our ethical obligations to the sick, the other in the primacy of self-interest and the marketplace. These two orders are not fundamentally reconcilable and, like it or not, the Academy and the profession will be forced to choose between them.*[31]

Pelligrino posed the key question: "Should we stand firm in the belief that being a physician imposes certain specific obligations that forbid turning ourselves primarily into entrepreneurs, businessmen, or agents of fiscal, social, or economic policy?"[31] This was not the first time that the medical profession was called to address this fundamental question, nor would it be the last time. For much of the 19th and 20th centuries, the medical and dental professions have confronted these issues in the hope of arriving at compromises that are mutually supported by the public and the professions.

Summary

In the period of fast-paced, unregulated growth in dentistry in America, the conflict between commercialism and professionalism caused much unease for many of the leading members of the newly formed ADA. In attempting to create a code of conduct for its members, it met with opposition from dentists who believed that there was no need for policing by an outside agency as long as men "acted as gentlemen." Local dental associations threatened to resign from the ADA if a code was forced upon them. After lengthy discussions, a code of ethics was adopted in 1847 in which the duties of the dentist to his patients and to fellow practitioners were spelled out. In explicitly banning all forms of advertising and quackery, it hoped to improve its image with the American public. Despite the fact that many dentists abided by the principles of the code, it was abundantly clear that the code was ignored by a good number of advertising dentists, most notably by the notorious "Painless" Parker. The ADA also agonized over the increasing commercialization of practice and the question of patents. The medical profession's position that holding a patent was unprofessional was finessed by organized dentistry and found no condemnation in its code of ethics. With the output of increasingly better educated dentists, grounded in the sciences and equipped with modern technologies, there occurred a gradual moderation of the flagrant misbehaviors of the early 20th century. But caution must be exercised to prevent the business of dentistry from eclipsing its humanistic element.

References

1. Parmly E. Introductory address [Extracts from the Transactions of the Third Annual Meeting of the American Society of Dental Surgeons]. Dent Cosmos 1842;3:1–17.
2. Starr P. The Social Transformation of American Medicine. New York: Basic Books, 1982.
3. Fitch CP. Professional ethics. Dent Cosmos 1861;3:60–62.
4. McCabe JD. Address before the Virginia Society of Surgeon Dentists. Am J Dent Sci 1844;4:99–115.
5. Essig CJ. The scientific spirit and the ethics of dental practice. Dent Cosmos 1895;37:494–499.
6. Horne WC. Transactions of the American Dental Association, at its sixth annual session. Dent Cosmos 1866;8:62–90.
7. Davis NS. History of Medicine with the Code of Medical Ethics. Chicago: Cleveland, 1907.
8. Stellwagen TC. Proceedings of the Odontographic Society of Pennsylvania. Dent Cosmos 1867;8:592–593.
9. Abbott JT. Northern Iowa Dental Association. Dent Cosmos 1868;10:429.
10. Smith CC. Illinois State Dental Society. Dent Cosmos 1871;13:409–416.
11. Union dental meeting with the New England Dental Society. Dent Cosmos 1890;32:954–969.
12. Burket JF. Ethics. Dent Cosmos 1895;37:230–237.
13. Ottolengui R. Proceedings of the Dental Society of the State of New York. Dent Cosmos 1895;37:680–684.
14. Harlan HE. Ethics—Professional. Pacifico Medico-Dental Gazette 1898;6:74–75.
15. Ottolengui R. The code of ethics in its relation to the present needs of the dental profession. Dent Cosmos 1892;34:366–373.
16. Waddington I. The development of medical ethics—A social analysis. Med Hist 1975;19:36–51.
17. Dean GS. Professional ethics. Dent Cosmos 1893;35:505–519.
18. Noyes E. Ethics and Jurisprudence for Dentists. Chicago: Tucker-Kenworthy, 1915.
19. Young JH. Patent medicines: An early example of competitive marketing. J Econ Hist 1960;20:648–656.
20. Ambler HL. History of Dentistry in Cleveland, Ohio. Cleveland: Evangelical Association, 1911.
21. Johnson CN. Report of the committee to revise the code of ethics. Bull Illinois State Dent Soc 1909;5:4–6.
22. Kingsley NW. Has legislation cured quackery? Dent Cosmos 1900;42:501–507.

23. Oldstein HJ. Dental legislation for the elimination of malpractice in dentistry. Dent Cosmos 1919;61:859–861.
24. Childs L. Law for the dentist. Dent Cosmos 1927;69:603–604.
25. Childs L. Law for the dentist. Dent Cosmos 1929;71:786–787.
26. Hubbard E. Advertising and popular credulity. In: Seventh Annual Convention of the Associated Advertising Clubs of America. Boston: Pilgrim Publicity, 1912:94–97.
27. Meriam HC. Professional atmosphere and morals; or, patents and secrets vs a liberal profession. Dent Cosmos 1889;31:413–429.
28. Unjustifiable patents. Dent Cosmos 1890;32:999.
29. Boardman WE. A historical view of patents and copyrights. Dent Cosmos 1890;32:690–694.
30. White JD. Dental patents. Dent Cosmos 1865;6:495–496.
31. Pellegrino ED. The medical profession as a moral community. Bull N Y Acad Med 1990;66:221–232.

16

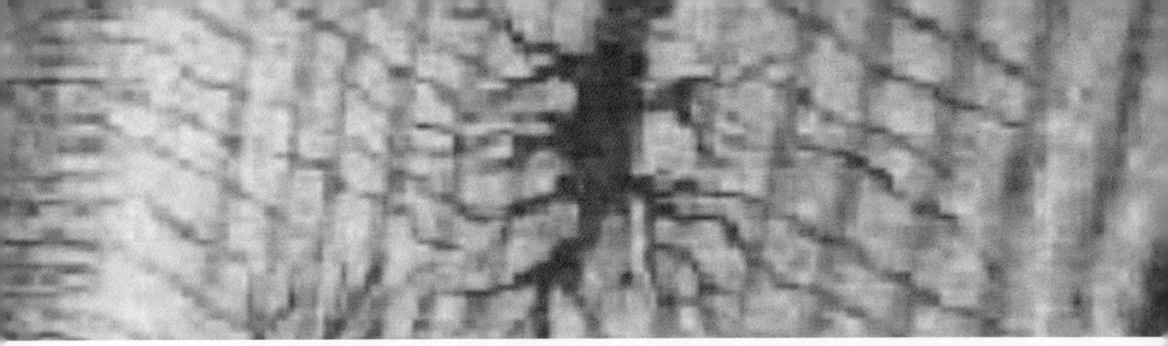

Early Dental Research

Until the 19th century, dental science had been dominated by anatomical studies of human teeth and their development, conducted primarily with simple magnifying lenses, but soon comparative anatomical studies of animal dentitions took on considerable popularity. The monumental works of Frédéric Cuvier and Richard Owen revealed the complexity and functional adaptations of animal dentitions, illustrated in beautiful engravings. Interest in the microscopic anatomy and the development of dental tissues increased in Europe along with the growth of the science of biology. Soon the perfection of the microscope brought with it a whole generation of scientists, who, particularly in France, Germany, and England, established the science of dental histology. The names of Retzius, Rashkow, Purkinje, Tomes, Hertwig, and Nasmyth are forever associated with dental histology. These same men, around the middle of the 19th century, were also actively engaged in elucidating the nature of the cell, the nucleus and protoplasm, and were establishing that extracellular matrices were formed from cellular precursors. Attempts to explain the mechanisms of the formation of enamel and dentin were intimately tied to concepts of the origin of cells and to their potential for generating tissues by conversion and/or secretion.

The Origin of Cells

A profound question facing biologists during the early years of the 19th century was how to explain the origin of cells and their role in forming tissues and organs. It was a difficult problem stemming from the fact that when tissues were examined at the highest microscopic power, they were observed to be made up of fibers, granules, and globules. The low resolving power of their microscopes limited their ability to probe any deeper into the nature of cells. Many biologists reasonably assumed that cells developed de novo from the aggregation of globules and granules in a process known as the investment theory. In 1858, Rudolf Virchow, the father of modern pathology, attacked the view that cells arose from the aggregation of elementary particles:

> *Even in pathology we can now go so far as to establish, as a general principle, that no development of any kind begins de novo, and consequently as to reject the theory of equivocal (spontaneous) generation just as much in the history of the development of individual parts as we do in that of entire organisms...equally little are we disposed to concede either in physiological or pathological histology, that a new cell can build itself up out of any non-cellular substance. Where a cell arises, there a cell must have previously existed (omnis cellula e cellula), just as an animal can spring only from an animal, a plant only from a plant.*[1]

For Virchow, cells gave rise to new cells in a continuous proliferation without discontinuity: "No developed tissues can be traced back either to any large or small simple element, unless it be unto a cell."[1] Virchow described how cells of various shapes gave rise to an intercellular substance through secretion to form tissues. Each cell created a zone (surrounding territory) of extracellular substance. How secretion was accomplished was unclear. Various tissues could be distinguished by the chemical composition of their extracellular substance. Connective tissues yielded gelatin when boiled, mucous tissues contained an acid precipitate called *mucin*, and cartilage contained a substance called *chondrine*.[1] The evidence that new cells originated from parent cells and that extracellular tissues were products of cellular activity swept away all sorts of imaginary notions of de novo cell formation, opening the way to a true understanding of biologic life.

Unlike the situation in Europe, there was little or no conduct of notable research in the newly formed United States, nor were there many institutions where such activities could be supported. However, as improved compound microscopes became increasingly available, and at prices affordable to individual investigators, microscopy clubs were formed where new discoveries, improvements in tissue preservation, and methods of tissue staining were reported. Medical and dental societies bought microscopes for the use of their members.

The perfection of magnifying lenses and the development of new methods of preserving and staining tissues for histologic analysis made between 1840 and 1870 led to rapid advances in describing the diversity of cells, their internal organization, and their participation in the structure and function of organs. Despite such progress, there was little unanimity in defining the structural characteristics of dental tissues or in explaining how they developed. Biologists were in disagreement as to what they saw in their microscopes, generating more controversy than enlightenment.[2]

According to Alexander Nasmyth:

> *Want of practice in the manipulation of materials, the precise nature of which has not been attended to; want of familiarity with microscopic appearances; ocular deception; the want of a well-defined magnifying power, and imperfect light in the microscope used, have been doubtless, also, causes of many of the conflicting conclusions to which almost all inquiries in this region of anatomy have arrived.*[3]

Theories of Tooth Structure and Dentin Development

Chapin Harris and Richard Owen

Chapin Harris and his colleagues, in founding the first dental school, recognized that if dentistry was to take its place next to medicine as a member of the learned professions, it needed to advance the dental science upon which its clinical practice was based. In his textbook *The Principles and Practice of Dental Surgery*, Harris discussed most of what represented the dental science of the mid 19th century, namely the anatomical basis of tooth development, the structure and physiology of bone, and the microscopic anatomy of oral mucosa and the salivary glands.[4] In reviewing what was then known of the formation of dentin and enamel, Harris noted that there was disagreement among leading anatomists as to the role of cells in elaborating the mineralized structure of both tissues.

Quoting extensively from Richard Owen's *Odontography*, Harris demonstrated his knowledge of contemporary science in reviewing early microscopic studies of dentinogenesis. Owen, author of the monumental work of comparative dental anatomy *Odontography*, published from 1840 to 1845, coined the word *dentine* (now referred to as *dentin*) to describe the major component of the tooth. Owen described that dentin was composed of three parts; minute tubes, cells, and "earthy particles." He attributed the discovery of the dentinal tubules to Leeuwenhoek and credited Jan E. Purkinje with confirming that dentin was comprised of tubular "fibres" arranged parallel to one another, oriented perpendicular to the surface of the pulp, and separated by an intertubular tissue. Purkinje verified the tubular nature of the dentinal fibers by demonstrating their capacity to imbibe ink through capillary attraction.[5] Owen suggested that the tubules and cells of dentin contained "a plasma, or liquor sanguine, and thus relate not only to the mechanical conditions of the tooth, but to the nutrition of the dentine."[5] The notion that dentin contained a nutritive fluid would take on significance in subsequent debates on whether dentin was a living tissue or a dead substance and whether it was capable of repair.

Owen began his research on tooth development in 1837 without any knowledge of the contemporaneous discoveries made by Purkinje and Anders Retzius.[1] In his studies of the comparative anatomy of teeth, Owen noted that in dentin formation the chief points that remained problematic were "the nature of the transition (from cell to mineralized matrix), and the relation of the cells to the dentinal tubes and the intertubular tissue." He reviewed the findings of Theodor Schwann, Isacus Raschkow, and Purkinje in identifying elongate, nucleated cells associated with a "preformative membrane" at the surface of the pulp. Summarizing the generally accepted model of dentinal development, Owen stated:

> *The main facts, then, which may be considered as established by the researches of Purkinje and Schwann, relative to the formation of dentine and the changes which the dentinal pulp undergoes during that process are the following: the proper tissue of the pulp consists of*

---

[1] Owen described his disappointment over learning that his research findings had been previously published as follows: "I exhibited the most characteristic of these specimens at my lectures on the teeth, at the Royal College of Surgeons, in May, 1837, and stated that: I had sections of these fragments prepared for the microscope; and stimulated by the amount of clearly defined and beautiful structure which they exhibited, I proceeded to examine similar sections of the human teeth and of those of many of the lower animals. The excitement of the research became heightened as the sphere of observation expanded, and I had collected extensive materials for a Treatise expressly on the Structure of Teeth, when the fourth number of Muller's *Archiv für Physiologie*, for the year 1837, containing an Analysis of Purkinje's and Fraenkel's Treatise, came into my hands, in December, 1837, and awoke me from the dream of discovery in which I had been indulging. I received, shortly after, the fifth number of the same volume of Muller's *Archiv*, containing Dr. Crepijn's German Translation of the treatise of Retzius, upon the perusal of which I abandoned my intention of publishing those general observations on the structure of the teeth which I had before deemed to be new, but now found to have been mainly anticipated by Purkinje and Retzius."

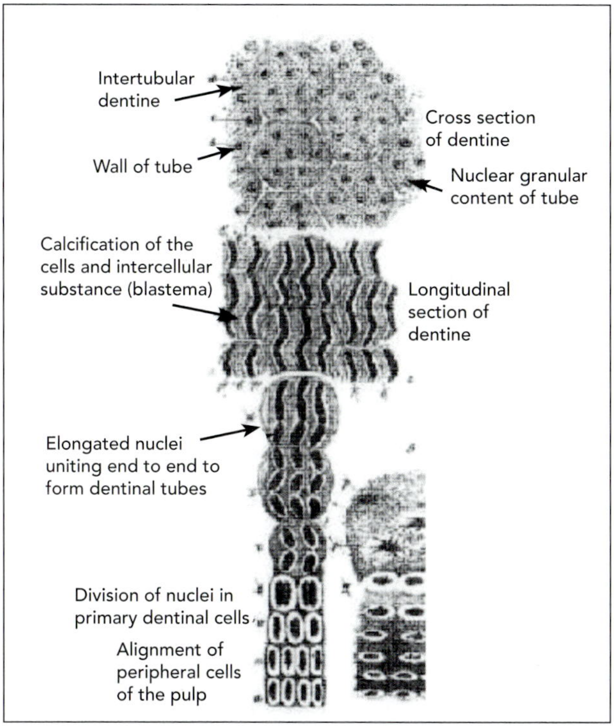

Fig 16-1 Owen's diagrammatic explanation of the formation of dentinal tubules by division and coalescence of nuclei and mineralization of intercellular substance. (From Owen.[5])

minute nucleated cells, with capillary vessels and nerves, invested by a dense structureless membrane which disappears during the formation of the dentine. The superficial pulp-cells assume an elongated form; they correspond in diameter and direction with the tubes of the contiguous cap of dentine. These or similar cells are observed, in a state of transition into dentine, in the interspace between the pulp and the previously formed cap of dentine; they adhere to the latter when it is displaced from the pulp.[5]

Owen proposed a mechanism to explain how the elongated cells at the surface of the pulp formed the dentinal tubes and the intertubular mineralized tissue through a process of nuclear division, elongation, and fusion at the interface between the pulp and the hardened dentin (Fig 16-1). Dentinal tubes were generated by the confluence and attachment of nuclear segments derived from the elongated cells. New

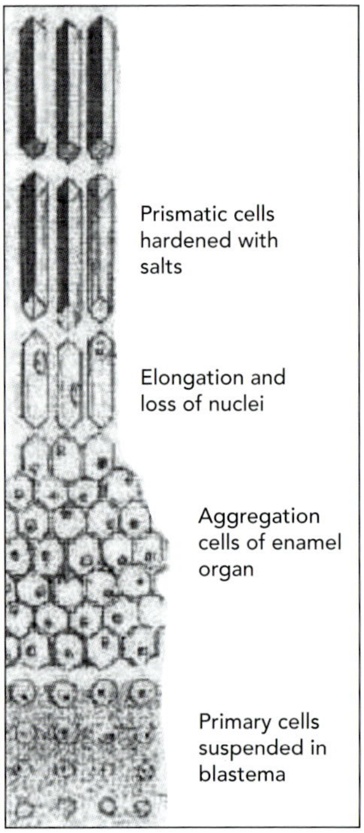

Fig 16-2 Owen's concept of the mechanism whereby enamel prisms arise by conversion and coalescence of cells. (From Owen.[5])

elongated cells arose from the pulp to replace the older transformed cells.[5] The ossified intertubular substance was thought to form in the spaces between the "metamorphosed nuclei" of the elongated cells.

Johannes Muller, employing an acid demineralization method, showed that the dentinal tubules had walls of a flexible "animal tissue" (ie, organic matrix) and that, in their normal state, they were impregnated by mineral (calcareous salts). Concurrently, Anders Retzius of Stockholm University observed that the dentinal tubules had fine anastomosing branches and terminal ramifications.[5]

When examining enamel at low magnification, Owen observed it to be composed of fibers, hexagonal in cross section, oriented with their long axis at right angles to the tooth surface, and packed in a honeycomb configuration (Fig 16-2). Owen described the presence of elongated cells in close contiguity with the surface of the dentinal pulp. These cells were reported to lose their nuclei before being "converted into long and slender cylinders...pressed by mutual contact into a prismatic form. These cylinders have the property of imbibing the calcareous salts of the enamel from the plasmatic fluid" (see Fig

16-2). As enamel grows, "the cells in the immediate contiguity with the calcified prisms undergo the same changes as their predecessors, and become united to them by their peripheral pointed extremities, while the fluid plasmatic contents of the cells are exchanged for the dense salts of which the enamel is chiefly composed."[5] Owen also proposed that the characteristic transverse striae of the enamel fibers might be produced by multiplication of "delicate nucleoli into compartments" within the elongated cells.[5]

Alexander Nasmyth

Alexander Nasmyth, an early contributor to the microscopic anatomy of tooth development, reported that the elongated peripheral cells of the pulp were transformed into the solid fibers of dentin. These fibers had the same dimensions of the dentinal tubules and were filled with "earthy matter" or calcareous salts. As for the dentinal tubules, Nasmyth dismissed their existence, stating: "The tubes have been said to be principally visible by means of their contents, the reason of which appears to me obviously to be, that these contents are the only part of them which actually exist." The interrupted or "baccated" appearance of the dentinal fibers, as visualized following partial acid demineralization, suggested to Nasmyth that the calcareous salts were accumulated in compartments (nuclei) elaborated in some fashion at the cellular forming front.[3]

Nasmyth illustrated the regular arrangement of the cells of the formative surface of the pulp,[2] noting their close correspondence to the arrangement and dimensions of the dentinal fibers, yet he was unable to elucidate the manner by which the cells gave rise to the fibers: "Although…it is demonstrated that the interfibrous substance of the ivory is formed by the deposition of osseous matter in the cells of the reticular surface of the pulp, I cannot boast of being able fully to unveil that interesting process." He suggested that "these cells (reticular) are subdivided into minute cellules," which become filled with granules and ossified to form the dentinal fibers. Although Nasmyth did not claim infallibility for his views, he did allow that they were "bold and novel."[3]

[2] It is apparent that Nasmyth was viewing the surface of the pulp "en face" after having lifted away the first layer of dentin from the pulp. In hindsight, we can interpret Nasmyth's reticular arrangement of "cells" (as represented in his drawings) as odontoblasts "cross-sectioned" at the level of the distal terminal web. Here the cell membranes contain a high concentration of zonula adherens and occludens junctional proteins, all serving to create a fairly rigid and optically refractive close attachment between neighboring cells.

Thomas H. Huxley and Albert Kölliker

Thomas H. Huxley, a rising star among English biologists, caused a stir in 1853 when he published a rejection of the Schleiden and Schwann cell theory. Huxley's opposition centered less on the anatomical cellular unit structure of animals (as outlined by Schwann) than on the physiologic interpretation of that concept.[6] In explaining his view, Huxley proposed that the animal body contained an all-encompassing living substance, the periplast, which was concentrated at nodal points or endoplasts. In contrast to the cell theory, wherein new cells arise through division of preexisting cells, Huxley's endoplasts were thought to form de novo within the periplast in a process analogous to crystallization or congealment.[7]

In the same year of his controversial publication, Huxley (jointly with G. Busk) completed an English translation of the German edition of Albert Kölliker's *Manual of Human Histology* (the most celebrated textbook of histology since Owen's *Odontography*). The Huxley and Busk translation was printed as a limited edition for members of the Sydenham Society. Kölliker, a highly respected biologist, was a strong supporter of the cell theory. In the process of translation, Huxley interjected his own contrarian opinions of the cell theory in the form of lengthy textual annotations.[6] In contrast to Kölliker, Huxley rejected the notion that the nucleus (endoplast) exerted a directive "force" upon the periplast and stated that nuclei could not be transformed into tissue structures. Huxley proposed that chemical transformation occurred in the periplast independent of the endoplast: "By chemical change or deposit it [the periplast] acquires Horn, Collagen, Chondrin, Syntonin, Fats, Calcareous Salts, according as it becomes Epithelium, Connective tissue, Cartilage, Muscle, Nerve or Bone."[7]

In 1853, in a paper reflecting his contrarian views on the cell theory, Huxley denied that cells played any role in forming enamel and dentin. Huxley proposed that dentin was formed "not by the ossification of the histological elements of the pulp, but by deposition in it"[8] (ie, within the matrix or periplast of the pulp and not within pulpal endoplasts). Similarly, enamel was formed by deposition of calcareous salts in an extracellular periplastic matrix, not by conversion of endoplasts. Epithelial cells played no role in the development of enamel. Huxley stated that the conversion theory of enamel formation was as incorrect as the excretion theory. In this, his only publication dealing with tooth development, Huxley placed importance on the presence of a "basement membrane" (Raschkow's membrana preformativa) covering the outer surface of the pulp. Huxley noted that although a layer of "cylindrical nucleated epithelial cells" adhered to the outer surface of this "basement membrane," the enamel was formed beneath this membrane in direct contact with the dentin.[8] Huxley concluded that the cylindric epithelial cells could not have undergone conversion into enamel.

Huxley's similar dismissal of direct conversion of pulp cells into dentin was attacked by Edouard Lent, a student and defender of his mentor, Albert Kölliker. Kölliker and Lent, proponents of the cellular origin of extracellular matrices, had proposed that dentinal tubules arose through conversion of the surface cells of the pulp.

Lent's criticisms were rebutted by Huxley in a new paper in which he leveled caustic accusations toward Kölliker for having encouraged "in a student a disingenuousness of which he himself, I hope, would be heartily ashamed."[9;3] Huxley's biographer, J. Davis, noted Huxley's propensity for being prickly toward his antagonists:

> *Huxley's many occasions for despondency began to be augmented in 1852 by professional jealousies, and by attempts, luckily unsuccessful, to retard his further progress. Then, as always, he proved himself a perfectly straightforward antagonist, but at the same time one whom it was decidedly unpleasant to tackle.*[10]

In the second English translation of his *Manual of Human Histology* (1860 Buchanan translation), Kölliker summarized his view of the development of dentin based in large measure on the results of

[3] Huxley's belligerent reply to Lent (and Kölliker) is not surprising in view of Huxley's criticisms in the first translation of Kölliker's textbook from the original German into English for the Sydenham Society, a limited edition for members only. According to Kölliker, there was interest in a wider circulation: "On this account, on my visit to the British Association at Glasgow in the year 1855, I was urged by several of my English friends to prepare an independent English edition, which should also have the advantage of a more compact form. After mature consideration, I resolved to act on this suggestion; and, in the same year, I succeeded in finding a publisher, Mr. J. W. Parker, ready to forward the work by all the means in his power. In carrying out my project, however, a considerable obstacle presented itself. The translation was executed under my own supervision by one of my pupils, who spared no pains or diligence upon it, but when submitted to English friends, on whose judgment I could thoroughly rely, it was pronounced to have followed too literally the German original. I was, therefore, obliged to abandon all idea of publishing the work in that condition. A complete revision of the manuscript, which almost amounted to a remodeling of the translation, was, however, undertaken by Dr. George Buchanan and another friend in England; and these gentlemen have done their part in a manner which merits my warmest thanks."[11] Huxley had no part in the second translation. It is also of interest that the Sydenham edition contained no description of oral and dental tissues, yet the 1860 edition contained a full section dealing with dental tissues and their development. Did this new section represent original work of the young Edouard Lent or had it been omitted from the earlier Huxley and Busk translation edition? It would seem that seeds of animosity had been planted between Kölliker and Huxley at that earlier time, no doubt regarding their differences concerning the cell theory.

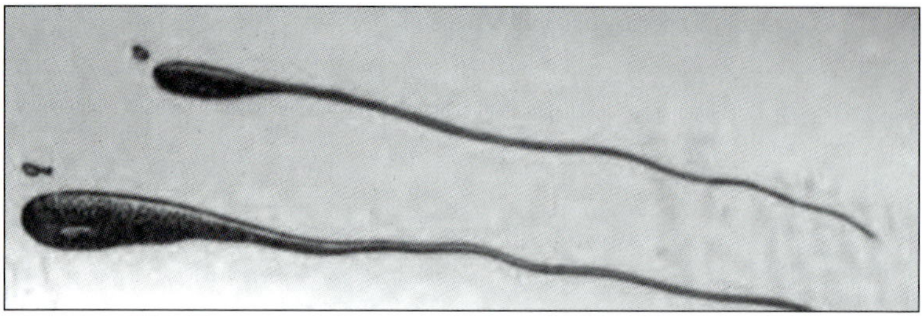

Fig 16-3 Lent's isolated dentinal cells. (From Kölliker.[11])

one of his pupils, E. Lent. Working with macerated pulp tissue, Lent was able to isolate cells that had long cytoplasmic extensions (Fig 16-3). He wrongly interpreted these extensions to be dentinal tubules or canals. Kölliker and Lent concluded that the formation of dentin proceeded as follows:

> *The dentinal canals are direct processes of the whole dentinal cells, which processes may send out subordinate branches, and anastomose by means of them. To all appearances, a single cell seems, in many cases, to be sufficient to form an entire dentinal canal, or at least a very large part of one. The matrix of the dentine is not formed of the dentine-cells, but is a secretion of these cells and of the tooth pulp: in other words, an intercellular substance.*[11]

This appears to be the first report that dentin matrix is a cellular secretion distinct from cellular conversion.

Kölliker concluded his discussion of dentin formation by venting his displeasure with Huxley: "With regard to the formation of the dentine from dentinal cells, it is certain, that no other tissue than the cells contributes anything to the result, and Huxley is decidedly wrong in maintaining that no histological element of the pulp is concerned in the formation of the tooth."[11]

Kölliker described dentin as consisting of a homogenous matrix with numerous tubules or canals running from the surface of the pulp cavity through the entire thickness of the dentin as far as the enamel and the cementum (Fig 16-4). Each dentinal tubule, lined by an apparent wall, underwent ramification in the form of fine branches, especially dense at their termination near the innermost surfaces of the enamel and cementum. The dentinal tubules with their walls intact

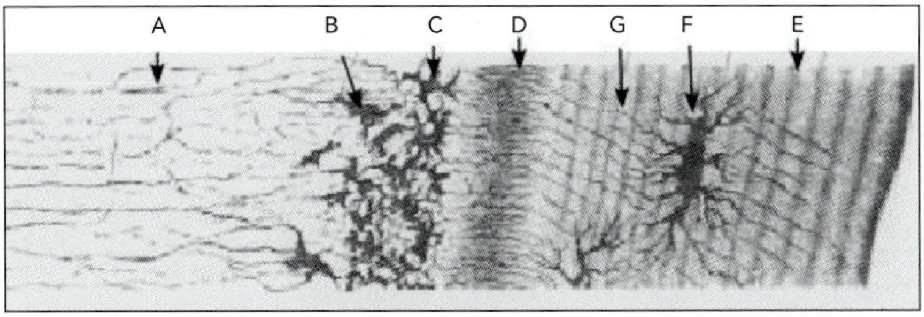

Fig 16-4 Dentin and cementum from the middle of the root depicting dentinal tubules (A), interglobular spaces (B and C), the innermost layer of cementum (D), cementum lamellae (E), lacunae (F), and canaliculi (G). (Adapted from Kölliker.[11])

could be isolated by macerating dentin in "acids or alkalies." In life, dentin, cementum, and to a lesser degree enamel were permeated by a nutritive fluid:

> *The functions of the lacunae of the bones and their canaliculi, are performed here by the dentinal canals and their ramifications, the lacunae and canaliculi in the cement, and the spaces between the prisms of the enamel. All these spaces, during life, contain a fluid which, on the one hand, comes from the vessels of the pulp, and, on the other, from those of the alveolar periosteum, and furnishes the conditions necessary for a change of material, slow though it be.*[11]

John Tomes

A major contribution to the structure of dentin was made by Dr John Tomes of London. He showed that the linear, elongated, formative cells located at the interface between the pulp and the mineralizing dentin underwent division, increased in length, and became aligned with the developing dentinal tubes. He proposed that mineral was concentrated within and around the cells to form the tubes and intertubular fibers.

Tomes reported that the anastomosis of the dentinal tubules, through branching side processes, was especially pronounced in root dentin. He described communication between the terminal branches of the dentinal tubules with the enamel and the lacunae of cementum. In agreement with Kölliker, he held the view that the tubules contained a fluid. Tomes found it difficult to reconcile the physiologic and nociceptive properties of dentin based solely on the fluid content of the dentinal tubules, and in further investigations he made a key discovery:

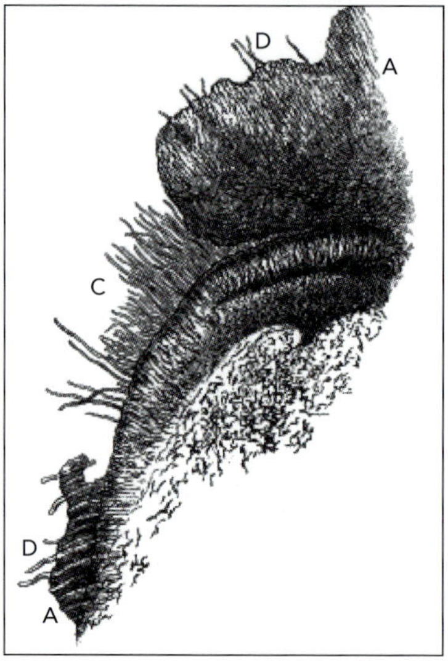

Fig 16-5 Dental pulp of an adult tooth depicting the dentinal fibrils protruding from peripheral cells (C) and the mineralized dentin (A and D). (From Tomes.[12])

> *I had, however, but little expectation of finding that one of the most important points in dental structure had been overlooked, namely, that each dentinal tube is permanently tenanted by a soft fibril,*[4] *which, after passing from the pulp into the tube, follows its ramifications....The end of the fibril, when accidentally broken across, exhibited a minute globule of transparent but dense fluid...gathered into a more or less spherical form. These appearances may be explained by assuming that the fibril consists of a sheath containing a semifluid matter, similar to the white fibrillae of nerves [Fig 16-5]; but whether such a conclusion can be justified admits of doubt.*[12]

Tomes gave credit to Kölliker, Lent, and Huxley as having observed short fibrils extending from the elongated cells at the surface of the pulp but noted that none of them had found fibrils to be "permanent" occupants of the dentinal tubules in fully formed dentin.

Although he failed to identify the origin or termination of the fibrils (now known as *odontoblastic processes*), Tomes stated:

[4] The dentinal fibril would later be identified as the odontoblastic process, a cytoplasmic extension of the odontoblast and the part of the cell from which dentin matrix is secreted.

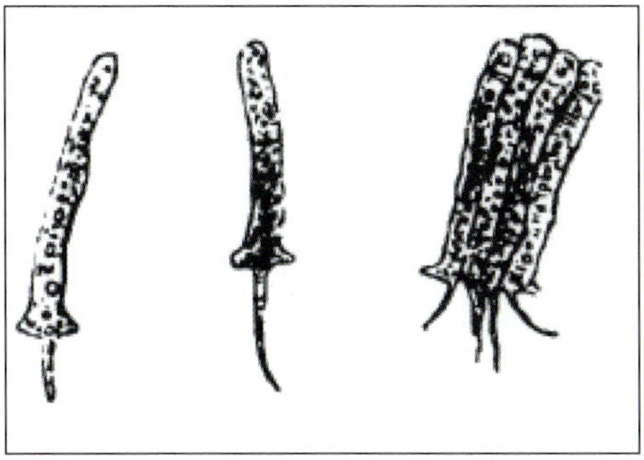

Fig 16-6 The columns (cylindric cells) of the enamel with their processes. (From Tomes.[13])

That the dentine owes its sensation to the presence of the dentinal fibrils cannot, I think, be readily doubted, seeing that if their connection with the pulp be cut off by the destruction of the latter, all sensation is at once lost... [concluding that] the dental fibrils are subservient not only to sensation in the dentine, but that they are also the channels by which nutrition is carried to that tissue; and that, like other organized tissues, they may become the seat of morbid action.[12]

In his investigations of enamel formation, Tomes made microscopic examinations of teased and macerated parts of enamel organs exposed to mild acid decalcification. Tomes demonstrated nucleated "cylindrical columns" (cells) attached to enamel fibers (now known as *rods* or *prisms*).[13] When isolated from the enamel, these cells "were terminated by delicate processes, which must at the time of separation have been withdrawn from the interior of the partially calcified fibres....Immediately above the point from which the process starts, each column has, when separated from its fellows, a slight circumferential dilation" (Fig 16-6).[13] Furthermore, Tomes demonstrated that the enamel-forming cells adhered laterally to adjacent cells by this "circumferential dilation." He described enamel as being constructed of parallel fibers that ran a wavy course from the surface of the dentin to the enamel surface. In thin sections, the enamel fibers were observed to be marked by regularly spaced transverse striae; when viewed on end, each fiber appeared to have a hexagonal to round

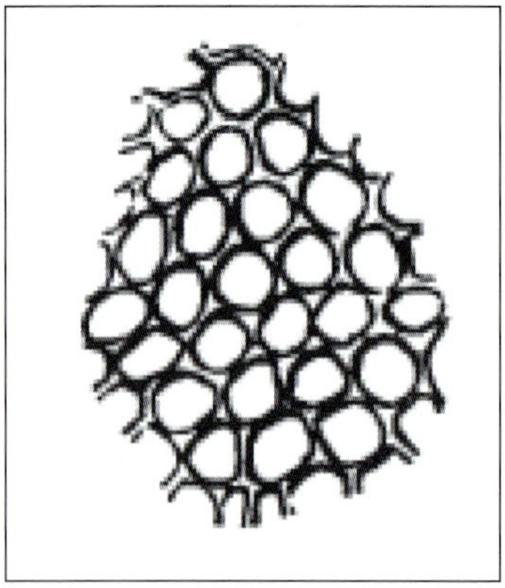

Fig 16-7 A transverse section of the enamel after the removal of granular masses by acid, showing the empty sheaths. (From Tomes.[13])

cross-sectional shape. This aspect was clearly demonstrated following a brief exposure to acid (Fig 16-7).

Tomes concluded that elongated columns (epithelial cells) gave rise to the enamel fibers:

> *The conversion of the one into the other taking place in the following manner—The proximal end of the column becomes calcified, not uniformly throughout its thickness, but the outer surface or sheath first receives the salts of lime, and at the same time the columns become united laterally. At this point the columns (cells) readily separate from the fibres and leave a surface which, when looked upon directly, has the appearance of a membrane.*[13]

Tomes detected that each enamel-forming cell contained a terminal process that could be withdrawn from the forming surface of the enamel. Many years later, this process would be called *Tomes process* and be identified as the secretory pole of the ameloblast.

Carl Heitzmann and Carl Bödecker

An interesting twist in the history of dental histology involves Carl Heitzmann, MD, author of the 1884 textbook *Microscopical Morphology of the Animal Body in Health and Disease*. In 1874, Heitzmann had emigrated from Vienna to New York City, where he established a laboratory for microscopic investigations. Heitzmann advertised courses in laboratory histology and microbiology: "six-weeks, six sessions per week, for a fee of twenty six dollars per course." In a speech before a dental convention, he claimed that over 700 individuals, including many physicians and dentists, came to take his courses. Heitzmann developed a strong following among dentists of New York City, stating:

> *It was your profession (thanks to noble-hearted men such as Dr. Atkinson) which first gave cordial recognition of my work. My laboratory was favored especially by dentists, and, without boasting, I can say that most of the work in the investigation of the anatomy of the teeth which has been done in the last few years, has emanated from thence.*[14]

Frank Abbott, William Atkinson, and Carl Bödecker were Heitzmann-trained contributors to his textbook and to numerous articles in *Dental Cosmos*.

Before coming to New York City, Heitzmann had been a lecturer in morbid anatomy at the University of Vienna. He held the view that "the body is by no means composed of isolated elements, so-called cells, as it was formerly thought to be...but that the tissues from the crown to the heel are one continuous mass of living matter, mainly in a reticular arrangement."[14] Like Huxley, Heitzmann rejected the cell theory. He developed a new terminology to communicate his theories, believing that a living principle or substance (*bioplasson*) permeated all tissues and was capable of forming distinct units, so-called bioplasson bodies or plastids. Furthermore, the bioplasson could take the form of minute fibers, penetrating throughout what he called the *basis-substance* (extracellular matrix) and interconnecting all bioplasson bodies.[14]

In announcing the cell theory dead, replaced by his living reticular substance, or bioplasson, Heitzmann found no support. Worse yet, and much to his disappointment, he was ignored: "Frey, of Zurich, who wrote a book, tried to ridicule the whole thing and to kill me off by placing me in a foot-note in his book." Ignored by the elite of biologic science, he left Europe in 1874 "in disgust and despair" and found "heartiest support and encouragement" in New York, where scientists, unlike those in Europe, were not "prejudiced by the teachings of the older masters."[14] Writing in 1882, he boasted that:

> *In the past seven years I have demonstrated all that to hundreds who were desirous to learn something about the new theory. It seems to me that what we have done in the past seven years in this country carries us quite ahead of the old world; we have become the leaders in this line of investigation.*[14]

Many of those who accepted his theories were dentists who had enrolled in his courses and were to play a significant role in the development of dental histology. Carl Bödecker, Heitzmann's pupil, in the chapter on the structure and development of teeth in Heitzmann's book, described the basis-substance of dentin (matrix) to be permeated by dentinal tubules or canaliculi[15] (Fig 16-8). Each tubule contained a dentinal fiber that gave off numerous lateral offshoots that penetrated into the adjacent basis-substance. The dentinal fibers are continuous with the "bioplasson bodies" of the pulp. Heitzmann and Bödecker, being cognizant of the well-known structure of bone, with its lacunae and its network of canaliculi containing living fibers, adopted it as a model and applied it to the structure of dentin, enamel, and cementum. Bödecker summarized their concept of the structure of dentine as follows:

> *The dentinal canaliculi are excavations in the basis-substance of the dentine, each containing in its center a fiber of living matter. Besides the dentinal canaliculi, there exists an extremely delicate net-work within the basis-substance of the dentine, into which innumerable offshoots of the dentinal fibers pass. Although we cannot trace the living matter throughout the whole net-work in the basis-substance, we are justified in assuming that not only the dental canaliculi, but the whole basis-substance of the dentine is also pierced by a delicate net-work of living matter. The living matter of the dentine is in direct union with that of the bioplasson bodies of the pulp, of the cementum, and the enamel.*[16]

Heitzmann claimed to have proven Tomes's suspicion that dentinal fibrils were connected with sensation:

> *This approaches our views, for we can prove living matter proper and nerve-tissue to be one and the same thing; and we can trace the ultimate fibrils of nerves to direct and indirect connection with the dentinal fibers. Any irritation of the dentinal fibrils is transmitted to the nerves which are present in the pulp tissue.*[14]

In a similar vein, Heitzmann proposed that the living matter (bioplasson) of cementum, consisting of lacunae harboring nucleated plastids, was interconnected by fibers within canaliculi, forming an "uninterrupted connection" with the dentin on one side and the pericementum on its other side[5] (see Fig 16-8).

---

[5] Figure 16-8, an illustration of the apparent interconnection of dentinal fibers with cells of the cementum (protoplasmic bodies) and their processes (offshoots), and Fig 16-9, an illustration of dentin formation, are drawings, not photomicrographs. R. R. Andrews stated that drawings were simply imaginary depictions whereas photomicrographs revealed the truth.

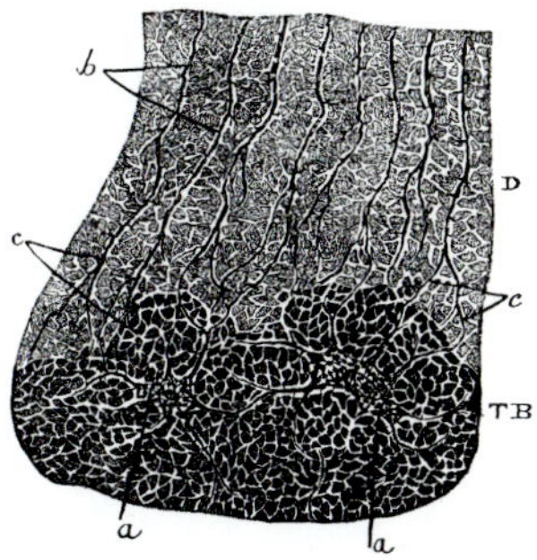

Fig 16-8 Cross section of a molar root. D—dentine; TB—cementum (tooth bone); A—protoplasmic bodies of the cementum; B—dentinal fibers with their transverse offshoots; C—dentinal fibers and their union with the offshoots of "cement-corpuscles." (From Heitzmann.[15])

Bödecker's description of the structure of enamel encompassed similar ideas. Enamel was described as being

> *traversed by fibers of living matter located in the interstices between the enamel rods. The fibers are connected with each other by delicate fibrillae, piercing the enamel rods in a vertical direction. The enamel fibers send conical thorns toward the enamel rods, and such thorns are visible in all interstices between the enamel rods...the enamel fibers are continuous with the dentinal fibers.*[16]

Thus, Heitzmann and his pupils proposed that all tissues of the tooth were interconnected by a living substance (bioplasson) connecting plastids (cellular-like bodies) through fine fibers and fibrillae (what today are described as *cytoplasmic processes*).

In concluding the section of his book dealing with teeth, Heitzmann stated the following:

> *The development of the teeth has for a number of years been studied in my laboratory by C. F. W. Bödecker, and these studies are not yet completed. One of the important facts gained by the researches of Bödecker is, that the views held by former observers, concerning the development of the enamel, is erroneous. It is true that the enamel starts as an epithelial prolongation of the oral cavity, but the epithelia themselves never participate in the formation of enamel. The epithelia break down into medullary corpuscles, from which arises the well-known graceful myxomatous tissue. This tissue again returns to the medullary condition before producing enamel, the process being identical to that by which dentine is produced. Dentine is formed of medullary corpuscles, which are arranged in rows at the periphery of*

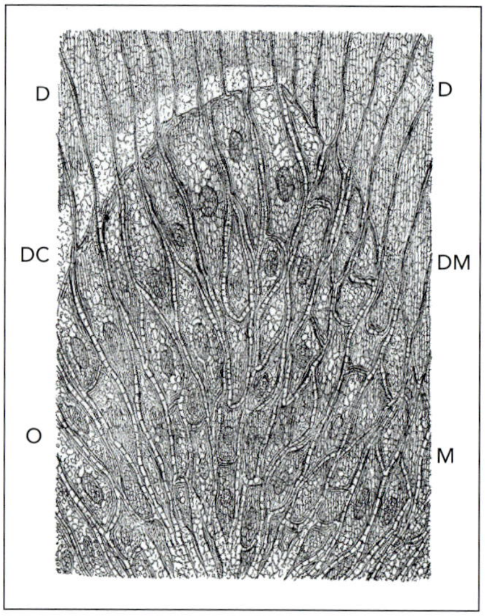

Fig 16-9 Peripheral region of the tooth pulp in a tooth from a pig fetus 10 cm in length (magnification ×800). D—calcified dentin; DC—noncalcified dentin; DM—dentin in the process of formation from medullary corpuscles; O—odontoblasts in multiple rows, with spindle-shaped elements wedged between the broad odontoblasts; M—medullary corpuscles arisen from odontoblasts, which attach to the distal ends of the odontoblasts. (From Abbott.[17])

> *the papilla, and which afterward change into the glue-yielding basis-substance, the seat of infiltration, with lime-salts. The canaliculi of the dentine are formed between the medullary corpuscles, and the dentinal fibers arise from a coalescence of the living matter which is present between the medullary corpuscles, termed "odontoblasts."*[15]

In 1888, Frank Abbott,[6] a student of the Heitzmann school of microscopy, found evidence in support of the transformation theory in dentin formation.[17] Abbott believed that primitive medullary cells, formed by agglomeration of the living substance of the pulp, were transformed into tall, elongated odontoblasts at the periphery of the pulp. In a subsequent step, the odontoblasts "split up into smaller portions of protoplasm which we term medullary or embryonal elements, and whenever this is the case we see the fibrils (dentinal) passing into the already formed basis-substance of dentine, between the rows of embryonal corpuscles."[17] Abbott described how "each odontoblast, while being reduced to medullary corpuscles at its distal or peripheral end, is being added to by an attachment of medullary corpuscles of the papillary tissue at its proximal or central end"[17] (Fig 16-9). Twenty years after Rudolf Virchow had denied the validity of the investment theory (that new cells developed by aggregation of elementary living units), Abbott held the view that the pulp contained a living matter,

[6] Frank Abbott was dean of the New York College of Dentistry (1869) and president of the American Dental Association (1888).

a "myxomatous basis-substance" able to produce protoplasmic bodies (medullary cells) that were continually added to the odontoblasts.

Heitzmann and his students were convinced that new embryonic "medullary" cells could arise from the aggregation of living particles of bioplasson. This process was thought to occur in the pulp and to contribute to the growth of dentin. It was also their belief that a living medullary substance was liberated from enamel and dentin during the progress of dental caries, forming a nutrient for the invading microorganisms. They viewed dental caries as "an inflammatory process which, beginning as a chemical process, in turn reduces the tissues of the tooth into embryonic or medullary elements, evidently the same as during the development of the tooth."[18] This idea was in direct contradiction to the microbial-acid demineralization theory of W. D. Miller.

Thirty years after Virchow's demonstration of the validity of the cell theory, Bödecker, Abbott, and William Atkinson, disciples of Heitzmann, found themselves far from the mainstream of cellular biology, refusing to accept the growing body of evidence that disproved the bioplasson concept of tissue structure and development. Perhaps it was their lack of predental education and the failure to master medical basic sciences that left them without the critical ability to evaluate scientific theories and thus open to acceptance of fringe ideas, such as Heitzmann's bioplasson theory.

Quack Science

In this nascent period of dental science, it was easy for self-promoting pseudoexperts to rise to prominence in the profession. For dentists who had followed the apprenticeship pathway or had been exposed to very little science in their short dental school curriculum, there was much to learn about the newly developing disciplines of physiology, histology, embryology, metallurgy, and electricity. For the average dentist, it was difficult and often impossible to distinguish real science from the obfuscations of egocentric imposters. It was common practice at regular dental association meetings in major cities, such as Boston, New York, and Philadelphia, to invite academics and self-educated investigators to lecture on new advances in science. A sterling example of the gibberish to which members of some dental societies were exposed is contained in the published lectures of William Atkinson, MD, as recorded in the New York Dental Association meetings of 1864 and 1865.[19,20] In two lectures on the microscopic structures of teeth and the origin and development of dental tissues, not one fact was put forth by Atkinson that was backed by experimental confirmation; all of his pronouncements were figments of his imagination. Atkinson, an ardent proponent of vitalism and Heitzmann's bioplasson school, rambled on about universal plasma, infusorial masses, nerve energies, and galvanoid and vital currents, in all likelihood thoroughly perplexing his unsophisticated listeners.[21] Atkinson's prominence as a clinician and his stature in organized dentistry gave him a false authority in fields (embryology and histology) in which he knew very little. Atkinson, like the vitalists and the proponents of the Heitzmann bioplasson theory, supported the idea that dental caries was produced from the pulp outward—a spread of some form of inflammation, or a loss of vital spirit, affecting the dentin and causing it to disintegrate. Vitalists continued to hold this idea in spite of the growing evidence that decay started on the surface of the tooth through a bacterial fermentation process.

Scientific Progress and Enamel Development

In this sea of amateurs, there were a few clear-sighted professionals who, through long observation and experimentation, made true progress. These men understood the cellular organization of tissues, and, although they did not yet fully understand the function of cells, they believed that ultimately these microscopic entities held an explanation of the mechanism of life, with no need to resort to universal vitalism. R. R. Andrews and G. V. Black demonstrated clear insights during a typical scientific presentation at the First District Dental Society of the State of New York held December 9, 1885. That evening, Dr R. R. Andrews of Cambridge, Massachusetts, having been invited to speak on the development of teeth, began with the following statement:

> *Having become personally interested in photography, I have been enabled to prepare specimens of my collection illustrating this subject; and from the negatives of these photographs I have produced the lantern slides which are to be exhibited to you this evening [Fig 16-10]. They do not show the details of a careful drawing; they do show the condition of the tissue as the microscope reveals it to us.*[22]

This was an attack on those who drew what they "saw" in the microscope (Heitzmann and Bödecker) as opposed to those who recorded the "truth" on photographic paper. It was indeed a very fine lecture

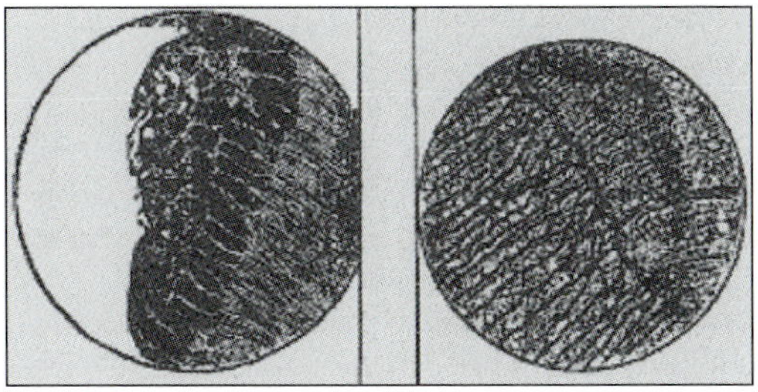

Fig 16-10 Photomicrographs of odontoblasts *(left)* and dentinal tubules *(right)* as prepared by R. R. Andrews, 1866.

with excellent micrographs depicting the cellular nature of the embryonic dental tissues. During a scholarly explanation of how cellular action was a fundamental mechanism operating in tooth formation, Andrews demonstrated the layers of ameloblasts and odontoblasts, the prismatic structure of enamel, and the tubular nature of dentin.

Following the completion of Dr Andrews's lecture, the session was open to review, during which Dr G. V. Black made lengthy comments supporting the findings of Dr Andrews. Black, an accomplished histologist in his own right (see chapter 8), provided a clear exposition of the cellular nature of the developing tooth, revealing his knowledge of the new biology and in the process discrediting vitalism as an explanation for organogenesis. Black spoke as follows:

> *This has been a funny meeting so far, and a funny discussion; but I hope you will not expect anything funny from me, because I am not a funny man. We have had here a repetition in its most essential phases of a discussion that occurred in London fifty years ago…one party was arguing for the vitality of the dentine, and the manifestation of that vitality in its diseases; while the other party was arguing as earnestly for the chemical nature of those diseases, and that vitality at most only modified them.*[22]

Black continued, arguing that vitalism failed to explain dental caries while the new concept of acid fermentation held much promise. Finally, Black concluded his long discussion as follows:

> *Physiology in its principal points is the same throughout all manifestations of life, and we must get down to bedrock in this matter—study physiological principals—if we would understand that which we see, and the diseases with which we must deal. Now I will*

get into trouble, for I know my friend over there [Atkinson] will not agree with me in what I am about to say. The cell is the unit of physical life. No matter whether that cell represents a complete individual as we see it in the ameba, or is a component of the complex individual, one among the multitude that make up the sum of the higher animal forms, or their individual parts, as we see it in the stellate reticulum of the enamel-organ as depicted by my friend [Andrews] here on the blackboard. But then this doctrine has been taught so long and so well that everybody understands it. [Here there were interjections from vitalists in the audience—"Not much," "Not in that way," "That theory is exploded."] Everybody understands it,—outside of New York. I have said the cell is the unit of physical life—I am not talking of spiritual life.—And it has certain characteristics in its dealings with matter which are common to all units of physical life that exist on this planet. These are its physiological attributes, and they may be summarized in four propositions. First each cell is capable, when in contact with certain material, of furnishing or elaborating a substance capable of digesting food material, or preparing it for absorption and assimilation. This you may call diastase, soluble ferment, unorganized ferment, enzyme, or by any of the words in use to represent the digestive agent. Second, it is capable of assimilating the food so prepared. Assimilation results in growth. Third, every individual unit of life is capable of de-nutrition. This consists in shedding out in the form of waste products, material that has once been formed into protoplasm, or used in connection with the nutritive process. Fourth, it has the power of reproduction in a definite line of forms. These four powers may be—yes, they are—varied widely among the different organisms with which we meet. They are capable of living on widely different foods, and the digestive agent elaborated is different—that is to say, adapted to the digestion of different foods. Then the waste products differ widely among the different organisms, and yet they have much in common, as we find them in the animal, the vegetable and the so-called third class, the kingdom of the microbes.[22]

Andrews and Black represented the new dental scientists, men who were abreast of the current state of physical, chemical, and biologic research and were capable of interpreting and applying new discoveries to the developing branch of dentistry. In the last two decades of the 19th century, dental histology in America was dominated by three men (J. L. Williams, R. R. Andrews, and W. X. Sudduth) who, through the application of photomicroscopy, helped to bring some order out of the existing confusion and tear down the erroneous ideas propagated by the Heitzmann School.

Employing a frozen, thin-sectioning technique, Williams

succeeded in obtaining a few specimens so thin that but a single layer of odontoblasts is shown, and with all of the tissues in their natural relations. The dentinal fibrillae were seen to be prolongations of the odontoblasts. From some of the cells but a single fiber could be traced,

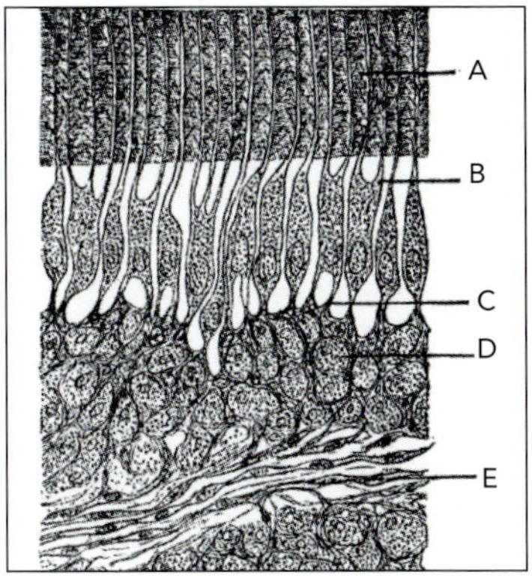

Fig 16-11 A—dentin; B—odontoblasts, showing the origin of dentinal fibrillae; C—connection of the odontoblasts with the reticulum of the pulp; D—large corpuscles held in the reticulum; E—nerve fibers. (From Williams.[23])

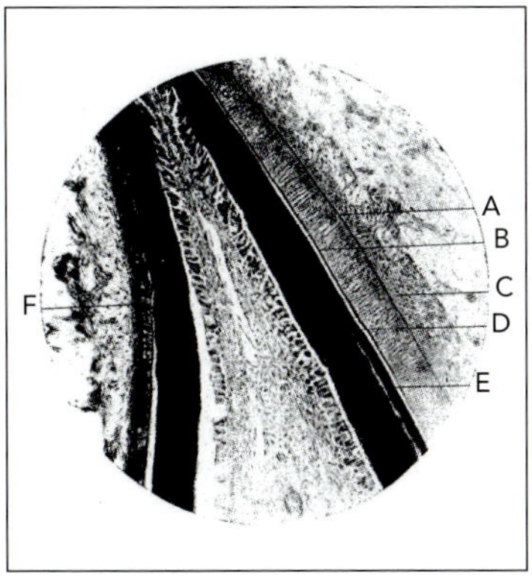

Fig 16-12 Photomicrograph of a section of a developing tooth in an embryo lamb (magnification ×150). A—outer ameloblastic membrane; B—inner ameloblastic membrane; C—cells of stratum intermedium; D—forming enamel; E—dentine; F—ameloblasts showing globular masses of calcoglobulin. (From Williams.[24])

> *while from others two and sometimes three fibers were seen to originate [Fig 16-11].... Delicate fibers are also seen to project from the ends of the cells lying next to the pulp-tissue.... Nerve fibers are seen to ramify everywhere near the surface of the pulp, and under high power can be seen to send terminal fibrillae into the reticulum [Fig 16-12], with which the roots of the odontoblasts are in immediate connection.*[23]

Williams came to conclude that the odontoblasts performed a dual function, secreting the material for the formation of dentin and performing a neural (ganglionic) function.

Turning his attention to the development of enamel, Williams declared that "The active elementary agents in the formation of enamel are the ameloblasts. It is probably formed, not by a change of these cells into a glue-yielding basis-substance which becomes infiltrated with lime-salts, but by a process of secretion and deposition."[23] Indicating a difference with Heitzmann, Williams stated the following:

> *If it is true, as taught by Prof. Heitzmann, that the building up of enamel proceeds by the successive formation of layers of ameloblasts or enamel-forming cells, which are changed into a glue-yielding basis-substance which becomes the seat of calcific infiltration, then it is*

> *strange that we are never able to discover but a single layer of cells. If there were successive layers formed, as there must be if the cell substance itself becomes the seat of calcific infiltration, why are we not able to discover these successive layers of cells in process of formation? So far as appearances teach us anything, it seems as though the ameloblasts were the active agents in depositing the lime-salts on the periphery of the dentine, and that they gradually recede with the progressive formation of the enamel.*[23]

In 1886, Williams published a critical review of the formation of dentin and enamel in which he demonstrated the impossibility of upholding the theories contained in the work of Heitzmann, Bödecker, and Abbott, namely their proposals that dentin and enamel are constructed by a conversion of "medullary corpuscles," that dentinal fibrils arise from the pulp, that enamel is permeated by a living system of fibrils, and that caries is a disease of inflammation. It was a carefully reasoned argument based on Williams's histologic studies.[25] He identified two schools of thought: *(1)* those who proposed a direct conversion of cells into calcified enamel (represented by Tomes, W. Waldeyer, and others) and *(2)* those who supported the secretion theory wherein the cells produced an extracellular matrix that underwent calcification (led by Edward Sharpey-Schafer, Ferdinand Graf von Spee, Andrews, and Sudduth).

Williams, using photomicrographs, described the stratum intermedium, a layer of cells between the ameloblasts and the reticulum of the enamel organ, associated in rodent teeth with epithelial papillae and a rich network of capillary loops. This anatomical configuration led him to propose that "In the development of enamel the cells of the stratum intermedium play the most important part in the selection from the blood of the material for the construction of this tissue."[24]

In 1884, Xavier Sudduth rejected the concept of the direct conversion of cells into calcified matrix, stating that there was no example in nature where this occurred in normal development. Taking bone as an example, Sudduth pointed out that osteoblasts did not become calcified: "Lime salts are deposited around the spherical osteoblasts in the form of spherules, increasing in thickness from within outward, and, thus approaching one another, they coalesce. The osteoblasts persist in the lacunae; their connection with neighboring lacunae forming the canaliculi."[26] Sudduth concluded that odontoblasts "do not become directly calcified, but send out rod-shaped fibrils, around which tubular dentine is formed; so also in the enamel we have the prismatic ameloblasts super-intending the deposit of prismatic enamel." He depicted elongated processes from the distal end of both ameloblasts and odontoblasts (Fig 16-13) but failed to recognize their significance in the formation of the calcified matrices.

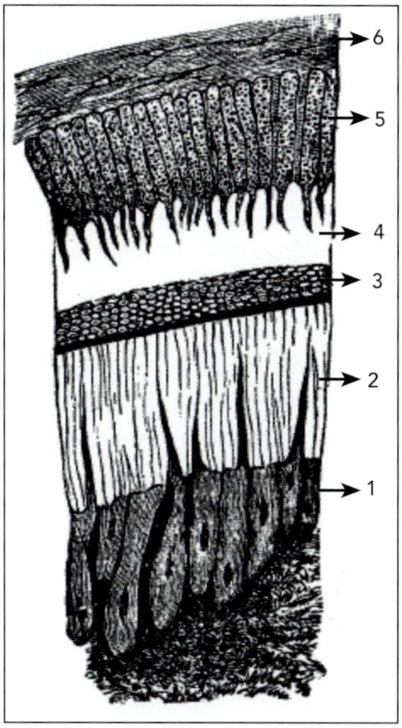

Fig 16-13 Forming enamel and dentin. 1—odontoblasts; 2—dentin; 3—thin layer of enamel showing pits; 4—space caused by shrinkage; 5—ameloblasts, with Tomes processes, extending into space 4; 6—stratum intermedium. (From Sudduth.[26])

R. R. Andrews of Harvard University, speaking before the International Medical Congress held in Berlin in 1890, reported that:

> *In teasing off portions of active enamel-cells from the forming enamel, I have found the surface of the dentine on which it is being formed covered with layers of globules that have been deposited there by the enamel-cells. These given out from the cell continually form, by coalescing, larger globules, and these become the enamel rods.*[27]

Furthermore, Andrews claimed that there existed in enamel a system of fibers "guiding and sustaining the globules that are excreted from the enamel-cells which are to form the future enamel rods, upholding and supporting them."[27] Andrews learned subsequently that a similar discovery had been made by Dr Spee in Germany. Spee had identified the enamel globules as "enamel-drops." Spee reported that spherical enamel-drops formed in the enamel cells near the nucleus and collected in great numbers at the periphery of the cells near the dentin.[7] Through a process of coalescence, the enamel-drops gave rise to the enamel rod.

---

[7] A view that would become confirmed in the latter half of the 20th century with the development of the electron microscope, as secretion granules containing the matrix of enamel and dentin were discovered to originate in the Golgi complex adjacent to the nucleus.

Williams shared the opinion of Sudduth, Andrews, and Spee that enamel was formed by droplets (calcoglobin) secreted by ameloblasts. His observation that enamel prisms formed at an angle (30 degrees or more) from the long axis of the ameloblasts raised a problem for the idea that the ameloblasts were converted into prisms. Williams identified two "membranes" located at either end of the layer of ameloblasts, one separating the ameloblasts from the enamel (which he named the *inner ameloblastic membrane*) and one at the end of the ameloblasts nearest to the stratum intermedium (the *outer ameloblastic membrane*).[8] He proposed a role for the stratum intermedium in cooperation with the ameloblasts in forming the calcoglobulin droplets. Williams also described a rich blood supply to the enamel organ.

Williams was emphatic in rejecting the bioplasson "reticulum" of Heitzmann and Bödecker:

> *In the untouched photographs which accompany this paper nature tells her own story of the structure of protoplasm, and it will be seen that the resemblance to the fanciful drawings which Heitzmann has made to illustrate a ridiculous theory is very remote. I cannot but regard the action of the National Association of Dental Faculties, in adopting Bödecker's work as a text-book, as altogether deplorable. It is deplorable because it is certain to greatly injure the scientific status of dentistry in America.*[24]

Here again, Williams emphasizes photographic evidence over sketches in documenting histologic research. His technique was perfect, and his micrographs were unsurpassed for clarity and detail (see Fig 16-12). Heitzmann had exceptional artistic talent, which he put to good use in illustrating his publications (as well as those of Abbott and Bödecker), but he was apparently unwilling to support his theories with photomicroscopy.

Heitzmann's concept of the interconnection of all cells into one living substance did not die easily; even as late as 1912, C. S. Minot, director of the Anatomical Laboratories of Harvard Medical School, delivered a series of lectures at the University of Jena in which he stated:

> *Cells have been considered for a long time as independent bodies. Quite slowly this view has been changing. Many years ago botanists made the observation that vegetable cells may be united by fine threads of living substance. Similar relations have been observed in animals. In the seventies of the last century J. Heitzmann, a Viennese physician who had immigrated to New York, affirmed that cells are*

[8] These "membranes" were later resolved by electron microscopy to be concentrations of cytoplasmic filaments associated with the proximal and distal terminal web apparatuses of the ameloblasts.

> *not definitely separated from one another. He advanced the statement that protoplasm is continuous and has scattered nuclei. The opinions expressed by Heitzmann remained in their time almost without notice. Very gradually his view met with wider acceptance.*[28]

Was Minot resurrecting Heitzmann, a graduate of Vienna's medical school, to flatter his Austrian audience?

In the Dental Cosmos obituary notice of Heitzmann's death, it was stated that:

> *The most pronounced of his theories and that which achieved much prominence was his so-called "reticulum theory" of protoplasmic matter as opposed to the cellular theory of Virchow and others. The acceptance which his reticulum theory gained among his pupils and readers was in great measure due to the aggressive personality of its originator. He not only urged its acceptance with an almost imperious forcefulness, but was correspondingly intolerant of views opposed to his own.*[29]

Despite these shortcomings, it was noted that his investigations "initiated and developed an interest in scientific research in dentistry which has been of incalculable benefit to our profession."[29]

Microbiology

Histology and embryology were just two of the newly developing sciences that affected dentistry. Another area, alluded to previously in Dr Black's comment (see page 436), was the incipient science of microbiology. For certain, one of the major areas of interest to the developing dental science was the discovery that the mouth was populated by enormous numbers of microorganisms. The prominent British physician Sir Thomas Watson expressed it in dramatic terms: "It is a notorious fact that numerous parasites do crawl over our surface, burrow beneath our skin, nestle in our entrails, and riot and propagate their kind in every corner of our frame; producing oftentimes such molestation and disturbance as require the interference of medicine."

The question then being asked was: Were living organisms harmful or simply parasitic microbes of little significance to oral health? Dr John McQuillen, professor of physiology in the Philadelphia Dental College, noted the following in the July 1875 edition of *Dental Cosmos*:

> *The prominent part assigned by some observers to the oral organisms, or parasites, so called by many, be they vegetal or animal, in the production of decay in the teeth, and, on the other hand, the emphatic denial by a*

> *number of careful and reliable investigators that they have anything at all to do with the matter, make it necessary that we should inquire into the origin of the belief that they are active agents, and ascertain for ourselves by actual observation whether that belief will stand the test of rigid investigation.*[30]

G. V. Black was among those dentists impressed with the growing importance of microorganisms as pathologic agents. In fact, his first book, *The Formation of Poisons by Micro-organisms*, published in 1884, was a compilation of his lectures given at the Chicago College of Dental Surgery, describing the development of the new science of microbiology.[31] In this book, Black demonstrated his knowledge of the research of Robert Koch, Edward Jenner, John Needham, Joseph Lister, and Louis Pasteur in reference to the propagation of microorganisms, the antiseptic technique, infection, and pathogenic secretions (poisons). In the last section of his book, Black included his own ideas of the potential importance of microbes and their products in the pathogenesis of disease. But the true founder of dental microbiology was Dr W. D. Miller, the first university-trained dental scientist (see chapter 8).

Electricity and Magnetism

Another science that captured the attention of dentists during the early 19th century was electricity and magnetism. Attempts to use electricity as a means of inducing local anesthesia were made in the mid 19th century. In 1859, Dr J. H. McQuillen, in his monthly "Review of Dental Literature and Art" in the *Dental Cosmos*, wrote that electricity as a mode of inducing local anesthesia had been embraced with "furor" by a certain portion of the Philadelphia dental community. He described how a committee, presumably of the Philadelphia Franklin Institute, had hastily concluded that electricity was an effective local anesthetic agent. A Philadelphia dentist, J. B. Francis, had applied for a patent and had been awarded a medal in honor of his discovery by the Franklin Institute of Philadelphia.[32] Francis described his method as follows:

> *The negative pole or wire of the ordinary electro-magnetic machine, which is a graduated battery, is attached to the forceps or to one handle of it, and then placing the metallic handle of the other pole in the hand of the patient; by this means a current is at once formed on the forceps coming in contact with the tooth...and the extraction is made at once.*

Soon after these testimonials of success, dental supply houses offered appliances of this nature for sale. But there was mounting evidence that the notion of galvanic anesthesia was not as effective as it was purported to be. The College of Dentists of England reported that the continuous current of electricity was inapplicable as a local anesthetic in dental operations. In their review of 65 cases in which the anesthetic value of electricity was tested, the outcome in 60 cases was negative, often causing more pain to the patient, while in the 5 cases in which there appeared to have been a benefit, it was attributed to other causes such as syncope or other positive mental effects.[33]

Another misapplication of this new technology was in the treatment of neuralgia. Numerous reports of the beneficial effects of constant galvanic currents in the treatment of facial neuralgia made it appear as such a simple procedure that every "modern" dentist should have the equipment to provide such treatments. For example, Dr Joseph Stead reported the following in *Dental Cosmos*:

> *My third case occurred on the 4th of this present October, to a valued female servant of an old patient of mine. She was a girl of about twenty-four years of age, and had been suffering from facial neuralgia of both sides for three months. For two nights previously to coming to me, she had been compelled to get up from bed and come downstairs and spend the night awake, and in great agony. Five minutes' application (of current) cured one side of the face, and a second five minutes' application cured the other, and then, to my surprise, she fell fast asleep in her chair at my house.*[34]

Stead's apparatus consisted of an eight-cell Weiss battery supplying current to two conical electrodes covered with small wet sponges. In the treatment of neuralgia, the electrodes were placed several inches apart over the painful area and current allowed to pass for several minutes.

In 1892, Dr A. C. Westlake of Elizabeth, New Jersey, in speaking before the annual meeting of the Dental Society of the State of New York, said that "the application of electricity in dental practice is destined to become popular after its principles are better known by the progressive dental surgeon."[35] For Westlake, the progressive dentist was to become an *electrologist*, introducing applications in electrosurgery and electromedication. Westlake described an apparatus constructed by his electrician for regulating currents to operate small instruments such as a mouth illuminator, mallet, hot-air syringe, and water heater. The device was also used for local electroanesthesia, electrocautery, and electromedication or cataphoresis. According to Westlake:

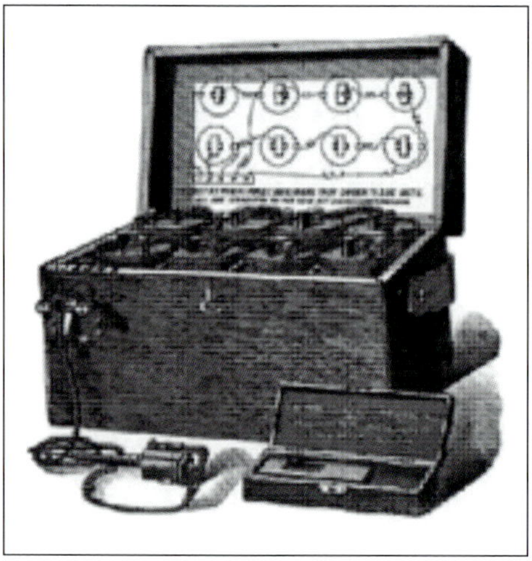

Fig 16-14 Battery-driven electro mallet. (From Custer.[36])

> *If the positive and negative poles are brought in firm contact on the gum at both sides of the root or tooth to be extracted, the end of these electrodes being in the form of a cup or saucer, within which is placed sponge or cotton saturated with a four or six per cent solution of cocaine, or absolute alcohol, ether and chloroform combined, or some other properly selected vegetable anesthetic, and the current turned on gently to the required degree, this preparation can be forced into the tissue sufficiently to cause local anesthesia.*[35]

He extolled the principle of driving medication into the tissues: "We must comprehend these things. We must have them, if we are going to practice anything but mechanics."[35] Electric motors were soon used to power laboratory lathes, operative mallets, intraoral lighting devices, and rotary dental engines, all of which made the mechanical aspects of dentistry more efficient[36] (Figs 16-14 to 16-16).

In 1895, Dr W. J. Morton, professor of diseases of the mind and nervous system and electrotherapeutics at The New York Postgraduate Medical School and Hospital, published a method for bleaching teeth based on the principle of cataphoresis. His apparatus consisted of a galvanic battery of 40 cells supplying at least 60 volts, a rheostat, a milliamp meter, and appropriate silver electrodes. Experimenting with extracted teeth, Morton reported that the bleaching power

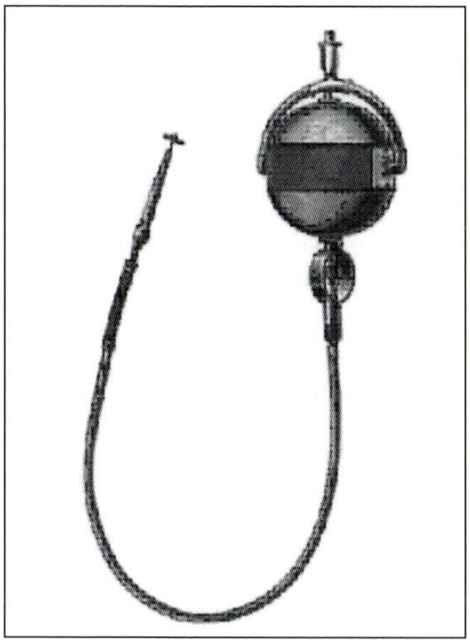

Fig 16-15 Electrically powered Ritter dental engine. (From Custer.[36])

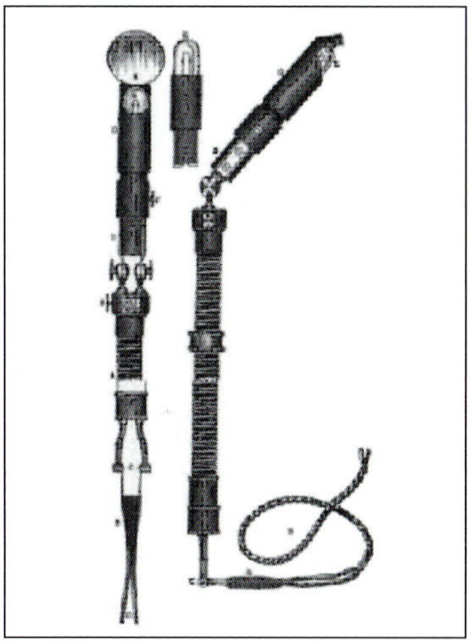

Fig 16-16 S. S. White mouth lamp. (From Custer.[36])

of a solution of hydrogen peroxide and sulfuric ether was enhanced by electricity in the form of a cataphoretic force.[37] Morton was well known on the speaker circuit for his promotion of the concept of "electromedicamental diffusion" of drugs in medical practice. Morton was well respected in dental circles because he was the son of Dr William J. Morton, famed for his introduction of ether anesthesia at the Massachusetts General Hospital. The editorial column *Dental Cosmos* confirmed the usefulness of the method for bleaching enamel when applied to pulpless teeth. In an address to the First District Dental Society of New York City, Morton described a new cataphoretic electrode for producing local dental anesthesia with a solution of guaiacol-cocaine. Dr Morton described its use in several cases involving cavity preparation, tooth implantation, and surgical removal of a nevus, demonstrating that profound dental anesthesia could be produced more rapidly by cataphoresis than with the older syringe method of injection.[38]

The physical and chemical properties of metals, gutta-percha, and rubber were also high on the list of research topics. Perhaps the greatest area of interest was in the discovery of x-rays and their potential application in dental diagnosis (see chapter 14).

Summary

Although the dental profession's early excursions in science were not entirely successful, it was clear that by the end of the 19th century, many dentists were convinced that its future development was tied to scientific research.

In 1913, the National Dental Association created the National Dental Scientific Foundation and Research Commission, whose duties were "to raise funds for carrying on exhaustive dental and oral research, to disseminate scientific knowledge, to support, establish, and encourage research, and such other duties as shall pertain to the furthering of this cause."[39] The commission was to form a corporation to collect, invest, and disburse moneys provided by the commission. Research was proposed in the following subject areas: "systemic infections having dental origins, pyorrhea alveolaris, etiology of caries, salivary analysis, etiology of dental erosion, dental amalgams, metallurgy for substitutes for platinum, etc., and the relation of foods to defective tooth structure." The commission announced that $4,000 per year was available to begin selecting scientists for a few of the previously named projects.[39] Although only a modest amount of money was raised, the foundation demonstrated a commitment among the dental association members and several dental colleges to embark on a formal research program. Momentum for the support of research grew with the 1926 Carnegie Foundation's report on the state of dental education, but it would take another 28 years before the development of the National Institute of Dental Research.

References

1. Virchow R. Cellular Pathology. London: John Churchill, 1860.
2. Baxter A, Farley J. Mendel and meiosis. J Hist Biol 1979;12:137–173.
3. Nasmyth A. Three Memoirs on the Development and Structure of the Teeth and Epithelium. London: John Churchill, 1841.
4. Harris CA. The Principles and Practice of Dental Surgery. Philadelphia: Lindsay and Blakiston, 1845.
5. Owen R. Odontography; Or, a Treatise on the Comparative Anatomy of the Teeth. London: H. Bailliere, 1840–1845.
6. Richmond ML. T. H. Huxley's criticism of German cell theory: An epigenetic and physiological interpretation of cell structure. J Hist Biol 2000;33:247–289.
7. Huxley TH. A lecture on the identity of structure of plants and animals. Q J Microsc Soc 1853;1:307–311.
8 Huxley TH. On the development of the teeth, and on the nature and import of Nasmyth's "Persistent Capsule." Q J Microsc Soc 1853;1:149–164.
9. Huxley TH. On the enamel and dentine of the teeth. Q J Microsc Soc 1855;3:127–130.

10. Davis JR. Thomas H. Huxley. London: J. M. Dent, 1907.
11. Kölliker A. A Manual of Human Microscopic Anatomy. London: John W. Parker and Son, 1860.
12. Tomes J. On the presence of fibrils of soft tissue in the dentinal tubes. Philos Trans Royal Soc London 1856;146:515–522.
13. Tomes J. A System of Dental Surgery. London: John Churchill, 1859.
14. Heitzmann C. The minute anatomy of the teeth in the light of the bioplasson theory. Dent Cosmos 1882;24:281–291.
15. Heitzmann C. Microscopical Morphology of the Animal Body in Health and Disease. London: Trubner, 1884.
16. Bödecker CF. The teeth. In: Heitzmann C (ed). Microscopical Morphology of the Animal Body in Health and Disease. London: Trubner, 1884.
17. Abbott F. Odontoblasts in their relation to developed dentine. Dent Cosmos 1888;30:773–783.
18. Abbott F. Caries of human teeth. Dent Cosmos 1879;21:177–184.
19. Atkinson WH. Origin and development of dental tissues. Dent Cosmos 1864;6:256–259.
20. Atkinson WH. Microscopic structures of teeth. Dent Cosmos 1865;6:419–422.
21. Atkinson WH. Career of the elements of tissues. Dent Cosmos 1872;14:65–70.
22. Andrews RR. First District Dental Society, State of New York. Dent Cosmos 1886;28:369–386.
23. Williams JL. Embryology: With special reference to the development of the teeth and contiguous parts. Dent Cosmos 1884;26:193–200,257–262.
24. Williams JL. On the formation and structure of dental enamel. Dent Cosmos 1896;38:101–127.
25. Williams JL. A critical essay on the development and minute anatomy of the teeth in health and disease. Dent Cosmos 1886;28:65–80.
26. Sudduth WX. Dento-embryonal histology and technology. Dent Cosmos 1884;26:658–665.
27. Andrews RR. A contribution to the study of the development of the enamel. Cambridge, MA: Harvard University, 1893.
28. Minot CS. Modern Problems of Biology. Philadelphia: P. Blakiston's Son, 1913.
29. Obituary. Carl Heitzmann, M.D. Dent Cosmos 1897;39:164–165.
30. McQuillen J. Oral organisms. Dent Cosmos 1875;17:571–577.
31. Black GV. The formation of poisons by micro-organisms. A biological study of the germ theory of disease. Philadelphia: P. Blakiston, Son, & Co, 1884.
32. Lufkin AW. A History of Dentistry. Philadelphia: Lea & Febiger, 1948.
33. McQuillen JH. Dental journals. Dent Cosmos 1859;1:135–137.
34. Stead J. Constant galvanic current in treatment of neuralgia. Dent Cosmos 1872;14:42–43.
35. Westlake A. Electricity: Its application in dental practice. Dent Cosmos 1892;34:887–892.
36. Custer LE. Dental Electricity. Dayton, OH: U. B. Publishing, 1901.
37. Morton WJ. Cataphoresis and solutions of H_2O_2 for bleaching teeth, etc. Dent Cosmos 1895;37:484–489.
38. Morton WJ. Guaiacol-cocain cataphoresis and local anesthesia: A new cataphoric electrode and the Wheeler fractional volt selector. Dent Cosmos 1896;38:48–53.
39. Price WA. Notes and announcements of the National Dental Association. Dent Cosmos 1913;55:1199–1201.

17

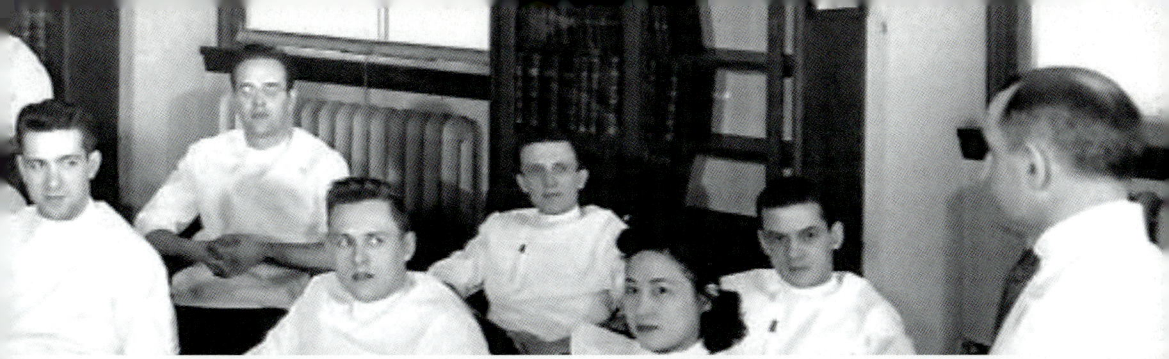

The Gies Report and Beyond

By the close of the 19th century, all elements essential to dentistry's acceptance as a member of the learned professions had been established: Dental schools were in operation in most states; dental literature was flourishing; state dental examiners ruled on who was qualified to practice; dental science was in its early stage of development; and practicing dentists were organized at local, state, and national levels. Two major institutions, the American Dental Association (ADA) and the National Institute of Dental Research (NIDR), dominated the history of dentistry during the 20th century. The rapid growth of dental science and technology led to a more thorough knowledge of dental and oral diseases and to improved methods of dental care. The story behind the discovery of the anticaries effect of fluoride and the resulting dramatic improvements in dental health is told as a further example of how individual determination and dedication made an impact on the profession.

Quality of Dental Schools

As the 19th century came to an end, a small number of university-affiliated schools sought to impose new standards on the increasing number of proprietary schools. There was pressure from the university-affiliated schools for adoption of stricter entrance requirements and more exposure to medical and basic sciences in the dental curriculum. Many dental educators, along with leaders within organized dentistry, recognized a need for reform within dental education. Comparisons made to the medical educational system showed that dentistry was lacking well-educated students and that unless more time was spent at the baccalaureate level, especially in science, there was no possibility of developing a cadre of dental scientists who could lead the way to better understanding of diseases and their treatment and prevention.

Significant reform was initiated when the Dental Educational Council of America was formed in 1909 by representatives from the National Association of Dental Examiners, the National Association of Dental Faculties, and the National Dental Association. The Council's primary aim was to develop standards by which all three of the parent organizations could advance dental education. Dr Henry Banzhaf, secretary of the Council, noted that it was the general opinion of the Council that: "there were some things wrong with dental education, that some dental colleges and state boards did not understand each other very well, and that by reason of their limited interchange of views these organizations were drifting farther apart instead of coming nearer together." Furthermore, in the profession there "was apathy, lack of interest and distrust of dental education."[1]

Dr W. E. Grant, chairman of the Council's Committee on Colleges, reporting on early inspections of dental schools, revealed that there was "great variance offered the dental student" and that

> *the lack of technic laboratory instruction and the entire absence of any equipment or facilities for instruction in the pure science branches, and the woeful neglect of practical and laboratory instruction, the equipment necessary to enable a student to properly do clinical work, insufficient clinical material, and the absence of competent demonstrators" noted in the past by state board examiners now required immediate remedial action.*[1]

Money and organizational support was needed to permit the Council's work to continue with its inspections of all dental schools. The Council also recognized the failure of dental schools to agree on uniform entrance requirements. One of the most problematic areas involved the issuance of certificates of equivalence of high school education by state superintendents of public instruction. These certificates were issued to individuals who had no high school education upon taking a simple 2- to 3-hour examination before a dental examiner.

The rift between the university-affiliated schools and the proprietary schools was laid wide open in an address to the Stomatological Section of the American Medical Association (AMA) by Dr J. G. Sharp, dean of the Dental School of the University of California. Taking aim at the proprietary schools as the major reason for the educational deficiencies of the dental profession, Sharp said:

> *Their [the commercial schools'] great weakness lies in the fact that most of them are self-supporting, which means that their success rests in their student enrolment and the successful operation of their infirmary, and here originates their commercial basis, which must be considered by them before any other factor—hence on this basis the standards of our schools differ according as they have few or many students. Such means of standardization lead to all manner of methods for keeping the treasury full. These include low preliminary qualifications, unethical advertising, misrepresentation of facts, etc., as an attraction of the unsuspecting candidate.*[2]

Sharp called for investigations and the establishment of national standards for all dental schools, recommending that dental colleges be placed under the control of "higher institutions of learning, our endowed and state universities, provided they themselves are further recognized by some higher and set standard, as by the Association of American Universities or Carnegie Foundation for the Advancement of Teaching [CFAT]."[2]

Sharp's views reflected the policies of the newly established Dental Faculties Association of American Universities.[1] Risking further alienation of dentists, Sharp faulted the state board of examiners and the National Association of Dental Faculties for "lacking courage" to improve the educational system and blamed the profession for its "total indifference" to the low standards of its colleges. He proposed the launch of a campaign to reform dental education by bringing it under university association and overview.[3]

He suggested that one route to standardization would be to permit existing dental schools to join the Dental Faculties Association of American Universities if they were to become affiliated with universities on the accepted list of the CFAT. In this regard, it was suggested that dentistry seek the assistance of the Carnegie Foundation in "clarifying the dental educational atmosphere as it is now doing

[1] The Association consisted of six schools in 1910: Harvard University Dental School, University of Michigan College of Dental Surgery, University of California College of Dentistry, University of Iowa College of Dentistry, University of Minnesota College of Dentistry, and the University of Pennsylvania School of Dentistry. Dr J. G. Sharp served as president in 1910.

for the medical profession."[3;2] Pressure for reform was coming not only from the academic elite but also from practicing members of the profession, such as William Lovett. Speaking before the Southern Branch of the National Dental Association in 1911, he called for abolishing half of the dental schools, identifying support for dental research, better medical education for dentists, and banishment of the advertising quack.[4]

Joseph Kauffmann of the Dental Department of the Bronx Hospital of New York City criticized new dental school graduates for their lack of scientific knowledge and for a lack of public spirit:

> *There are two noticeable deficiencies in the poorly educated dentist of today. One is a lack of scientific concept and knowledge, as manifested by a persistence of the purely mechanical outlook. The other is a scarcity of public-spirited endeavor, as seen in the slouchy attitude toward high professional ideals concomitant with a failure to be imbued with what may be termed the spirit of public service.*[5]

He laid the blame for these shortcomings upon the commercialized dental schools. He recommended the complete abolition of commercialized dental schools and the placement of the oversight of dental education in state universities. Kauffmann went so far as to disapprove of the philanthropically endowed schools for their "lack of academic independence." The "money-begging" of the endowed schools was just as bad as the moneymaking of the proprietary schools. As a firm believer in the public-spirited interests of the state, he viewed the future of dental education to reside in the newly state-supported dental schools such as had been established in California, Illinois, Iowa, Michigan, and Minnesota.[5]

At the Third Annual Meeting of the Dental Faculties Association of American Universities, it was ruled that dental schools under the supervision of universities approved by the Carnegie Foundation were eligible for admission to the association. Furthermore, a motion was

---

[2] Based on Sharp's proposal, the Dental Faculties Association of American Universities approved the following resolution: "Whereas, The Carnegie Foundation for the Advancement of Teaching has done more than any other organization in determining and maintaining a proper standard of entrance requirement for admission to colleges and universities; and Whereas, The investigation that has been and is being conducted in medical educational institutions, with regard to admission requirements and facilities for giving instruction, has done much to elevate the standards of medical education; therefore be it Resolved, That schools or colleges of dentistry that are an integral part of and under the direct supervision of universities accepted by the Carnegie Foundation for the Advancement of Teaching may be eligible to hold membership in the Dental Faculties Association of American Universities."

approved to invite the Carnegie Foundation to make an investigation of dental schools such as it had made of medical schools.[6]

Medical education had been faced with similar problems at the turn of the century as nearly 150 medical schools were churning out over 5,000 graduates per year. Many of the medical schools were commercial ventures aimed to generate income for the owners, with no concern for advancing patient care or the state of the art. In 1906, the AMA conducted a study of all medical schools, reporting that more than 50% of the schools were deficient in meeting standards of the AMA. It graded schools on their performance in state licensing examinations and curriculum content. Eighty out of 160 medical schools were classified as Class A schools, while most Class B and Class C schools were considered beyond salvation. The AMA, reluctant to make this information public, approached the CFAT for assistance in conducting an "independent" survey of medical education with the ultimate aim of exposing and eliminating its inferior proprietary colleges.[7,8]

The Flexner Report

The Carnegie Foundation appointed Abraham Flexner, a graduate of Johns Hopkins University and well-known educational reformer, to lead this project. Flexner, not being a physician, brought no medical baggage along, but he did bring his own personal elitist attitudes to bear in rooting out the riffraff in medical education. His model institution was the Johns Hopkins Medical School, a four-year research-oriented, hospital-based clinical program.

Flexner visited all 160 medical schools, exposing deplorable conditions in most proprietary schools. Flexner reported that "laboratories were nowhere to be found, or consisted of a few vagrant test tubes squirreled away in a cigar box; corpses reeked because of the failure to use disinfectant in the dissecting rooms; libraries had no books; faculty members were busily occupied in private practice."[7] Flexner demonstrated his contempt of the commercial element by stating that it contaminated medical education and that "mercenary concerns that trade on ignorance and disease" needed to be eliminated.[8] Abraham Flexner was attacked by many physicians (most notably by Sir William Osler of Oxford University) as an outsider and a nonclinician, with no right to dictate how medical education was to be delivered.[9] But physicians at university-based medical schools welcomed the Flexner Report because, if implemented, it would mean better conditions of employment and more resources for academic pursuits.

Furthermore, the graduates of established medical schools (Class A) looked forward to eliminating competition from poorly trained practitioners.[8] No longer were the ranks of the medical profession to be filled by lower middle–class riffraff who jeopardized medicine's status in society.[7] In addition, the average physician viewed overcrowding as the cause of a decline in his income and loss of social status and was entirely supportive of reducing medical school enrollments.[10] By 1920, the number of US medical schools had been reduced to 85, while the number of new graduates had shrunk to 3,535, down from over 5,000 in 1910.

Flexner was successful in reforming medical education because many leading educators and clinicians were making similar appeals for higher standards in scientific knowledge and clinical proficiencies, both privately and within organizations such as the Association of American Medical Colleges and the AMA. As early as 1870, the medical schools at Harvard, the University of Pennsylvania, and the University of Michigan instituted laboratory exercises and exposure to medical research, a movement reaching full realization at Johns Hopkins in 1893.[11] The Flexner Report concluded that the university was the optimal environment for medical education, with clinical training conducted in university-owned or -affiliated hospitals by full-time medical faculty. The Johns Hopkins Medical School became the model program copied by the most elite medical schools. By the turn of the 20th century, university medical schools became the top choice for aspiring medical candidates, while the commercial schools declined in popularity, with many closing due to lack of applicants.[11]

The Gies Report

The Flexner Report of 1910 generated increased activity in dental educational circles for a similar survey of dental schools with the aim of eliminating the "defects of commercialism" from dental education.[12] With the Flexner Report as its example, the dental profession received support from the Carnegie Foundation for a similar study of dental schools in the United States and Canada. Dr William Gies (Fig 17-1), a professor of biochemistry at Columbia University, was selected to lead the study. Although Gies was not a dentist, he did have insight into dental education as a member of the Biochemistry Department at Columbia University and as an investigator of the composition of saliva in relation to dental caries. He was also the founding editor of the *Journal of Dental Research*, the first journal specifically dedicated to oral and dental science.

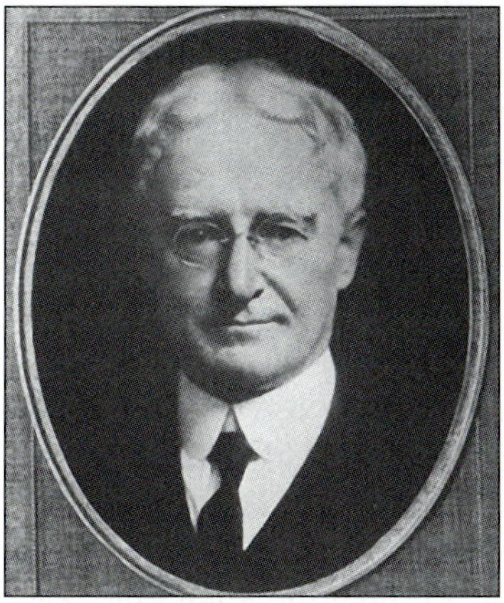

Fig 17-1 William Gies.

In 1926, concluding a 5-year survey of the dental educational system in the United States and Canada, Gies published a lengthy report that was to shape dental education for the remainder of the 20th century.[13] In compiling data for the report, Gies inspected 49 schools and interviewed hundreds of dental educators. The Gies Report revealed weaknesses in the great majority of dental schools when measured against the best of the university-based schools such as those at Harvard and Columbia. The essential conclusion of the Gies Report was that if dentistry was to achieve equality with medicine, it had to be a university-based program taught by full-time educators capable of advancing the discipline through research, and it must interact with other units within the university to enrich its academic and scientific base.

Gies stated unequivocally that:

> *The type of training afforded by most of the dental schools does not promise to make the practice of dentistry the health-service equivalent of an oral specialty of the practice of medicine, and important general improvements of dental education are required for the attainment of that objective. Appreciation by dental teachers of the necessity for thorough instruction in the mechanical aspects of the practice of dentistry has seldom been accompanied by due comprehension of the need for intimate understanding of the pathological involvements and the health-service relationships of such practice. Consequently, in most dental schools, instruction of dental students in the medical sciences has been unwisely directed, indifferently given, and poorly assimilated; and the practice of dentistry has failed, from lack of knowledge, ability, and vision, to measure up to its opportunity in health service.*[13]

In recommending that dentistry continue as an independent profession "equivalent of an oral specialty of medicine," Gies stated that the weakest schools would have to achieve conditions already in place in the best university-affiliated schools—ie, *(1)* require at least 2 years of preprofessional college education; *(2)* reorganize the curriculum to contain courses in medicine; *(3)* offer a 1- to 2-year graduate program for specialty training, including research, leading to the MS or PhD degree; *(4)* develop combined dental/medical training programs in maxillofacial surgery; *(5)* establish dental internships in hospitals; *(6)* provide continuing dental education and training for hygienists, technicians, and assistants; *(7)* create adequate libraries in dental schools; *(8)* promote research; *(9)* discontinue all independent dental schools that fail to meet the higher standards of the university-affiliated schools; and *(10)* be affiliated with university medical schools.[13]

On the age-old question of dentistry as a specialty of medicine, Gies concluded that:

> *Owing to the need for exceptional digital facility in the manifold intra-oral procedures of dental practice, and for the esthetic felicity in their execution, the extensive technical training and the clinical instruction and practice peculiar to dentistry cannot be superimposed upon a conventional medical curriculum, leading to the degree of M.D., without making the period of dental training prohibitive in length for most prospective general practitioners.*[13]

Dentistry required independent programs but with cooperative arrangements with medical schools whereby dental students were exposed to basic medical science and medical students were exposed to the dental and oral diseases that were known to have systemic consequences. A much-needed mutual understanding and respect would arise from such interactions.

Gies believed that if these reforms were to take place, then dental practitioners

> *would be trained to give the service not only of dental surgeons and dental engineers as at present, but of oral sanitarians and oral physicians as well. Instead of examining only the teeth and mouth of a patient, as is now usually the case in a restricted view of their responsibility, they would also suitably enquire into and keep careful records of the state of the patient's health, particularly as it affects or is modified by conditions of the teeth and mouth. Dentists would plan their procedures to meet not only the local indications but also the possible requirements of extra-oral relationships; would also recognize and note the significance of outstanding symptoms of systemic disease, and warn or advise the patient accordingly, or explain his need for a*

physician's attention; and could effectively discuss, with a physician, the oral conditions in their relation to the patient's general welfare.[13]

A prerequisite for such changes was better preprofessional education of dental students. In 1924, only 22 dental schools out of 43 required any prior college attendance. Only the better schools required a minimum of 1 year in an academic college. Nearly every medical school at that time required entering students to have graduated from high school and completed 2 years of college study. Gies recommended that dentistry match medicine's prerequisites in preprofessional education.

Gies emphasized that reforming dental education would require increased funding:

> *A dental school cannot develop the highest degree of educational quality, or the greatest measure of humanitarian service, from a financial soil consisting solely of the fees paid by students and patients, on which most of the schools are now obliged to subsist...hitherto, in an era notable for the generous financial support deservedly accorded to medicine, the similar needs of oral-health-service have been almost wholly ignored.*[13]

Dental schools were urgently in need of endowments.

By the time the Gies Report was made public, there were 44 dental schools in the United States and five in Canada, and all but 8 were university affiliated.[13] Many proprietary dental schools moved to affiliate with universities or folded before the Gies Report was published. The university-affiliated dental school model, based on the Flexner medical school model, became the standard in the United States and Canada.

The American Dental Association

Armed with the Gies Report, the ADA assumed greater control of dental education by setting standards and evaluating performance through accreditation reviews. In 1938, the ADA established the Council on Dental Education (CDE), whose board contained representation from the ADA, the American Association of Dental Schools (AADS), and the National Association of Dental Examiners (NADE). The aim of the CDE was to set standards for entrance requirements, curricular content, and licensure examination protocols. Soon US and Canadian dental schools would undergo periodic (7-year cycle) accreditation reviews that included on-site inspections and evaluations of curriculum and patient care operations.

The period from the publication of the Gies Report in 1926 to the end of the 20th century was marked by profound and rapid changes in dentistry, dental education, dental science, and in the way dental care was provided. Many changes were fostered by governmental policies at both the state and national levels. Dentists earned greater respect from the public, and a career in dentistry became prized by an increasingly well-educated applicant. In his history of the Hillenbrand era of the ADA, Dummett labeled the period from 1930 to 1970 as the "Glanzperiode" of American dentistry.[14] The ADA grew in prominence and influence in the post-World War II period under the leadership of its executive director, Dr Harold Hillenbrand (Fig 17-2). From 1946 to 1969, Hillenbrand managed the affairs of the ADA with organizational efficiency and skilled diplomacy during a time of social change in health care delivery and increasing involvement of the federal government.[14] A symbol of the increasing stature of the ADA in the American health enterprise was its new high-rise central headquarters in downtown Chicago (Fig 17-3). The new headquarters, completed in 1965 at a cost of $14.6 million, brought together under one roof a staff of 200 and the various components of organized dentistry. Its modernistic style was featured in the magazine *Interior Architecture*, and its interior spaces were adorned with many works of art acquired by the ADA Fine Arts Fund.[14]

Hillenbrand also exercised leadership in guiding the ADA in successfully managing the conflict between the excessive claims of dental manufacturers for their products and the dental profession's desire for truth and honesty in advertising. Throughout this controversial issue, he supported the evaluation of dental products by the ADA's chemical laboratory, followed by review by its Council on Dental Therapeutics and its authority to grant the ADA's Seal of Acceptance to products found to be safe and effective.[14] The ADA's Seal of Acceptance was hailed as a significant benefit to the public, not only in helping them make appropriate choices but also in stimulating dental manufacturers to back their claims with research results.

The oral health of Americans improved significantly during the last half of the 20th century. There was a double-digit drop in the percentage of edentulous adults and a sharp decline in the number of decayed, missing, or filled teeth in children. These improvements were due to a number of factors, most importantly the introduction of fluoridation, the use of antibiotics, improved methods of treating periodontal disease, and the retention of teeth by new endodontic techniques. Improvements in the provision of care, such as infiltration and block anesthesia, high-speed cutting drills, and new filling materials, helped to reduce the unpleasantness and fear of the dental visit.

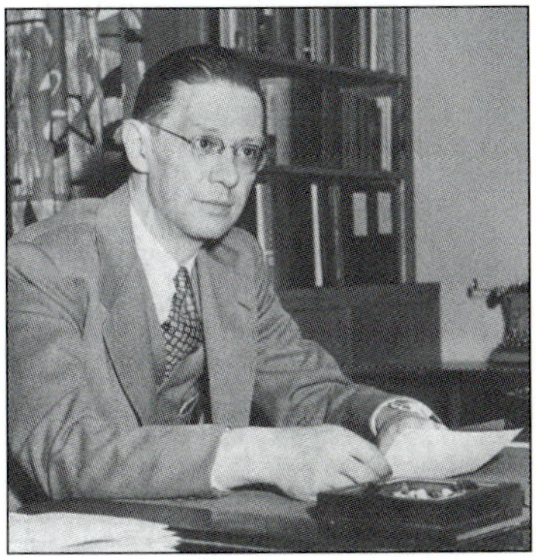

Fig 17-2 Harold Hillenbrand.

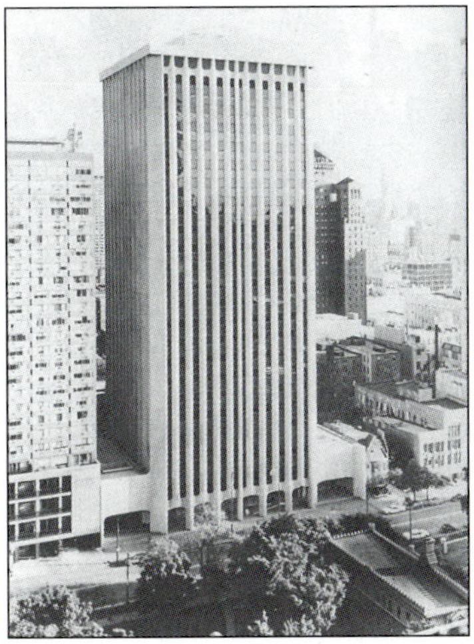

Fig 17-3 ADA headquarters in Chicago.

Greater awareness of the relationship of good oral health to overall health and the social importance of a pleasing facial and dental image led to an increased demand for dental care. Visits to the family dentist became a regular event in upper- and middle-class families, but for those who could not afford those visits it meant neglect, pain, early tooth loss, and the potential harm to overall health.

In a study of dental and medical care utilization in New York City, it was shown that the utilization of dental services was highly related to socioeconomic status.[15] In a 1-year period (1858–1959), two-thirds of all dental services were performed for one-tenth of the US population. Prepaid insurance programs, along with federal and state Medicare/Medicaid programs, helped to correct this imbalance during the last decades of the 20th century.

Specialized branches of dentistry became recognized by the ADA, beginning with oral and maxillofacial surgery, orthodontics, pediatric dentistry, periodontics, and prosthodontics in 1947; oral pathology in 1949; dental public health in 1950; and endodontics in 1963.

Licensure Examinations

Throughout the 20th century, state licensure examination was a source of controversy, pitting dental educators against practicing dentists in determining who should control the right to practice. Dental examiners, usually prominent members of the dental professional community, are political appointees who by state law have the obligation to examine and determine the competency of dental graduates to practice dentistry; thus, they are final gatekeepers of the profession. Traditionally, state licensure examinations included a written examination dealing with scientific and clinical facts and a proficiency examination involving the performance of clinical procedures on live patients during a specified time period in which the dental examiners evaluate the student at each step of the dental operation. These examinations, which take place over several days, are a source of great anxiety and financial expense for the students as well as for the faculty, who see the outcome as a reflection of their effectiveness.

Faculty may view the licensure examination as an unnecessary intrusion on their evaluation of students. They point out that, in granting the dental degree, they have affirmed the graduate to have achieved proficiency in all aspects of general dentistry and to be ready to undertake independent practice. They point out that dentistry is the only profession that requires demonstration of a manual exercise (other than a written examination). The medical and nursing professions have no requirement for a clinical examination. Despite such criticisms, it is clear that the existence of board examinations have had a net positive effect on dental school operations.

Up until 1967, each state had its own written and clinical examinations and mobility from state to state was restricted by the need to pass the examinations of each state. However, in 1967 there began a cooperative movement when New York State and the District of Columbia agreed to administer a single examination. This was followed by several eastern states in the formation of the Northeastern Regional Board Examination, permitting those who pass the examinations to practice in all member states. Central, Western, and Southern Dental Regional Boards soon followed.

Dental Science and Research

A limited initiative in research, especially in microscopic anatomy and in microbiology, occurred during the last few decades of the 19th century, conducted primarily by academics such as G. V. Black and funded mostly at their own expense. At the start of the new century, small research programs were developing at university-based dental schools, but dental research never achieved significance until the formation of the NIDR in 1948 and the resulting infusion of federal aid for research.

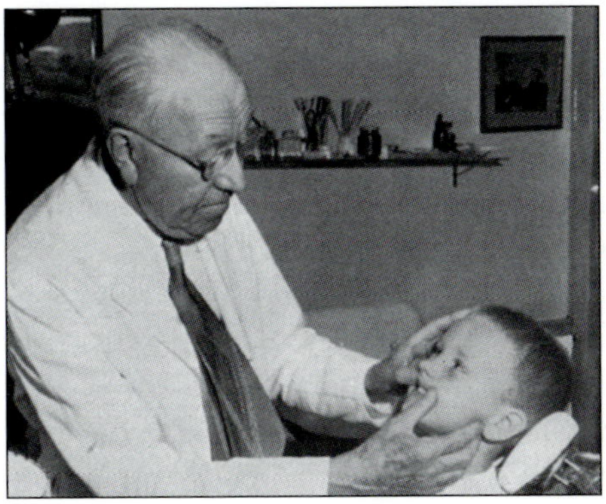

Fig 17-4 Dr Frederick McKay examining a young patient.

Frederick McKay and H. Trendly Dean

An inspiring story in the history of dental research concerns the discovery of the damaging effects of high fluoride intake and the paradoxical benefits of the intake of fluoride in lower amounts. Two men, Dr Frederick McKay (Fig 17-4) and Dr H. Trendly Dean (see Fig 17-5), deserve most of the credit for bringing to light the importance of fluoride in dental health. As a general practitioner in Colorado Springs in 1901, McKay[3] noted that many patients had discolored and abnormally developed teeth. This common disorder was characterized by white and brownish stains, mostly present on the labial surfaces of the anterior teeth but sometimes present in the form of horizontal bands. McKay learned that the problem was widespread and had been known for some time as the "Colorado Brown Stain." The cause of this abnormality was unknown, but speculation centered on a possible dietary origin, perhaps a deficiency in calcium consumption.

Colorado Springs was a boom town, a result of the discovery of gold and silver deposits in the surrounding mountains. Fortunes were being made in gold, silver, and other mining operations. The population of Colorado Springs grew from 11,000 in 1890 to 23,000 in 1900. On a per-capita basis, it became the wealthiest city in the United States and a magnet for dentists and physicians.[16] By 1902, the El Paso County Odontological Society was formed, later changing its name to the Colorado Springs Dental Society.

[3] McKay was a native of Lawrence, Massachusetts, and a graduate of the University of Pennsylvania, class of 1900.

McKay was perplexed by the lack of interest among the members of the local odontological society to investigate the cause of this disfiguring disease. In 1908, McKay and a few members of the El Paso Odontological Society presented a clinical case at the annual meeting of the Colorado Dental Association in Denver and were successful in getting the El Paso Odontological Society to allocate $21 to support dental examination of the public school children of Colorado Springs. With school board approval, McKay examined 2,945 children and found that 87.5% of the children showed some degree of the Colorado Brown Stain, or *mottled enamel*, as he preferred to call it.

In November 1908, prior to compiling this surprising data, McKay had written to Dr G. V. Black, professor of pathology at Northwestern University Dental School, inviting him to speak at the Colorado State Dental Society and trying to persuade Black to help in dealing with the issue of mottling of enamel (McKay to Black, 11/17/08).[17] In the same letter to Black, dated November 17, 1908, McKay discussed his conviction that enamel mottling was a local condition and that as far as he knew there was no report of it in the recent dental literature. McKay hoped to pique Black's enthusiasm by pointing out that "we have a splendid field for an original assay, and of a most scientific nature." As if that were not sufficient, McKay noted that Colorado's wonderful climate and beauties of nature would be great remedies for Black, a relief "after the heat and smoke of Chicago."

Black responded in the affirmative and requested samples of mottled enamel from extracted teeth, promising to have histologic reports prior to his visit to Colorado. Later that year, McKay shared with Black the surprising finding that nearly 90% of 2,945 Colorado Springs school children had mottled enamel (McKay to Black, 5/14/09).[17] For Black, these numbers represented a challenge to define the histopathogenesis of the lesions. In a preliminary report, he noted that in white lesions he had detected an absence of cementing substance between the enamel rods (Black to McKay, 2/23/09).[17] Black's preliminary histopathologic report gave McKay clout in enlisting financial support from the Colorado Springs Chamber of Commerce and the City Council.

It soon became apparent that the subject of mottled enamel was a hot potato for the local dental society as well as for the Chamber of Commerce; McKay was advised to use caution in revealing his data to the public. The dental society feared that its members would be embarrassed by the revelation that a widespread dental problem affecting the residents of the community had gone unreported and neglected. The Chamber of Commerce and city officials worried that publicity over mottled enamel could tarnish Colorado Springs's image as a capital of good health.

Meanwhile, McKay continued to examine the teeth of children throughout the Colorado region, taking water samples and submitting them to chemical analysis. McKay developed a detailed report on mottled enamel in collaboration with Black, which was published in the 1916 issue of *Dental Cosmos*.[18] According to McKay:

> *The remarkable thing about the lesion is that it is practically, if not absolutely limited in its distribution, in any large way, to certain well-defined geographical areas, in which it occurs in the teeth of only those individuals who were either actually born or lived continuously in any of these areas during the years of enamel formation; or in those who although being born elsewhere, were brought into such districts for a continuous residence during the years of enamel formation.*[18]

Furthermore, he observed that "this mottled condition, in itself, does not seem to increase the susceptibility of the teeth to decay, which is perhaps contrary to what might be expected, because the enamel surface is much more corrugated and rougher than normal enamel."

Over the next several years, Dr Black, in his laboratory at Northwestern University Dental School in Chicago, continued his microscopic investigations of ground sections of mottled teeth. In another article published in 1916 in *Dental Cosmos*, Black noted that many enamel rods floated free from the surface of the specimen, suggesting "that there was a failure of the deposit of the cementing substance between the enamel rods."[19] In the white lesions, the spaces between the enamel rods appeared to be empty, while in the dark-colored enamel the interrod spaces were filled with a brownish substance he called "brownin," having none of the translucency of normal enamel.[19] Both men had arrived at the conclusion that the white spots were developmental lesions, discolored after the teeth erupted into the oral cavity. The possible cause of the developmental lesion was generally believed to involve the drinking water. In McKay's words:

> *Even from the very beginning of the notice taken of this lesion and before any definite steps were taken to study it, the sentiment of both the profession and the laity in the areas of susceptibility was that the water was in some way responsible. Black urged again and again that the water theory be followed to some conclusion.*[18]

After several years of clinical examinations and "standard" chemical analysis of water samples from both immune and endemic communities, no solid conclusions were forthcoming. In concluding his 1916 article in *Dental Cosmos*, McKay noted:

> *Our complete Table of Analyses has been submitted to chemists for examination, and their opinions have been that no definite conclusion can be reached from it. Notably, Professor Strieby of Colorado College declares that the analyses arrive at nothing, but are contradictory. It is to be explained that these analyses as herein given were made according to the standard quantitative form.... In waters certain other elements of rarer varieties exist only in traces, the determination of which requires much more elaborate technique and spectroscopic and polariscopic tests, which are beyond the capacities of the ordinary chemical laboratories. Strieby declares that in future chemical examinations of waters, the "standard" analyses should be abandoned, and the work confined chiefly to searching for "traces" of these rarer elements.*[18]

After the death of G. V. Black in 1915, McKay single-handedly sought to enlist the US Public Health Service (USPHS) to take an interest in solving the problem of mottled enamel. Success was not achieved until 1926.

When McKay began his investigations of mottled enamel in 1901, he was unaware that Dr J. M. Eager of the USPHS had reported to the surgeon general of the United States that many Italian emigrants embarking in Naples for the United States were affected by severely discolored teeth.[16] The condition, known in Italy as "denti di Chiaie," was especially prevalent in the Chiaia quarter of Naples. The crowns of the affected teeth had many brown spots and horizontal black lines. The highest number of cases occurred along the Neapolitan coast, an area dominated by volcanic soil and sulfuric waters that drained from the nearby volcanic peaks. Upon learning of the Eager report, McKay lost no time in corresponding to Dr Vincenze Guerini, a noted dental historian and Neapolitan dentist, who confirmed McKay's suspicion that the condition was similar to Colorado Brown Stain.[16]

But it was not until 1927 that McKay was able to visit Naples in the hope of gaining an answer to the cause of this enamel defect. He learned that the condition in Naples had been corrected by a recent change in the water supply.[16] In an effort to obtain additional evidence of the key role of water, he conducted dental examinations in the populations of nearby villages. The "Eureka event" came in the small city of Resina, located at the base of Mt Vesuvius. Here he was astonished to learn that all adults had mottled teeth, while all the children had normal enamel. McKay recorded: "I was shown case after case of adult natives of this city who presented teeth typically marked, while we were not able one single native child who had anything but normal enamel." When he inquired about the water supply, he learned that the adults had been raised on water from deep wells, sunk hundreds of years ago into the ancient lava beds of Mt Vesuvius, while the children had been raised on new water piped from the slopes of the volcanic mountains. McKay was now certain that a waterborne substance caused the enamel defects.

McKay had also gained evidence that that the answer to mottled enamel resided in the drinking water from his experience in Oakley, Idaho. In 1925, the Women's Civic League of Oakley, bent on preventing any further discoloration of their children's teeth and after consultation with McKay, pressured the town to obtain its water supply from a nearby village whose children had perfect enamel. Seven years later, McKay found complete absence of mottled enamel in the children of Oakley.

In 1909, Dr F. Robertson, a dentist in Benton, Arkansas, had reported an almost 100% incidence of mottled enamel in children of nearby Bauxite, Arkansas, an aluminum mining town operated by the Aluminum Company of America (ALCOA). In the process of producing aluminum, Bauxite ore was mixed with a flux containing fluoride. In 1926, the Arkansas State Health Department requested that the Bauxite water supply be investigated by the USPHS. The mining company superintendent, Luther Branting, had contacted Dr McKay to enlist his help in investigating the cause of high incidence of mottled teeth in the local population. McKay urged the Bureau of Child Hygiene in Washington to conduct a study of the Bauxite water supply.[20] Two years later, the USPHS survey was conducted with Dr McKay acting as a consultant. The results of the survey were not made public until 1930, when McKay presented the data at a section meeting of the International Association for Dental Research. Nearly every child in the mining town of Bauxite had mottled enamel, while those in the nearby town of Benton had normal teeth. The water analysis conducted by the Public Health Service laboratory revealed no cause for the condition. Although McKay had previously agreed with ALCOA chemists and the USPHS to "avoid direct reference to the community," he did divulge that the investigation concerned the town of Bauxite, Arkansas, a major site for the production of aluminum. This posed a problem for ALCOA, who for many years had been conducting a campaign to establish the safety of aluminum products.[16]

Over the course of several years, it had been determined that the affected children had been raised on water from a deep well in Bauxite. In 1930, the ALCOA chemists had acquired a new quartz spectroscope that enabled them to measure extremely small amounts of minerals. When water from the Bauxite deep well was analyzed, it was found to contain surprisingly high levels of fluoride. After comparing water samples from numerous sites provided by Dr McKay, Harry Churchill of ALCOA's laboratories reported before a meeting of the American Chemical Society that the long-sought cause of mottled enamel might be the level of fluoride in the local drinking water.[20]

Within the space of a few years, fluoride was identified as the "toxic" factor in the drinking water that caused mottled enamel. The first experimental evidence came from a group of scientists at the Arizona Agricultural Experimentation Station. As in other medical advancements, the white rat was to play a key role. Husband and wife scientists M. Smith and H. Smith, along with E. Lantz, reported that concentrated water from St David, Arizona, a town plagued by mottled enamel, caused enamel defects in the teeth of white rats after one month of daily consumption. Based on prior reports from other sources that dietary fluoride produced dental defects, the Arizona researchers confirmed that feeding fluoride to rats caused enamel lesions similar to mottled enamel in human teeth.[16]

When C. H. Boissevain (1933) and H. T. Dean and E. Elvove (1935) analyzed the water supply to Colorado Springs with more sensitive instruments, they reported that the water contained at least 3.0 ppm of fluoride.[16]

In 1931, the USPHS appointed one of its young officers, H. Trendly Dean (Fig 17-5), to the newly formed National Institute of Health (NIH) with an assignment to conduct further studies of the relationship between mottled enamel and fluoride. In consultation with the older McKay, now practicing in New York, Dean applied his skills as a budding epidemiologist to analyzing additional data collected from several sites. In less than a year, Dean not only confirmed the close correlation between mottled enamel and high fluoride intake but also recognized that children affected with mottled enamel had significantly fewer caries: "Individuals in an endemic area show a lower incidence of caries than individuals in some nearby nonendemic area. Consequently, the study of mottled enamel may disclose some lead applicable to the vastly more important problem, dental caries."[4]

By 1936, Dean had assembled data from 335 endemic areas in 25 states, along with new chemical analyses by NIH chemists that showed no mottled enamel at 1.0 ppm and below in the drinking water.[20] In 1938, Dean, supported by statistical data, confirmed that nontoxic amounts of fluoride in drinking water were effective in reducing dental caries. This work led to the Grand Rapids Project, a

[4] Dean quoted in Harris.[20]

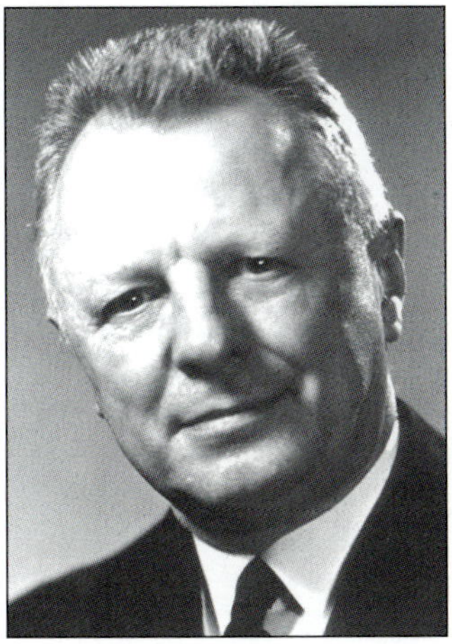

Fig 17-5 H. Trendly Dean.

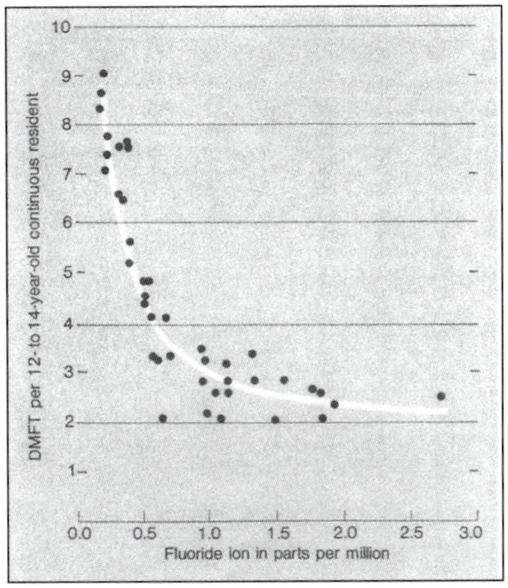

Fig 17-6 Number of decayed, missing, and filled teeth (DMFT) per 12- to 14-year-old continuous resident compared with the fluoride content of drinking water of 41 US cities. (From Eklund and Striffler.[21])

long-term clinical study of the effect of adding fluoride to the public water supply of the city of Grand Rapids, Michigan, compared with the neighboring nonfluoridated community of Muskegon. Beginning in 1945, 32,000 children in Grand Rapids and 8,000 in Muskegon were examined and followed for the next 15 years. When the final results were compiled, Dr David Scott, a member of the research team, experienced "one of the biggest thrills in my life." Grand Rapids children showed a reduction in dental caries of 50% to 63% in the 12- to 14-year-old group compared with the Muskegon children.[20] By 1980, the dental health of young children in the United States, as measured by the number of decayed, missing, and filled teeth had improved dramatically as a result of the fluoridation of water supplies[21] (Fig 17-6). United States Surgeon General Luther Terry hailed the study as a great preventive measure, equal with the pasteurization of milk, purification of water, and immunization against disease. McKay and Dean were the first dentists to receive the Lasker Health Award from the American Public Health Association in 1952. The search for the cause of mottled enamel and the resulting discovery of the anticaries effect of fluoride intake underlined the importance of dental research in providing better dental health to the public and helped to promote national support for dental research within the NIH.

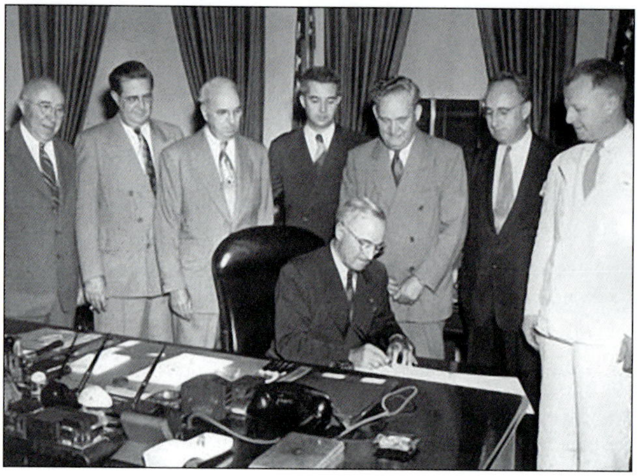

Fig 17-7 President Truman signing the bill establishing the NIDR. *(standing left to right)*: Dr C. W. Camalier, Congressman W. E. Brehm, ADA president Dr H. B. Washburn, Dr B. D. Forsyth, Dr C. O. Flagstad, Dr D. E. Lynch, and Dr H. T. Dean.

National Institute of Dental Research

A movement to create the NIDR was initiated in 1945 by Senator James E. Murray of Montana. The bill passed the senate in 1946 but was postponed in the House of Representatives. It would not be until 1948, after strong ADA lobbying of both legislative branches, including a White House meeting of ADA president H. B. Washburn with President Harry Truman, that a revised bill passed both houses and was signed into law by President Truman on June 24, 1948[20] (Fig 17-7). The law also created the National Advisory Dental Research Council (NADRC), a panel of scientists and lay members with responsibility for oversight of dental research and training. Dr H. Trendly Dean was appointed the director of NIDR and executive officer of the NADRC. Dean's priorities were to expand the number of dental researchers and to stimulate research in the nation's dental schools through grants.[20] As Dean took the directorship of NIDR, there was a great deficiency in dental research manpower: Only 11 dentists compared with 188 physicians were enrolled in the NIH postdoctoral fellowships.

The Korean War led to disruption of progress at the NIH as funding for the construction of its laboratory building was postponed and appropriations for research grants and training programs were severely reduced.[20] Approval of funding for the building was pushed into the Eisenhower administration and was nearly terminated in 1957 by Sputnik; Eisenhower's assistant, Sherman Adams, announced that national security programs necessitated postponement of the project.[20] In 1959, after 11 years of delay, construction of the NIDR laboratory building was finally underway. Trendly Dean had retired and been replaced by Dr Francis Arnold, a research colleague in the fluoride investigations. By the time of its dedication in 1961, the building was already too small for the dental research staff, which had expanded to 258 under Arnold's directorship.

In the latter half of the 20th century, the ADA and the NIDR dominated the dental landscape. Under their leadership, dental education and dental research advanced along the outlines contained in the Gies Report.

Dental Education

The full integration of dental schools into university centers marked the most important advance in dental education from the period following the Gies Report to the end of the 20th century. Of equal importance was the development of formally accredited training programs in the dental specialties. Acceptance within the university brought with it special responsibilities: maintenance of high educational standards, productivity in research and scholarly activities, and unique community health services.

The American Council on Education's 1961 Survey of Dentistry underscored a growing shortage of dentists and called for an increase in the number of dental schools as well as an increased enrollment at existing schools.[22] As a result, 14 new schools were started from 1960 to 1970, and with increased enrollments at already established schools, the number of dental graduates rose to just over 6,000 per year.[23] The cost of this expansion was funded at the federal and state levels. During the 1980s, fear of an oversupply of dentists and a decline in patient visits, coupled with the perception that dental caries was being eliminated by the use of fluoride, led to a significant reduction in public funding for dental education and a campaign by practicing dentists to tighten the pipeline of new dentists, even if it meant eliminating some schools. Six private dental schools were closed during the period from 1984 to 1994, and several other schools came under scrutiny and barely survived retrenchment. At the end of the 20th century, there were 54 dental schools (35 public and 19 private) in the United States.[24] Nineteen states had no publicly supported dental schools. Funding provided by the NIDR's extramural

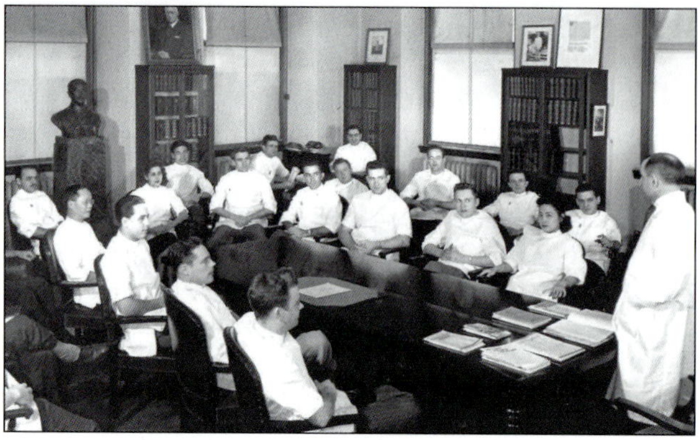

Fig 17-8 Dr Basil Bibby, director of the Eastman Dental Center, lecturing before a group of dental interns. Bibby was a noted expert on the cariogenicity of foods and the protective role of fluorides. (Courtesy of the Edward G. Miner Library at the University of Rochester.)

research program fueled the growth of research programs at many dental schools throughout the country. Postdoctoral studies coupling advanced clinical science with basic and applied research grew rapidly at major universities and at privately endowed institutes, such as the Eastman Dental Center (Fig 17-8) in Rochester, New York, and the Forsyth Dental Research Institute in Boston, Massachusetts.

All dental schools faced mounting financial strain as the 20th century came to a close. It is generally accepted that dental schools are the most expensive units within the university, largely due to the fact that the operation of a clinical facility must be borne by the dental school; in contrast, medical students receive clinical training within hospitals whose finances are separated from the medical school. In 2000, the average state expenditure per dental student was $49,347, 68% lower than for medical students. Bailit noted that if the actual cost of medical student clinical training (hospitals and other sites) were added to the cost of medical schools, the true cost of public support for medical education would be nearly twice as much as that for dental education.[24]

A breakdown of the sources of operational revenues for all schools in the year 2000 showed that state and federal support amounted to 32% and 9%, respectively, while tuition (27%), clinic income (19%), and other (13%) accounted for the balance.[24] Private dental schools relied more on tuition and clinic income (74%) compared with publicly supported schools (32%). During the period from 1990 to 2000, the level of public funding for dental education in inflation-adjusted dollars declined by 14%. The shortfall was made up by increases in tuition of about 10% per year. Bailit suggested that the private schools, by virtue of their larger class size, higher tuitions, and more efficient operation, were better equipped to manage the reduction in public funding.

The decline in public funding placed further stress on the ability of dental schools to achieve all aspects of their mission, especially in research and scholarly activity, as more faculty effort must be devoted to supervision of student clinics and teaching larger class sizes. At the start of the 21st century, public dental schools faced raising tuition costs, shortages of full-time clinical faculty, and an inability to cover the costs of maintaining and upgrading clinical centers. Current data reveal that faculty salaries have fallen well below the income of private practitioners,[5] creating an increase in open positions at most schools. The research mission of the dental school is at risk because of the increased difficulty of recruiting research faculty (holding both the DDS and PhD degrees). This problem is compounded by the increasing debt load of the dental graduate, who must now seek the best path to financial independence through private practice.

Discovery through research is an essential responsibility of the university that falls upon every one of its units. The dental school must demonstrate fulfillment of this mission through research grants and peer-reviewed scholarly publications. By 1993, dental school revenues from research averaged about 10% of the total school revenues. Over 78% came from federal, state, and local governmental sources. Total research expenditures for all schools were $113,764,118 (with the public schools at $92,633,697 and the private schools at $21,130,419).

The 2004 ADA report *The Economics of Dental Education* noted that:

> *Over the past two decades the number of basic science hours has declined among the curricula of U.S. dental schools. The concern voiced is that the commitment to basic science has become perilously low, compared to the preparation needed for dentists to practice effectively in an environment of increasingly complicated co-morbidities and complex therapeutic regimens. The dental practice of the future will require a sound foundation in the basic sciences to allow dentists to integrate a variety of clinical and laboratory information and to effectively collaborate with the entire health care team.*[25]

[5] It has been projected that general dentists and dental specialists will out-earn clinical faculty annually by $100,000 and $200,000, respectively, by 2015.[24]

Dental schools have not been uniformly successful in fulfilling these missions and as a result are isolated within the university. Nevertheless, there arose many outstanding examples of university-based dental schools that contribute positively to all components of the university's mission. The Institute of Medicine's (IOM) report on dental education stated as a basic premise that "dental schools must remain part of the university rather than once again become independent institutions—essentially trade schools—without the relationships to other professional, scientific, and humanities programs provided by universities."[26]

When public and private support for universities decline, dental schools are the most likely component to be placed under the microscope. The ability to cut costs and/or increase income in dental schools is problematic because the schools *(1)* must maintain and renew clinical facilities to keep pace with rapid advances in technology, *(2)* are often limited by state-mandated caps on tuition, and *(3)* must keep high faculty-to-student ratios in clinical disciplines where close supervision of patient care is required. Out of 54 dental deans surveyed for the IOM report, 47 stated that the major issue they faced was insufficient financial income. The IOM report noted that during the last decades of the 20th century, the average dental school was running about a $1 million shortfall in its clinic operation.[26] The report concluded that there were no "silver bullets" to remedy the financial crisis in dental schools.

To partially solve their financial problems, many schools have developed new approaches to deliver clinical care and to increase efficiency in operations. Outsourcing clinical education to extramural sites, such as community-based care centers, exploiting new simulation programs, and increasing the efficiency of faculty have been suggested.[25] As noted in a recent ADA evaluation of dental education: "One thing is clear—dental education is experiencing severe systemic difficulties. These difficulties are unlikely to disappear on their own. Fundamental changes in the structure and management of dental education will be required."

In *The Economics of Dental Education*, the ADA stated that:

> *Practitioners, educators, researchers, and the public have a vital stake in securing that bright future for dental education. Without a high quality, economically viable education system, the nation cannot replenish its supply of dental professionals. Without such a system, the public will not have continued access to the world's best oral health services. And without such a system, the chances of future scientific breakthroughs are diminished. Too much is at stake. We cannot afford to let dental education fail, even in part. Nor can we afford to let it*

> *decline in quality until it is considered more a trade than a learned profession.... Many schools have found it difficult to offset ebbing revenues with major cost economies without threatening important educational programs. This has created a financial hardship for dental schools and placed them under grave pressure to limit costs of operation and delay capital improvements. Skyrocketing tuition, high student debt, vacant faculty positions and aging physical facilities now have led many concerned and knowledgeable individuals to now believe we have approached the crisis stage in dental education.*[25]

In a recent white paper on the dental health professions, D. DePaola and H. Slavkin, in outlining the need for reform, stated that action is required among many areas, including the continued integration of dental schools in academic health centers, implementation of measures to reduce the cost of education, improvement of the clinical productivity of schools, increased access to dental care, and increasing diversity in the profession.[27]

Despite the progress made during the 20th century, calls for reevaluation of dental education surfaced as the century came to a close. Dental schools were faced with declining financial support and a declining applicant pool and internally stressed by the need for curricular reform driven by rapid growth of basic science and new technologies of patient care. Dental education for the 21st century must include greater exposure to the newest developments in basic sciences (genetics, immunology, and tissue regeneration) and medical sciences (systems physiology and pathology).

At the outset of the 21st century, the escalating costs of dental education, the imbalance in access to dental care, the evidence that oral health is linked to systemic health, and the ever-rapid pace of scientific discovery came together to create a sense of urgency for dental educators and the dental profession to find new models for educating dentists and for providing expanded care to all segments of the community. Change is in order, but a return to the "private for-profit model" without a strong research component and university oversight would be wrong.

Summary

In concluding this journey through the ages, it must be apparent that the evolution of dental practice has been marked by difficulties, many overcome by the intelligence, originality, and dedication of special individuals who added to the technology and science of the discipline and defined how dental practice was to be taught and regulated. They built a remarkable system in a relatively short time; now it is to be preserved. Saluting the outstanding advances that have been made since the founding of the first dental school in Baltimore, we recognize that there remains much to do.

Success of the profession in raising standards of practice, levels of education, and the application of ethical principles in managing the commercial side of health care has been accomplished through organized dentistry. The ADA and its many component societies at the state and local levels in concert with dental examining boards and the American Dental Education Association have forged a system that has worked well in producing highly competent dental practitioners.

From the earliest times, dental and oral diseases have always been included in the classical medical treatises. History explains how dentistry came to be a separate practice from medicine, more closely related in its mechanical aspects to the early practice of surgery. Although dentistry has thrived as a separate educational and patient care system, it is now more than ever evident that there can be no fundamental separation between it and medicine. What the future holds is unclear, yet everyone who has examined its current status is in agreement that the dental profession must be part of the university, must contribute to biomedical science through research, and must prepare graduates who as part of an interdisciplinary team can meet the demands of new health delivery systems.

References

1. Banzhaf HL. Dental Educational Council of America (secretary's annual report). Dent Cosmos 1912;54:363–369.
2. Sharp JG. Dental Faculties Association of American Universities (proceedings of the second annual meeting). Dent Cosmos 1910;52:1399–1404.
3. Sharp JG. A new era in dental educational standards. Dent Cosmos 1910; 52:1211–1217.
4. Lovett WA. Microscopical introspection: A review of the present status of dental education. Dent Cosmos 1911;53:1015–1023.
5. Kauffmann JE. Commercialized dental education. J Dent Res 1921;3:391–395.
6. Dental Faculties Association of American Universities (report of the third annual meeting). Dent Cosmos 1911;53:817–825.
7. Starr P. The Social Transformation of American Medicine. New York: Basic Books, 1982.
8. Rutkow I. Seeking the Cure: A History of Medicine in America. New York: Scribner, 2010.
9. Chambers DA. Flexner at 100. Perspect Bio Med 2011;54:3–7.
10. Markowitz GE, Rosner DK. Doctors in crisis: A study of the use of medical education reform to establish modern professional elitism in medicine. Am Q 1973;25:83–107.
11. Ludmerer KM. Abraham Flexner and medical education. Perspect Bio Med 2011;54:8–16.

12. Gillett HW. Fifty years of dental progress; the development of medical-dental relations. Dent Cosmos 1936;78:160–166.
13. Gies WJ. Dental education in the United States and Canada: A report to the Carnegie Foundation for the advancement of teaching. New York: Carnegie Foundation, 1926.
14. Dummett CO, Dummett LD. The Hillenbrand Era. Organized Dentistry's Glanzperiode. Bethesda, MD: American College of Dentists, 1986.
15. Suchman EA, Rothman AA. The utilization of dental services. Milbank Memorial Fund Q 1969;47:56–63.
16. McClure FJ. Water Fluoridation: The Search and the Victory. Bethesda, MD: U.S. Department of Health, Education, and Welfare, 1970.
17. Black GV. G. V. Black Digitized Collection of Manuscripts, Correspondence and Photographs in the Galter Health Sciences Library, Northwestern University. Evanston, IL: Northwestern University, 1867–1915.
18. McKay FS. An investigation of mottled teeth: An endemic developmental imperfection of the enamel of the teeth, heretofore unknown in the literature of dentistry. Dent Cosmos 1916;58:477–484,627–644,781–792,894–904.
19. Black GV. Mottled teeth: An endemic developmental imperfection of the enamel of the teeth heretofore unknown in the literature of dentistry. Dent Cosmos 1916;58:129–156.
20. Harris RR. Dental Science in a New Age: A History of the National Institute of Dental Research. Rockville, MD: Montrose, 1989.
21. Eklund SA, Striffler DF. Anticaries effect of various concentrations of fluoride in drinking water: Evaluation of empirical evidence. Public Health Rep 1980;95:486–490.
22. Hollinshead BE. The Survey of Dentistry. Washington, DC: American Council on Education, 1961.
23. Walker MP, Duley SI, Beach MM, et al. Dental education economics: Challenges and innovative strategies. J Dent Educ 2008;72:1440–1449.
24. Bailit HL, Beazoglou TJ. State financing of dental education: Impact on supply of dentists. J Dent Educ 2003;67:1278–1285.
25. Brown LJ, Meskin LH (eds). The Economics of Dental Education. Chicago: American Dental Association, Health Policy Resources Center, 2004.
26. Field MJ (ed). Dental Education at the Crossroads: Challenges and Change. Institute of Medicine Report. Washington, DC: National Academy, 1995.
27. DePaola DP, Slavkin HC. Reforming dental health professions education: A white paper. J Dent Educ 2004;68:1139–1150.

Index

C

D

E

F

G

H

I

J

K

L

M

N

O

P

Q

R

S

T

U